ADVANCE PRAISE FOR

The Case Against Fluoride

"For anyone who has ever wondered why cities add fluoride to water—and questioned whether they should. Written with clear and easy-to-read prose, and supporting citations, *The Case Against Fluoride* carefully lays out the arguments against fluoridation and reasons why it should be discontinued. The authors examine the evidence on fluoridation and conclude convincingly that it should now be considered 'harmful and ineffective.'"

—DR. HARDY LIMEBACK, Professor and Head of Preventive Dentistry, University of Toronto

"Sweden rejected fluoridation in the 1970s, and in this excellent book these three scientists have confirmed the wisdom of that decision. Our children have not suffered greater tooth decay, as World Health Organization figures attest, and in turn our citizens have not borne the other hazards fluoride may cause. In any case, since fluoride is readily available in toothpaste, you don't have to force it on people."

—ARVID CARLSSON, Nobel Laureate in Medicine or Physiology (2000) and Emeritus Professor of Pharmacology, University of Gothenburg

"This book clearly shows that water fluoridation is poor public policy and must end. As a concerned citizen, I applaud the authors for bringing this issue to the world's attention."

—ED ASNER

"Alfred North Whitehead said the scientific method means leaving 'options open for revision.' An ancient Roman adage says that 'whatever touches all must be approved by all.' These characterizations of science and democracy are the reasons for reading this book. Especially if you and your family are drinking administratively mandated fluoridated water."

—RALPH NADER

THE CASE AGAINST
Fluoride

How Hazardous Waste
Ended Up in Our Drinking Water
and the Bad Science and
Powerful Politics
That Keep It There

PAUL CONNETT, PhD
JAMES BECK, MD, PhD | H. S. MICKLEM, DPhil

Foreword by
Albert W. Burgstahler, PhD

CHELSEA GREEN PUBLISHING
WHITE RIVER JUNCTION, VERMONT

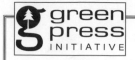

Project Manager: Patricia Stone
Developmental Editor: Jill Mason
Copy Editor: Jill Mason
Proofreader: Nancy Ringer
Indexer: Peggy Holloway
Designer: Peter Holm, Sterling Hill Productions

Printed in the United States of America
First printing September, 2010
10 9 8 7 6 5 4 3 2 1   10 11 12 13 14

Our Commitment to Green Publishing

Library of Congress Cataloging-in-Publication Data
Connett, P. H. (Paul H.)
  The case against fluoride : how hazardous waste ended up in our drinking
water and the bad science and powerful politics that keep it there / Paul
Connett, James Beck, H. Spedding Micklem.
      p. ; cm.
  Includes index.
  ISBN 978-1-60358-287-2
  1. Water--Fluoridation--Health aspects--United States. 2.
Water--Fluoridation--United States--History. 3. Fluorides--Toxicology. I.
Beck, James S. II. Micklem, H. S. III. Title.
  [DNLM: 1. Fluoridation--adverse effects--United States. 2.
Fluorides--adverse effects--United States. 3. Health Policy--United States.
4. Water--adverse effects--United States. WU 270 C752c 2010]

  RA591.7.C67 2010
  363.739'4--dc22

                                            2010024925

Chelsea Green Publishing Company
Post Office Box 428
White River Junction, VT 05001
(802) 295-6300
www.chelseagreen.com

CONTENTS

FOREWORD

In an age of increased awareness of the hidden, often insidious, hazards of many environmental pollutants, it is tragically ironic that fluoride—one of industry's most widely dispersed and persistent effluents—is inadequately assessed and poorly understood.

No doubt one of the main reasons why the toxicity of the continual exposure to comparatively low levels of fluoride is not better known is because of the generally favorable image that still surrounds the fluoridation of drinking water. Even though much contradictory evidence exists, dental and public officials persist in promoting and upholding the procedure because they evidently continue to believe "it is medically safe for all people."

Fluoridation is motivated by the well-intentioned desire for better teeth and less tooth decay, but even that result is questionable or, at best, marginal. A laudable dental goal has been allowed to outweigh the extensive, well-verified medical evidence collected in this book. . . .

The above words are from the description of a book, *Fluoridation: The Great Dilemma*, I coauthored in 1978. That text, and the personal context behind its writing, informs the historical significance of this current text by professors Paul Connett, James Beck, and Spedding Micklem (with important support from Peter Meiers on the historical details) and deserve a quick reflection.

While working at the University of Kansas in Lawrence, KS, starting in the mid-1950s, I developed a low-thyroid condition that was not relieved by taking thyroid extracts. In 1964, I became aware of clinical reports of verified illness from fluoridated water by the distinguished Michigan allergist George L. Waldbott, MD (1898–1982), appearing mostly in specialized foreign journals. From these reports I learned that fluoride in drinking water at the recommended level of 1 part per million (or 1 mg of fluoride per liter of water) could cause a wide variety of reversible toxic effects, including excessive tiredness, aching joints, neuromuscular pains, and other symptoms often associated with hypothyroidism. Knowing that Lawrence had fluoridated water and that I was consuming four or five times the amount mentioned by Waldbott, I switched to distilled water and found that my low-thyroid symptoms quickly began to disappear. My wife, Patricia, who had been experiencing back pain for some years, also found her discomfort was completely relieved after she also changed to distilled water.

With these experiences fresh in mind, I contacted Dr. Waldbott and arranged to visit him, and we soon became close friends. In 1966 he founded the International Society for Fluoride Research and, in 1968, inaugurated its journal, *Fluoride Quarterly Reports* (now simply *Fluoride*). Waldbott started the new journal because major U.S. medical journals, due to unqualified endorsement of fluoridation by the U.S. Public Health Service in 1950, had systematically declined to publish reports of adverse ill effects from fluoridated water.

In 1957, Dr. Waldbott collaborated on a preliminary account of his research on fluoride in *The American Fluoridation Experiment* (Devin-Adair, 1957; revised 1961). Eight years later he published his monograph *A Struggle With Titans—Forces Behind Fluoridation* (Carlton Press, New York, 1965). However, he also wanted to write a more comprehensive book dealing with the ever-growing body of research on adverse health effects of fluoride.

When he sent me drafts of this new book, my late colleague Professor H. Lewis McKinney (1935–2004), who taught the history of science at the University of Kansas, and I began editing the book that became, with McKinney and me as collaborating coauthors, *Fluoridation: The Great Dilemma* (Coronado Press, Lawrence, KS, 1978). This book probably helped set the stage for later books on fluoridation, including *The Fluoride Deception* by journalist Christopher Bryson (Seven Stories Press, NY, 2004) and now the present book, *The Case Against Fluoride*, by my good friend Paul Connett and his coauthors Drs. Beck and Micklem.

In this new book, the authors have assembled their wide-ranging backgrounds in several scientific disciplines to explore the controversy of water fluoridation. Like Dr. Waldbott and others before them, they have followed the best science wherever it leads. Doing this has inevitably led them to conclude, as I have, that on ethical grounds water fluoridation never should have been started, and on scientific grounds it should be ended as soon as possible. Anyone reading this text *with an open mind* will reach the same conclusion.

It is my hope that this book will enable good science to prevail over dogma on this issue. This is important not only to end a significant health threat to fluoridated populations but also because it is critical for a civil society to be informed by honest science. This change can occur only if enough people—especially new generations of scientists, doctors, and dentists—want it to happen.

Albert W. Burgstahler, PhD
Professor Emeritus of Chemistry
The University of Kansas
Editor, *Fluoride*
www.fluorideresearch.org

ACKNOWLEDGMENTS

First and foremost we would like to acknowledge the solid foundation provided to us by the Health Effects Database of the Fluoride Action Network (FAN; www.FluorideAlert.org). This comprehensive summary was compiled by author Paul Connett's son Michael, who ran the FAN Web site from 2000 to 2008. Michael also provided additional help in his coauthorship of many reports published by FAN, including submissions to both the NRC fluoride review panel in 2003–2006 and the EPA's Office of Pesticides. With all these, the authors have taken full advantage of what former BBC journalist Christopher Bryson has called Michael's "encyclopedic knowledge of the scientific literature on fluoride." FAN's research director, Chris Neurath, also helped with these submissions and has been particularly helpful in reviewing the literature on fluoride and osteosarcoma (see chapter 18), as well as preparing a graphical summary of the World Health Organization data on tooth decay discussed in chapters 5 and 6. The FAN critique of the use of sulfuryl fluoride was masterminded by Paul's wife, Ellen, and sprang from her work in maintaining the world's largest database on the dangers posed by fluorinated pesticides and other fluorinated products (http://www.fluoridealert.org/ f-pesticides.htm). Ellen has also provided huge support in the monumental task of compiling the endnotes, as well as making key supporting documents available on the FAN site, which she manages.

We are also greatly appreciative of the help given to us on various aspects of the book by the following individuals: Peter Meiers, who shared his unique knowledge of the early history of fluoridation—we are especially grateful that he coauthored chapters 7, 9, 10, and 11; Dr. Kathleen Thiessen, to whom we are particularly grateful for allowing us to reproduce in chapter 14 excerpts from her public statements refuting claims by the ADA and the CDC that the 2006 NRC review (on whose panel she sat) was not relevant to water fluoridation; Jack Cook, who helped in many ways, ranging from preparing most of the graphics and tables to offering sage advice on many aspects of the book; Wendy Varney, who assisted greatly in our understanding of the history of fluoridation in Australia, first through her text *Fluoride in Australia: A Case to Answer* and, second, through an updated essay on the subject that she kindly sent to us; and Gail Cooper, who expertly edited the text pro bono, prior to submission to the publisher. Many members of the Fluoride Action Network around the world have provided all kinds of help to us, ranging from moral support to very specific suggestions on the text. They include Ailsa Boyden, David McRae, Philip Robertson, and Daniel Zalec (Australia); Carole Clinch, David Hill, and Hardy Limeback (Canada); Robert Pocock (Ireland); Miriam Westerman (Israel); Mark Atkins, Mary Byrne, and Bruce Spittle (New Zealand); John Graham, Vyvyan Howard, Elizabeth McDonagh, and Stephen Peckham (United Kingdom); and Jeanette Bajorek, Albert Burgstahler, Doug Cragoe, Mike Dolan, Danny Gottlieb, Bette Hileman, Bob Isaacson, Maureen Jones, David Kennedy, Carol Kopf, and Eleanor Krinsky (U.S.A). Notwithstanding all this, any errors in the text remain the sole responsibility of the authors.

We also would like to thank our publisher, Chelsea Green, for having the courage to take on this project. Brianne, Pati, Susan, and Joni have been a joy to work with. We would also like to acknowledge the herculean feat accomplished by our final copy editor, Jill Mason.

Finally, we would like to thank our wives, Elia Beck, Ellen Connett, and Damaris Micklem, for their patience and support during the many hours spent writing this text.

INTRODUCTION

If you picked up a book that described a government plan to put a hazardous industrial waste product into the public water supply to deliver a topical medical treatment, without fully investigating its long-term health effects and without receiving the informed consent of all the citizens involved, you might well think you had picked up a science-fiction novel. But this is not Orwell, or Kafka, or even Hans Christian Anderson; it is a matter of historical fact. We are talking about water fluoridation.

Yet fluoridation has the wholehearted support of the United States Department of Health and Human Services (DHHS) and most professional dental and health bodies in the English-speaking world. How can this be?

In this book we do not argue against the use of *fluoride* in toothpaste or dental dressings and sealants; but we explain how *fluoridation*—the addition of fluoride to the public water supply—is a house of cards, propped up by very poor ethics and very poor science, and waiting to fall.

The Structure of the Book

The book is written in six parts: "The Ethical and General Arguments against Fluoridation," "The Evidence That Fluoridation Is Ineffective," "The Great Fluoridation Gamble," "The Evidence of Harm," "Margin of Safety and the Precautionary Principle," and "The Promoters and the Techniques of Promotion."

We do not presuppose any great scientific knowledge on the part of the reader. Numerous references to the primary scientific literature and other sources are provided, but attention to those is entirely optional: The text is intended to be intelligible and sufficiently comprehensive on its own.

Politics versus Science

From its inception, fluoridation has been more about politics than about science. That is not unusual. Politics and science have to rub shoulders in many contexts; the contact can be abrasive, and the result is rarely beneficial to the conduct and quality of science. Two consequences of this are (1) that the amount and type of science that is done can be largely determined by political influences; and (2) that the relatively rational discourse that usually accompanies scientific disagreements, at least in public, may be replaced by outright hostility even to the point of personal abuse and discrimination. In the case of fluoridation, political influence has ensured that remarkably little scientific work has been done on the issue, and it has generated a high degree of animosity between promoters and opponents. Not for nothing was a recent book titled *The Fluoride Wars*.[1] The sections "A Little History" and "Endorsements versus Science" below hint at the extent to which science has been sidelined and emasculated. Later in the book, we shall also see many examples of how science has been manipulated and misrepresented to serve an essentially political end.

The Issue Examined

Water fluoridation is the deliberate addition of a fluoride compound to the public water supply for the purpose of reducing tooth decay. It can come as a shock to find that the chemicals used to fluoridate the water are not pharmaceutical grade, like those used in fluoridated toothpaste and other dental products, but are mainly hazardous waste products of the phosphate fertilizer industry (chapter 3). An even greater shock is to find that while many agencies promote the practice of water fluoridation in the United States, no federal agency accepts responsibility for it (see chapter 4).

Currently, over 180 million Americans and about another 200 million people worldwide are drinking artificially fluoridated water. In the United States and several other fluoridating countries, the so-called optimal concentration of fluoride is 1 milligram per liter, or 1 part per million (ppm; it actually ranges from 0.7 to 1.2 ppm, depending on average ambient temperatures).

Proponents claim that 1 ppm is an extremely small concentration and could not possibly cause any harm. In fact, however, it is not at all small for a substance of fluoride's known toxicity; it is 25–250 times more than the range of concentrations of fluoride found in mother's milk (chapter 12). This means that a bottle-fed baby in a fluoridated community is getting up to 250 times more fluoride than a breast-fed baby (chapters 1 and 12). Meanwhile, according to the U.S. Centers for Disease Control and Prevention (CDC),[2] 32 percent of children in the U.S. have a condition called *dental fluorosis*, a mottling or discoloration of the tooth enamel caused by excessive exposure to fluoride before the secondary teeth have erupted (see chapter 11).

One of the surprises for independent reviewers of this issue is that the scientific evidence that fluoridation works to reduce tooth decay is actually very weak (see chapters 6–8). According to World Health Organization statistics,[3] rates of tooth decay in twelve-year-olds have been coming down as fast in non-fluoridated countries as in fluoridated ones (chapters 5 and 6). Meanwhile, the scientific evidence indicating that fluoridation may be causing harm gets stronger with each passing year (see chapters 10–19).

A Little History

Fluoridation trials began in 1945, but in 1950, before any trials had been completed, and before any comprehensive health studies had been published, the practice was endorsed by the Public Health Service (PHS). Endorsements from the American Dental Association (ADA), the American Public Health Association (APHA), the American Medical Association (AMA), and others quickly followed but still without any solid scientific information to judge the efficacy and safety of the practice. We dub this abandonment of the normal procedures for determining the safety and efficacy of a medical practice "The Great Fluoridation Gamble" (see chapters 9 and 10).

Endorsements versus Science

Since 1950, endorsements have been routinely used to promote fluoridation. Citizens have been lured into accepting water fluoridation on the basis of "authority," not on the basis of any substantial scientific evidence of effectiveness or safety. Because that authority includes the PHS (now the DHHS), as well as professional dental and medical bodies, the endorsements have proved very effective in distracting attention from the absence of rigorous, well-designed, and controlled studies. From a scientific point of view, such a superficial approach to a serious issue is unusual. From a public relations point of view, however, endorsements have proved to be a very effective tool in the promotion of fluoridation for over fifty years. We examine the techniques used in the promotion of water fluoridation in more detail in chapter 23.

Another aspect of the inadequate scientific approach to fluoridation is how poorly potential health effects have been investigated and fluoride exposure monitored. Even the most basic studies have not been attempted (see chapter 22).

From time to time the governments of fluoridating countries have set up panels to review the safety and effectiveness of fluoridation, but by virtue of the selective makeup of these panels, their conclusions are frequently little more than rubber stamps for a long-entrenched government policy (see chapter 24). A notable exception to the self-serving reports is the review by the U.S. National Research Council (NRC) of the National Academies (formerly the National Academy of Science),[4] which we discuss below (see the section "The NRC Review" and chapter 14).

Why This Book Is Necessary Now

Some may wonder why we have written this book now. It may appear that fluoridation is a peripheral issue compared with the major economic, environmental, and political threats facing our planet today. That is true, but we would argue that, unlike those many other problems, this one is as easy to end as turning off a spigot, if the political will can be found. Only a complete change of attitude can generate such political will, however, and only a sober assessment of scientific reality is likely to shift the prevailing attitude.

Another reason for writing now is that promoters of fluoridation seem to be becoming increasingly aggressive in their activities, pressing for mandatory statewide fluoridation in the U.S.A., Canada, and Australia and passing laws to indemnify water providers against legal liabilities in the UK.

Finally, the recent publication of the NRC review—the first scientific review relevant to fluoridation that is both comprehensive and impartial—was a landmark.[5] Promoters of fluoridation have argued on specious grounds that the review is not, in fact, relevant to fluoridation. We intend to set the record straight on that point.

The NRC Review

The comprehensive review by the U.S. National Research Council of the National Academies, published in 2006, was carried out in response to a request from the Office of Drinking Water of the United States Environmental Protection Agency (EPA) to consider whether the EPA's safe drinking water level for fluoride, currently 4 ppm, needed to be changed. The NRC review contained 507 pages and approximately 1,100 citations to the primary literature.[6] For most scientific opponents of fluoridation, this review looked like the final victory in the long battle to expose the health dangers inherent in this practice, and, from the point of view of a former risk assessment specialist at the EPA, it was.[7] However, the agencies that continue to promote this program (e.g., the CDC and the ADA) are extremely influential, and with the help of a largely acquiescent media, they have managed to convince many decision makers—erroneously—that the NRC report can be ignored in discussions about fluoridation. Even the supposedly unbiased book *The Fluoride Wars* seems to have bought into this view. It scarcely mentions the review, which (along with other aspects of the book) throws the authors' claim of impartiality into serious doubt.

The NRC panel concluded that the current EPA safe drinking water standard of 4 ppm was not protective of health and recommended that the EPA

Office of Drinking Water perform a health risk assessment to determine a new MCLG (maximum contaminant level goal) for fluoride.[8] As of July 2010 (over four years after the NRC review was published), that had not been done.

In this book we review many of the findings of the NRC report (see chapters 15–19), along with those of some more recent scientific studies, so that these important health issues, and their vital relevance to the practice of water fluoridation, do not remain hidden either from the lay public or from open-minded professionals.

We do not believe that we are overstating the seriousness of the possible downside of fluoridation: People with impaired kidney function accumulate more fluoride in their bones and are more vulnerable to its toxic effects on those tissues and possibly others (chapter 19); some young men may be losing their lives to a fatal bone cancer because of this practice (chapter 18); millions of citizens may be having their bones weakened (chapter 17) and their thyroid function lowered (chapter 16); millions of infants may be having their mental development subtly impaired (chapter 15); and many adults may be suffering from a series of common complaints—from arthritic symptoms to tiredness not relieved by sleep to gastrointestinal problems—that could be reversed if the fluoride was removed (chapter 13).

Note the word "may." We do not claim that all these harms have been conclusively proven. What we can say, however, is that much existing information points clearly to *a variety of serious risks* inherent in the fluoridation program. We argue that these risks are far too high when we are considering the mass medication of millions of people, the more so since the benefits are now seen to be so small and achievable by other means in dozens of non-fluoridating countries.

Reliance on the ADA and the CDC

The vast majority of rank-and-file proponents of water fluoridation have received little encouragement to read the scientific literature concerning either fluoride's toxicity or the efficacy of fluoridation. They, as well as the media, rely on pro-fluoridation pronouncements from the ADA and the CDC. For example, nearly every day someone, somewhere is quoting the CDC's claim that "fluoridation is one of the top ten public health achievements of the 20th century,"[9, 10] without realizing that that agency is fundamentally biased on the issue. In essence, on the issue of fluoridation, the CDC's Oral Health Division behaves like an adjunct of the ADA. Indeed, the two bodies often work together on their fluoridation promotional activities—at taxpayers' expense (see chapter 4).

Bias

In the following pages, we concentrate on arguments against fluoridation, basing them clearly on the existing scientific data, while attempting to acknowledge weaknesses and recognize the existence of counterarguments. We make no apology for our bias; it is a necessary corrective and counterbalance to the contrary bias and obfuscation seen in the many pro-fluoridation statements that have appeared.

The Promoters' Motivations

Because the pro-fluoridation case is so unsatisfactory scientifically, we have been forced to address some of the possible motivations behind the continued push to fluoridate the water of more towns and states in the United States and other fluoridated countries (see chapter 26). We have been tempted to paddle into rough waters here (who of us really knows what motivates others?) because it is so puzzling to witness the efforts of proponents to step up the fluoridation of more and more water supplies, even as the evidence for the effectiveness and safety of this program gets less and less convincing. If this evidence is so weak, what can explain the continued zealous promotion of fluoridation?

Risk

What is important to remember is that we are talking about *mass medication,* not a drug that is prescribed after due consultation for an individual. A risk of harm estimated at say 1 in 10,000 may be considered entirely acceptable in the latter case; in fact, we accept far higher risks of undesirable side effects if we are seriously ill. But if we are giving a drug to nearly 400 million people worldwide, that risk of 1 in 10,000 translates into 40,000 cases of harm from one cause. The risks for some harms due to fluoridation are probably much higher. For example, 1 in 100 may be hypersensitive to fluoride (see chapter 13).

So proponents and opponents carry different burdens of proof. Proponents need to have conclusive proof of substantial benefit and very strong evidence for an extraordinarily low risk of harm (they have neither). For opponents, on the other hand, it should suffice to show that there is an identifiable risk of serious harm; conclusive evidence is not necessary. Even small risks are indefensible when deliberately imposed on a large population. This may seem like common sense, but it seems to elude proponents of fluoridation, who continue to talk about small risks as if they were acceptable and to insist that opponents provide conclusive proof (chapter 21).

This distinction lies at the very heart of the fluoridation dispute and comes up again and again. It is the touchstone. Proponents say that unless there is direct and conclusive evidence that fluoridation, as opposed to fluoride, harms anyone, then it is all right to carry on fluoridating. They are zealous in trying to dismiss any relevant evidence as having methodological flaws and claiming that it is "junk science"[11] or doesn't meet "normal scientific standards."[12] Opponents say that this demand for absolute scientific proof violates the precautionary principle, and the violation is extreme.

Even proponents of fluoridation do not deny that high levels of fluoride cause harm. In fact, millions of people living in areas of India and China with moderate to high levels of fluoride levels in their drinking water have suffered serious health consequences. Therefore, the onus is on the proponents to demonstrate that there is an adequate margin of safety between the doses that cause harm and the huge range of doses that may be experienced by those drinking uncontrolled amounts of fluoridated water and at the same time receiving unknown amounts of fluoride from other sources. Moreover, such a margin of safety should be large enough to protect *everyone* in society, not just the *average* person. Those who need protecting include the very young, the very old, those with poor nutrition, those in poor health, and those with impaired kidney function. Proponents have not demonstrated this. Worse, they seldom even address this key issue. We examine this further in chapter 20.

No Debate?

For many years proponents have tried to insulate themselves from discussion and from the obligation to investigate by claiming that "there is no debate" on fluoridation.[13] They argue that the evidence for fluoridation's benefits and lack of harm is so clear that it is not worth bothering with a handful of "ill-informed" critics. Such a simplistic (and conveniently self-serving) view is easily rebutted. It is long past time that proponents began to engage in this debate in a serious, transparent, and scientific manner.

As Thomas Huxley said, "Many a beautiful theory was killed by an ugly fact." As far as fluoridation is concerned, there are many ugly facts; they are revealed in the pages of this book.

ABBREVIATIONS

Organizations

AAAS	American Association for the Advancement of Science
ACSH	American Council on Science and Health
ADA	American Dental Association
Alcoa	Aluminum Company of America
AMA	American Medical Association
BFS	British Fluoridation Society
CDC	Centers for Disease Control and Prevention (US)
DHHS	Department of Health and Human Services (US)
EPA	Environmental Protection Agency (US)
FDA	Food and Drug Administration (US)
IPCS	International Programme on Chemical Safety
JADA	Journal of the American Dental Association
JAMA	Journal of the American Medical Association
NAS	National Academy of Sciences (US)
NCI	National Cancer Institute (US)
NHMRC	National Health and Medical Research Council (Australia)
NIH	National Institutes of Health (US)
NID(C)R	National Institute of Dental (and Craniofacial) Research
NRC	National Research Council (US)
NSF	National Sanitation Foundation International (US)
NTP	National Toxicology Program (US)
NYDOH	New York State Department of Health (US)
PHS	Public Health Service (US)
SEER	Surveillance, Epidemiology and End Results (US)

Technical terms

AMP	Adenosine monophosphate
DMFS	Decayed Missing and Filled Surfaces in the secondary teeth
DMFT	Decayed Missing and Filled secondary Teeth
IRIS	Integrated Risk Information System (EPA, US)
LOAEL	Lowest Observable Adverse Effect Level
MCL	Maximum Contaminant Level
MCLG	Maximum Contaminant Level Goal
ppb	parts per billion
ppm	parts per million
T3	Triiodothyronine
T4	Thyroxin

· PART ONE ·

Ethical and General Arguments against Fluoridation

In chapter 1, we examine aspects of fluoridation that make it a very poor medical practice. This discussion includes the "alpha and omega" argument against fluoridation—namely, that government does not have the right to force individuals to take a medication against their wishes. We show that this idea, which many citizens believe intuitively, is actually sanctified in a European convention and in modern medical ethics.

In chapter 2, we further argue that water fluoridation, even if it were a sound medical practice, is not an efficient or appropriate way to achieve the desired end.

In chapter 3, we examine the nature of the chemicals used in the fluoridation program. The shock to many is to find that these chemicals are not pharmaceutical grade, as used in dental products, but hazardous waste derived largely from the phosphate fertilizer industry.

In chapter 4, we examine just who is in charge of the American fluoridation program. We ask who ultimately has responsibility if harm is demonstrated. The answer to this question will probably shock the reader as much as it did us.

In chapter 5, we examine the experimental nature of the fluoridation program. Even after sixty years of the program there have been no rigorous studies demonstrating it's effectiveness, and many unanswered questions remain over health risks. Most countries do not fluoridate their water, yet their children's teeth are no worse than the teeth of children in fluoridated countries.

• 1 •

Poor Medical Practice

At a public meeting held on October 17, 2009, in Yellow Springs, Ohio, a community that was considering halting its fluoridation program, Paul Connett gave a twenty-minute presentation on the scientific arguments against the practice. After a county health commissioner and local dentist responded, a woman in the audience said, "Whether this practice is safe or not, or beneficial or not, I want freedom of choice. It is *my* right to choose what substances I put into my body, not *some governmental agency's.*"

This woman echoed what many opponents of fluoridation have believed and articulated for over sixty years: Government has no right to force anyone to take a medicine. Thus, while in the effort to end this practice worldwide it is helpful to provide scientific evidence that the program is neither effective nor safe, this commonsense position remains the crux of the argument against fluoridation.

The Need for Informed Consent
Every doctor knows, or should know, that he or she cannot force an individual to take medicine without that patient's informed consent. Doctors must tell their patients the benefits of any medicine prescribed and warn of any possible side effects. After they have done this, it is the patient—and only the patient—who should make the final decision as to whether to take the medicine.

This is what the American Medical Association (AMA) has to say about *informed consent*:

> Informed consent is more than simply getting a patient to sign a written consent form. It is a process of communication between a patient and physician that results in the patient's authorization or agreement to undergo a specific medical intervention.
>
> In the communications process, you, as the physician providing or performing the treatment and/or procedure (not a delegated representative), should disclose and discuss with your patient:
> * the patient's diagnosis, if known;
> * the nature and purpose of a proposed treatment or procedure;
> * the risks and benefits of a proposed treatment or procedure;

- alternatives (regardless of their cost or the extent to which the treatment options are covered by health insurance);
- the risks and benefits of the alternative treatment or procedure; and
- the risks and benefits of not receiving or undergoing a treatment or procedure.

In turn, your patient should have an opportunity to ask questions to elicit a better understanding of the treatment or procedure, so that he or she can make an informed decision to proceed or to refuse a particular course of medical intervention.

This communications process, or a variation thereof, is both an ethical obligation and a legal requirement spelled out in statutes and case law in all fifty states of the United States.[1]

By violating the individual patient's right to informed consent, fluoridation allows decision makers, without medical qualifications, to do to the whole community what an individual doctor is not allowed to do to his or her individual patients.

Counterargument 1: It Is Unethical *Not* to Fluoridate

Proponents respond to this ethical argument by turning it upside down. They argue that it is unethical to deprive children of a benefit that might reduce pain and help them lead healthier lives, especially children from low-income families.

However, by not putting fluoride in the water, you are not depriving anyone of access to fluoride: It is available in tablet form and in fluoridated toothpaste. (For a discussion about topical versus systemic benefits, see chapters 2 and 6.)

From an economic perspective, avoiding fluoride in water is an expensive business, whether it involves purchasing bottled water for cooking and drinking or the use of distillation equipment or reverse osmosis systems. Thus, low-income families are disproportionately burdened by fluoridation since by and large they cannot afford avoidance measures.

In the United States, dental decay is concentrated in poor and minority families. Fifty-five years after fluoridation began, the U.S. surgeon general stated in his 2000 report, *Oral Health in America*: "There are profound and consequential disparities in the oral health of our citizens. Indeed, what amounts to a 'silent epidemic' of dental and oral diseases is affecting some population groups. Those who suffer the worst oral health are found among the poor of all ages, with poor children and poor older Americans particularly vulnerable. Members of racial and ethnic minority groups also experience a disproportionate level of oral health problems."[2]

The motivation for targeting poor children for extra help is highly laudable, but adding fluoride to the drinking water to do so is misguided. In fact, it makes an inequitable situation even worse. This is because in Western countries the children most likely to suffer from poor nutrition come from low-income families, and we will see in chapter 13 that people with inadequate diets are those most vulnerable to fluoride's toxic effects. In our view, children from low-income families are the very last children who should be exposed to ingested fluoride.

Counterargument 2: No One Is "Forced" to Drink the Water

Proponents of fluoridation further counter the notion that fluoridation in the public water system violates the individual's right to informed consent to medication by arguing that fluoridated water is only delivered to the tap and no one is actually forced to drink it.

This argument certainly does not apply to low-income families. Their economic circumstances do force them to drink the water coming out of the tap. Thus, a program that is billed as equitable is actually inequitable, since families of low income are trapped by a practice that may cause them harm (see chapters 11, 13–19).

Moreover, even for families with the means to buy bottled water for drinking and cooking, or equipment to remove the fluoride at the tap, it is very difficult to avoid fluoride once it has been put in the community's water supply. It will be in every glass of water and cup of coffee or tea consumed in town—at work and in friends' homes. It will also be in the water that is used to water the garden and in the shower and bath water.

Counterargument 3: Fluoride Is a Nutrient, Not a Drug

Proponents have tried to muddy the waters in the argument of violation of informed consent and unacceptability of "mass medication" by insisting that fluoride is not a medicine or drug, but a nutrient. We examine the evidence for their claims.

Is Fluoride an Essential Nutrient?

There is little or no evidence that fluoride is an essential nutrient. To demonstrate that a substance is an essential nutrient one has to demonstrate that some disease results from depriving an animal or a human of this substance. This has never been done for fluoride (see chapter 12).

In a 1998 letter by Bruce Alberts, president of the National Academy of Sciences, and Kenneth Shine, president of the Institute of Medicine, to Professor Albert Burgstahler, editor of the journal *Fluoride* and several other scientists, in response to their complaint to the National Academy about the Institute of Medicine's inclusion of fluoride in the list of *nutrients* in its report *Dietary Reference Intakes for Calcium, Phosphorus, Magnesium, Vitamin D, and Fluoride*,[3] the following quote appeared:

> First, let us reassure you with regard to one concern. Nowhere in the report is it stated that fluoride is an essential nutrient. If any speaker or panel member at the September 23rd workshop referred to fluoride as such, they misspoke. As was stated in *Recommended Dietary Allowances 10th Edition*, which we published in 1989: "These contradictory results do not justify a classification of fluoride as an essential element, according to accepted standards. Nonetheless, because of its valuable effects on dental health, fluoride is a beneficial element for humans."[4]

What Alberts and Shine do not discuss here is whether the supposed benefits of this "beneficial element" are obtained from some internal biological process or via some nonbiological interaction of the fluoride with the surface of the tooth enamel. This is a crucial difference when considering water fluoridation, since the former would necessitate swallowing fluoride and the latter would not (see chapter 2).

While there is no solid scientific evidence supporting the notion that fluoride is a nutrient, strenuous attempts have been made by a number of proponents throughout the history of fluoridation to try to establish this notion in the public mind. In chapter 26 we examine these efforts, in particular the effort by Harvard researcher Dr. Frederick Stare and the aid given to him by the sugar and food lobbies.

Is Fluoride a Drug?

In a letter sent in December 2000 to Congressman Kenneth Calvert, chairman of the Subcommittee on Energy and the Environment, of the Committee on Science, the U.S. Food and Drug Administration (FDA) stated, "Fluoride, when used in the diagnosis, cure, mitigation, treatment, or prevention of disease in man or animal, is a drug that is subject to Food and Drug Administration regulation."[5] The National Association of Pharmacy Regulatory Authorities in Canada lists "sodium fluoride" and "fluoride and its salts" as drugs.[6]

According to Cheng et al. in an article appearing in the *British Medical Journal*, "The legal definition of a medicinal product in the European Union (Codified Pharmaceutical Directive 2004/27/EC, Article 1.2) is any substance or combination of substances 'presented as having properties for treating or preventing disease in human beings.'"[7]

Both the Centers for Disease Control and Prevention (CDC)[8] and the American Dental Association (ADA),[9] the main proponents of fluoridation in the United States, describe dental caries (tooth decay) as a "chronic infectious disease" and recommend fluoride to prevent the disease.

If fluoride is a drug or medicinal product, fluoridation is medication delivered on a massive scale.

An *Unapproved* Drug

In a June 3, 1993, letter to FDA commissioner Dr. David Kessler, former New Jersey assemblyman John V. Kelly wrote, "The Food and Drug Administration Office of Prescription Drug Compliance has confirmed, to my surprise, that there are no studies to demonstrate either the safety or effectiveness of these drugs [fluorides], which FDA classified as unapproved new drugs."[10]

It goes without saying that it would be highly questionable to deliver *any* drug via the public water system—let alone fluoride, which the FDA calls an *unapproved* drug. The designation "unapproved drug" means that it has not gone through rigorous trials to establish either its effectiveness or its safety. This designation also puts into question the ethics and legality of school nurses and teachers administering fluoride pills and/or rinses to students in U.S. schools located in non-fluoridated areas.

Other Arguments

Violating the modern medical ethic of informed consent is not the only feature of fluoridation that makes it a poor medical practice. In a recent videotaped interview, Earl Baldwin, a member of the British House of Lords and one of the advisory board members for the York Review, the UK-sponsored review of fluoridation,[11] explained why he thought fluoridation was a bad idea: "What physician do you know, who in his or her right mind, would treat someone he does not know and has never met, with a substance that's meant to do change in their bodies, with the advice: 'Take as much, or as little, as you like, but take it for a lifetime because it may help someone's teeth'?"[12]

Independent observers have been saying similar things since the inception of fluoridation, but these arguments have fallen largely on deaf ears. This is not because the reasoning lacks merit, but because those who promote fluoridation have the power to ignore both common sense and scientific argument. We examine the strategies and tactics used in the promotion of fluoridation in chapter 23. In the following sections we examine some of the commonsense arguments of opponents such as Earl Baldwin in more detail.

No Control over Who Gets the Medicine

For those who promote fluoridation, one of its attractions is that it delivers fluoride to everyone indiscriminately. But for opponents this is one of its greatest weaknesses. When fluoride is added to the water supply, it goes to everyone, including those most vulnerable to fluoride's known toxic effects. These include above-average water consumers; the very young; the very old; those with diabetes; those with low thyroid function or kidney disorder; and those with an inadequate diet, including those suffering from outright or borderline iodine deficiency (see chapter 16). Also, as we indicated above, it goes to families of low income who cannot afford avoidance measures.

No Control of Dose

A critical problem with delivering a medicine via the water supply is that there is no control over the dose. Dr. Arvid Carlsson discussed this issue in a letter he wrote in February 2009:

> Fluoridation is an obsolete practice. It goes against all principles of modern pharmacology. The use of the public drinking water supply to administer the same dose of fluoride to everyone, from the infant to those who consume copious amounts of water (such as diabetics), goes against all principles of science because individuals respond very differently to one and the same dose and there are huge variations in the consumption of this drug.[13]

Concentration versus Dose (from water and other sources)

Proponents of fluoridation stress how well engineers can control and monitor the concentration of the fluoridating agent added to the water supply. However, controlling *concentration*, measured in the case of fluoride in milligrams per liter (mg/liter), is not the same as controlling *dose*, which is measured in milligrams consumed per day (mg/day).

If someone drinks 1 liter of water containing fluoride at 1 mg/liter (i.e., 1 ppm, which is the concentration at which it is administered), they will ingest 1 mg of fluoride. If they drink 2 liters, they will receive 2 mg of fluoride, and so on. The dose gets larger the more water is drunk; and the larger the dose, the more likely it will cause harm. This is particularly serious for a substance like fluoride, which is known to be highly toxic at moderate to high doses, which accumulates in the bone, and for which there is little, if any, margin of safety to protect the most vulnerable against known health risks (see chapter 20).

We also receive fluoride from sources other than the water supply, and this amount varies from individual to individual. *Thus, it is the total dose from all sources we should be concerned about.*

To determine potential harm, we also have to take into account the body weight of the consumer. We discuss the difference between *dose* and *dosage* below.

Dose versus *Dosage*

The dose of aspirin or any other drug considered safe for a grown-up is not a safe dose for a baby. Similarly, a safe dose of fluoride for an adult cannot be considered safe for a baby. Thus it is alarming when one discovers that, over the course of the day, bottle-fed babies can receive nearly as much fluoride as an adult who drinks 1 liter of fluoridated water. According to the U.S. Environmental Protection Agency in a 2008 article on why children may be especially sensitive to pesticides, "In relation to their body weight, infants and children eat and drink more than adults."[14] The way toxicologists determine the safe dose for different ages is to adjust for the average body weight of the age range in question.

According to the EPA's 1986 calculation of a safe drinking water standard, a safe daily dose of fluoride for a 70-kg (154-lb) adult is supposed to be 8 mg per day.[15] In chapter 20, we challenge the faulty reasoning that led to this high figure. But in the meantime, if we adjust this figure of 8 mg per day for body weight, that would mean that only 0.8 mg per day would be safe for a 7-kg (15-lb) infant (i.e., a ten times lower dose because the baby's body weight is ten times lower). Even that dose may be too high for a baby, however, because a baby's developing tissues, particularly the brain, are much more vulnerable to toxic agents than an adult's. An infant is not simply a miniature adult.

Dose divided by a person's body weight is called *dosage* and is measured in milligrams per kilogram of body weight per day (mg/kg/day). The safe dose for an adult divided by an adult's body weight (assumed to be 70 kg) is called the *reference dose*, or RfD. Strictly speaking, we should call this a reference *dosage*, but people seldom do. Note the different units here. If we are talking about *dose*, we are speaking about mg/day, but if we are talking about a *reference dose*, or *dosage*, we are speaking about mg/kg/day. This is a big difference.

Now let's look at a real-life example of using a reference dose. The EPA lists IRIS reference doses for a number of toxic substances. IRIS stands for Integrated Risk Information System; it is used for health-risk assessments. The EPA's RfD for fluoride listed in IRIS is 0.06 mg/kg/day.[16]

It is worrying to see that this IRIS RfD is easily exceeded by a baby consuming formula made with fluoridated water. For example, a 10-kg infant drinking each day 1 liter of water containing fluoride at 1 ppm will get a *dosage* of 0.10 mg/kg/day (1 mg/day divided by 10 kg). That is almost twice the IRIS RfD.

It was after the 2006 U.S. National Research Council report[17] made it clear that bottle-fed babies were exceeding the IRIS RfD that the ADA finally recommended to its membership, in November 2006, that they advise their patients not to use fluoridated water to make baby formula.[18] The CDC followed suit,[19] but neither has made much of an effort to get this information to parents.

Different Responses to Same Dose

It is well known that there is a very wide range of sensitivity across the human population to any drug or toxic substance. Some people will be very resistant, while others will be very vulnerable or sensitive to the same substance. Most of us will have an average tolerance; however, we can anticipate that the most sensitive will be at least ten times more vulnerable than the average responder. Those who promote fluoridation gloss over the insufficient margin of safety to protect all citizens, especially the most sensitive, from the known adverse health effects of fluoride (see chapters 13 and 20).

Warnings, Help, and Compensation

One thing that is generally accepted about water fluoridation is that where it is implemented, the rates of dental fluorosis (mottling and discoloration of the enamel; see chapter 11) in children will rise. Very little warning is being given about this, especially to low-income families who bottle-feed their babies with formula made with fluoridated tap water. Nor is any financial help being provided to those families whose children are so affected. It can cost up to $1,000 to treat a fluorosed tooth with veneers—more when the veneers have to be replaced in subsequent years.

According to the CDC, 32 percent of American children are affected by dental fluorosis.[20] While most of those children have the *very mild* condition, those with the *mild, moderate*, or *severe* condition make up about 10 percent of the total, and many of those may need treatment (see chapter 11). Ten percent being affected would mean some 32,000 children in a city of one million needing cosmetic treatment that few families can afford. Public and media concern is growing on this issue; for example, see the transcript of a TV news clip from CBS in Atlanta, Georgia, broadcast in March 2010, at http://www.cbsatlanta.com/health/22776266/detail.html.[21]

Mandatory Fluoridation

The imposition of fluoridation on individuals without their informed consent becomes even more egregious when legislation is introduced to mandate the practice for whole states, provinces, or countries. While we do not consider that a local referendum is ethically satisfactory, since the medicine we take should not be determined by our neighbors, such a process may allow discussion, deliberation, and the opportunity for people to express their concerns—at least at the local level. When the practice of adding fluoride to the public water system becomes mandatory at the state, provincial, or even national level, the vast majority of the population has little idea of what is going on, either during the passage of the legislation or subsequently, when the measure is enforced. Informed citizens are usually dispersed in large jurisdictions and have few resources to match the lobbying power of either the national dental associations or governmental health bodies hell-bent on introducing this measure. Those who hold the ethical requirement of informed consent to be the final argument on this matter will continue to battle at the national and international levels to insist on this principle being recognized. But in practice, in today's world, local democracy—when it is allowed to operate—probably offers citizens a greater chance of protecting themselves against forced fluoridation.

A number of legislatures have introduced mandatory fluoridation legislation in various states within countries and sometimes for the whole country. These include the states of Victoria and Queensland in Australia; the states of California, Connecticut, Georgia, Illinois, Indiana, Louisiana, Michigan, Minnesota, Nebraska, Nevada, Ohio, and Tennessee (as well as Washington, D.C.) in the United States; and the countries of Singapore and the Republic of Ireland. As we write, efforts to introduce mandatory fluoridation are under way in the U.S. states of New Jersey, Oregon, and Pennsylvania

Mandatory fluoridation measures violate the principle of the crucial role of community participation in health measures outlined in the Ottawa Charter for Health Promotion.[22] Mandatory fluoridation also violates the Council of Europe's Convention on Human Rights and Biomedicine, whose article 5 states, "An intervention in the health field may only be carried out after the person concerned has given free and informed consent to it. This person shall beforehand be given appropriate information as to the purpose and nature of the intervention as well as on its consequences and risks. The person concerned may freely withdraw at any time."[23]

No local, state, or federal government—no matter how well intentioned—has the right to force anyone to take a medicine for a disease that is neither contagious (in a communal sense) nor life threatening.

Summary

Fluoridation—the deliberate addition of fluoride to the public water supply—is a poor medical practice because it violates the principle of informed consent to medication. It is indiscriminate and offers no control over the dose received by an individual. It makes inadequate allowance for differing sensitivity to toxic effects, or for the size and body mass of recipients; this last point is particularly important for young children who may receive proportionately much higher dosages than adults at a time when their bodies are far more vulnerable to toxic agents. Fluoride used in the fluoridation of drinking water is considered to be a drug, not a nutrient. It is chronically toxic at moderate doses. As a drug, it has not been rigorously tested and has not been approved by the U.S. FDA. Fluoridation increases the chances that a child will develop fluorosis of the permanent teeth, which can be disfiguring and require expensive cosmetic treatment in a minority of cases. The notion that fluoridation is equitable is misplaced for two reasons: Children from low-income families are more likely to have poor nutrition, making them more vulnerable to fluoride's toxic effects; and low-income families are least able to afford avoidance measures.

An Inappropriate and Inefficient Practice

Inappropriate Practice

When water fluoridation first began, in the 1940s, dental researchers believed that fluoride's main benefit came from ingesting it during the early years of life. They thought that fluoride worked systemically—specifically, that it built up in the enamel inside the growing tooth cells before the teeth erupted. They believed that early absorption of fluoride made the enamel more resistant to acids (the acids generated by bacteria breaking down sugars) when the teeth emerge into the oral cavity. However, starting in the early 1980s, as a result of new epidemiological and laboratory studies, many leading dental researchers and fluoridation promoters changed their position on fluoride's mechanism of action.

In 1999, the U.S. Centers for Disease Control and Prevention finally conceded what many dental researchers had been reporting over the previous two decades: Fluoride's predominant mechanism of action was *topical*, not *systemic*.[1] In other words, if fluoride works at all, it does so via direct exposure to the outside of the tooth and not from inside the body.[2–12] Here is the quote from the CDC report:

> Fluoride's caries-preventive properties initially were attributed to changes in enamel during tooth development because of the association between fluoride and cosmetic changes in enamel and a belief that fluoride incorporated into enamel during tooth development would result in a more acid-resistant mineral. However, laboratory and epidemiologic research suggests that fluoride prevents dental caries predominantly after eruption of the tooth into the mouth, and its actions primarily are topical for both adults and children.[13]

The acceptance by the CDC that fluoride works mainly in a topical fashion undermines the argument for swallowing fluoride and greatly strengthens the argument against mandatory fluoridation, especially if there is a hint of any health problems involved in the latter (and there are many hints in chapters

11–19). Since fluoride works largely on the outside of the teeth, and fluoridated toothpaste is universally available, there is simply not a strong enough reason to force people (often against their will) to drink fluoride because it is in their water supply. This position was clearly stated by Dr. Douglas Carnall, associate editor of the *British Medical Journal,* shortly after the publication of the York Review in October 2000.[14] He wrote, "Professionals who propose compulsory preventive measures for a whole population have a different weight of responsibility on their shoulders than those who respond to the requests of individuals for help. Previously neutral on the issue, I am now persuaded by the arguments that those who wish to take fluoride (like me) had better get it from toothpaste rather than the water supply."[15]

The point was recently echoed by Nobel laureate Dr. Arvid Carlsson. In a videotaped interview with Michael Connett in 2005, Carlsson stated, "In pharmacology, if the effect is local [topical], it's awkward to use it in any other way than as a local treatment. I mean this is obvious. You have the teeth there, they're available for you, why drink the stuff?"[16]

Using fluoridated toothpaste, instead of swallowing fluoridated water, does not eliminate systemic exposure completely, especially in young children who have not mastered their swallowing reflex. Even in adults some fluoride may be absorbed through the gums. However, this would be better than exposing every tissue in the body to fluoride with every glass of water that is drunk.

Inefficient Practice

Even if it could be demonstrated that ingesting fluoride produced more benefits than risks, using the public water supply to deliver the medicine is an extremely inefficient and clumsy method of distribution. Most of the medicine (over 99.5 percent) is thus used for washing the dishes, flushing the toilet, and watering the garden. Very, very little goes anywhere near the target, the teeth; the rest merely adds to environmental pollution. This process is very wasteful except for the phosphate fertilizer industry, which is probably happy to get rid of waste chemicals in this way. Without a purchaser manufacturers would have to arrange for costly disposal of this hazardous waste (see chapter 3).

In his PhD thesis, the late Dr. John Colquhoun outlined the argument that education had been more important than fluoridation in fighting tooth decay in children in New Zealand.[17] The same message was reiterated by a dentist in a recent editorial published in a California newspaper. He wrote, "Poverty and ignorance are the culprits responsible for rampant dental decay, not the lack of fluoride in the water. That's where our efforts should be directed, not toward mass medicating the entire population in order to serve a few. Education, education, and more education on oral hygiene, diet, and habits, along with easier access to preventive care, are the ultimate solutions."[18]

The writer is talking about educating not just children and parents but also dentists when he argues, "Dentists have been denied the education necessary to make a truly informed opinion regarding fluoride and community water fluoridation. They simply do not know the truth. Altruistic in aim, misguided in direction, led by many of our nation's finest servants, the dental profession has been ambling down the wrong path. It is time to correct our direction from mass medication to mass education."[19]

The miscalculation of opting for fluoridation over education has produced another horrible dividend. Many parents have taken their eyes off the important goal of limiting the sugar content of their children's meals, as well as the junk-food snacks and endless gallons of sweetened soft drinks consumed between meals. As a result, we are seeing a huge increase in obesity in children. Besides the health effects of obesity, it threatens to overwhelm the health care system with the massive costs of treating diabetes and other complications. According to a 2009 CNN report, the cost for treating diabetes is currently about $113 billion a year in the United States. In 2034, it is projected to be $336 billion.[20]

The money that is currently misspent on fluoridating chemicals, fluoridating equipment, and the whole apparatus of fluoridation promotion would be better devoted to a joint educational effort to fight obesity and tooth decay.

Summary

For many years, fluoride was believed to act *systemically* to prevent caries— tooth decay—by being incorporated into the enamel of the developing teeth. However, it is now known to act *topically*—that is, at the surface of the tooth. Thus, the main reason for ingesting fluoride has disappeared, but the increased risk of dental fluorosis and other possible health risks associated with the accumulation of fluoride remain. Even if fluoride worked via ingestion, using the water supply to deliver the drug would be highly inefficient since over 99.5 percent of the public water supply is not ingested, and most of the fluoride ends up in the environment. Education, not fluoridation, is what is needed to fight not only tooth decay but also the related and much larger problem of childhood obesity.

The Chemicals Used

It comes as a surprise to many people that the chemicals used to fluoridate drinking water in the United States are not pharmaceutical grade, meaning that they are not of the same purity used in dental products. Instead, the bulk of the chemicals used come from the wet-scrubbing systems of the phosphate fertilizer industry.

The Phosphate Fertilizer Industry

Wet scrubbers were introduced into the phosphate manufacturing process to remove two highly toxic gases: hydrogen fluoride (HF) and silicon tetrafluoride (SiF_4). For many years these gases had damaged vegetation in the vicinity of phosphate plants, as well as crippling cattle on local farms. Fortunately, a spray of water is able to capture the gases and convert them to a solution of hexafluorosilicic acid (H_2SiF_6). When this resulting solution has reached a concentration of about 23 percent, it is shipped untreated in large tanker trucks to chemical companies that then send it around the country to be used as a fluoridating agent in over 90 percent of the water supplies fluoridated in the United States. Sodium fluoride is used as a fluoridating agent in less than 10 percent of the water fluoridated.

This is how a research report from the Florida Institute of Phosphate described the history of the situation:

> In the late 1960s the state of Florida passed laws restricting air emissions in part because *fluorine [actually silicon tetrafluoride and hydrogen fluoride]* from the phosphate industry had begun to harm citrus trees and there were cases of *fluorosis* in cattle. Since that time phosphate companies have improved the techniques they use to remove contaminants before they are released into the air— such as scrubbing the stacks that processing plants use to release steam. Today *fluoride emissions are not considered to be a problem. It is scrubbed from the stack and is either recovered to make fluorosilicic acid, which can be sold for uses such as water fluoridation,* or is sent to the cooling ponds where losses to the air are within regulatory limits.[1] [emphasis added]

In 1975, there came perhaps one of the biggest regulatory changes for the phosphate industry: The U.S. Environmental Protection Agency required *mandatory reclamation* of the industry's waste products. For example, Florida's typical phosphate rock, which is mined to produce the phosphate used in the fertilizer industry, contains naturally occurring uranium-238 and radium-226, the latter of which gives birth to radon—an odorless, colorless gas that is known to cause lung cancer. Indeed, the same rock that is mined for phosphate is also mined for uranium.

Just how much of this radioactive material ends up in the bulk liquids used in fluoridation is not known. Nor is it known, outside the industry, whether any measures are taken to remove it prior to shipment. It would appear that the promoters of this practice rely on the dilution of approximately 180,000 to 1 at the waterworks to bring all the contaminants in the wet-scrubbing liquor (including arsenic and lead, for example) below regulatory levels (see "Other Contaminants in the Hexafluorosilic Acid Solution" below).

"An Ideal Solution"

For some regulatory officials, the use of the scrubbing liquor from phosphate plants for water fluoridation is considered a positive development. In 1983, Rebecca Hanmer, the deputy assistant administrator for water at the EPA, described the practice as "an ideal solution to a long standing problem. By recovering by-product fluosilicic acid from fertilizer manufacturing, water and air pollution are minimized, and water authorities have a low-cost source of fluoride available to them."[2]

However, William Hirzy, PhD, an EPA scientist, argues that the public water supply should not be used as a means of getting rid of hazardous waste, and in testimony before the U.S. Senate in 2000 he described Hanmer's views as "linguistic de-toxification."[3]

Clearly, being able to convert a hazardous waste material into a saleable product is very attractive for the phosphate industry. It would be extremely expensive to send this material to hazardous waste treatment facilities, but once this contaminated hexafluorosilicic acid waste product is purchased by someone, it becomes a "product" and no longer has to meet the stringent EPA legal requirements for handling hazardous waste. In this case, the purchasers are the public water utilities. Ironically, these hazardous waste products cannot be dumped into the sea by international law, nor can they be dumped locally, because they are too concentrated.

As Rebecca Hanmer pointed out, this practice does allow local communities access to a "low-cost" source of fluoride. Indeed, the alternative of using pharmaceutical-grade fluoride compounds in community fluoridation programs would be cost prohibitive. One of the reasons that is the case is because, as pointed out in chapter 2, over 99.5 percent of the fluoridating chemical goes nowhere near the teeth but gets used for washing, cleaning the car, and flushing the toilet.

Spinning the Fluoridating Chemicals

Because proponents of fluoridation are worried about the public's perception of adding a hazardous industrial waste to the public water supply, some of them have gone to tortuous lengths in an attempt to persuade citizens that the fluoridating chemicals are not captured hazardous waste products. Here is an example of some extraordinary spin from a Q&A pamphlet distributed by the Department of Human Services in Victoria, Australia, in 2009:

Does fluoride come from the fertiliser industry?

Scrubbers can also be used to reduce atmospheric pollution by gases, leading some people to conclude that because a scrubber is used to extract fluoride from rocks, fluoride must be a pollutant, but this is not the case.

Fluoride is not a waste product of the fertiliser manufacturing process, but rather, a co-product. If fluoride is not actively collected during the refining process for water fluoridation purposes, it remains in the phosphate fertiliser. However, due to the widespread practice of water fluoridation in Australia, fluoride is commonly extracted during the refining process.[4] [numbered references removed from excerpt]

Maybe this "health" agency is happier using the word "co-product" rather than "hazardous by-product," but the simple truth, as indicated previously, is that the captured gases (hydrogen fluoride and silicon fluoride) did enormous damage to crops and cattle surrounding phosphate fertilizer plants for about a hundred years before the industry was forced to put on wet scrubbers to capture those "co-products." Substances that cause damage to plants, animals, or humans are called pollutants. It is also not true, as this fluoridation-promoting health agency claims, that the captured gases would magically return to the phosphate fertilizer if they were not scrubbed from the air emissions. These claims are nonsense.

Other Contaminants in the Hexafluorosilicic Acid Solution

There is no question that the fluoridating agents are contaminated with other toxic pollutants. However, proponents claim that by the time a 23 percent solution of hexafluorosilicic acid is diluted by about 180,000 to 1 (to reach a fluoride concentration of 1 ppm), the contaminant levels will be below regulatory concern. However, this may not be true of arsenic.

Testing by the National Sanitation Foundation (NSF) International suggests that the levels of arsenic in these chemicals, after dilution into public water, can be as high as 1.66 ppb (parts per billion) and are of potential concern.[5,6] The current safe drinking water standard (alias the maximum contaminant level, or MCL) for arsenic is 10 ppb, and the American Water Works Association (AWWA) does not permit chemicals in the water to reach one-tenth of that standard. Clearly, fluoride is an exception to the rule, since AWWA allows and supports the addition of fluoride at 1 ppm, even though the MCL for fluoride is 4 ppm.

Moreover, as far as regulatory standards are concerned, it should be remembered that a number of water standards for contaminants are set at compromise levels. To determine the federally enforceable standard (i.e., the MCL), considerations of the cost of removal are set against an ideal safety goal (the MCLG, or maximum contaminant level *goal*). The MCLG for arsenic is set at zero, while the MCL is 10 ppb. Although it can be appreciated that a compromise has to be reached when considering how much money it costs to *remove* a naturally occurring contaminant like arsenic, it is more difficult to justify the deliberate *addition* of *any* level of arsenic to the drinking water, as occurs when industrial-grade fluoridating agents are used, thereby exceeding arsenic's MCLG of zero.

The EPA sets the MCLG for arsenic at zero because arsenic is known to be a human carcinogen, and for the EPA there is no safe consumption level for a cancer-causing chemical. By allowing the use of arsenic-contaminated fluoridating chemicals, we are sanctioning an increased cancer risk for the whole population in an effort to reduce tooth decay by a small amount. Most people are unaware that that is the trade-off that has been made.

The lack of oversight of the fluoridation program by the FDA partially explains why the chemicals used have not been tested in their pure, let alone their contaminated, form. The chemical usually tested in animal studies is pharmaceutical-grade sodium fluoride, not industrial-grade hexafluorosilicic acid. When the switch was made from sodium fluoride to the silicon fluorides (either hexafluorosilicic acid or its sodium salt), the crude assumption was made that, once it was diluted and the solution brought to a neutral pH, a solution of hexafluorosilicic acid would be equivalent in all respects to a solution of sodium fluoride. This assumed two things: (1) that hexafluorosilicic acid completely dissociated to free fluoride ions, hydrogen ions, and hydrated silica; and (2) that the presence of hydrated silica would have negligible significance. The notion of complete dissociation was based on theoretical calculations, not on real-life testing. This reasoning also neglects the possibility that the hexafluorosilicate ion (or some other silicon-fluoride species) might be reformed in the acidic conditions of the stomach (see the next section).

The Chemistry and Toxicology of Artificially Fluoridated Water
Before we embark on this discussion, it is important to stress that there is plenty of evidence (particularly from India and China) that moderate to high levels of *natural* fluoride in water cause a litany of health problems (see chapters 14–19). Just because a substance appears naturally in water does not mean the water is safe to drink. Arsenic, for example, occurs naturally in water, but it is highly toxic, and some communities are spending a lot of money removing it to meet regulatory standards.

The possible difference between the biological effects of free fluoride ions and the biological effects of silicon fluorides has been the subject of a lively debate between Coplan and Masters on the one hand and Urbansky and Schock on the other. The recent debate was sparked when studies by Masters et al. reported an association between the use of fluorosilicic acid (or its sodium salt) to fluoridate water and an increased uptake of lead into children's blood.[7, 8] They did not find the association when sodium fluoride was used, and they hypothesized that the silicon fluorides facilitated the uptake of lead present in the stomach (from any other environmental source) into the child's bloodstream. Because of lead's acknowledged ability to damage a child's developing brain, this is a very serious finding, yet it is being largely ignored by fluoridating countries. See the next section, "Fluoridating Agents and Lead," for a discussion of corroborating findings in a 2010 animal study.

Urbansky and Schock have argued on theoretical grounds that with the dilutions used in fluoridation, the dissociation of the silicon fluorides would be complete.[9, 10] The EPA financed a research study at the University of Michigan to investigate the dissociation of hexafluorosilicic acid at high dilution. The authors reported that at pH 7 the dissociation was virtually complete, but that at pH 3 most of the fluoride appeared in a silicon-fluoride complex containing five bound fluoride ions.[11] This raises the question of whether, when the hydrated silicon and fluoride ions enter the stomach at pH 1–2, they recombine to form this complex, resulting in a species with different chemical and biological properties from those of a bare fluoride ion.

Fluoridating Agents and Lead

A recent study by Maas et al. indicates that fluoridating chemicals alone, and in conjunction with other chemicals added to water (such as chloramine), have the ability to increase the leaching of lead from brass fittings.[12] Also, Masters and Coplan's suggestion that hexafluorosilicic acid increases uptake of lead into children's blood received strong support from an important animal study performed by researchers from Brazil and published in the April 2010 edition of the journal *Toxicology*.[13]

In that study the authors designed an animal experiment to see whether Masters and Coplan's hypothesis was biologically feasible. They investigated whether fluoride (as hexafluorosilicic acid) co-administered with lead increased the uptake of lead into blood and calcified tissues in rats, over lead administered alone. Blood lead concentrations over three times higher were found in the rats exposed to *fluoride plus lead* compared with those exposed to *lead only*, and the difference was statistically significant ($p<0.001^{*}$).

Lead concentrations were found to be 2.5 times higher in the superficial enamel, 3 times higher in surface bone, 2 times higher in whole bone, and 1.7 times higher in the dentine when the animals were co-exposed to fluoride.

The authors concluded, "These findings show that fluoride consistently increases blood lead and calcified tissues lead concentrations in animals exposed to low levels of lead and suggest that a biological effect not yet recognized may underlie the epidemiological association between increased blood lead levels in children living in water-fluoridated communities."[14] In essence, these authors have provided a well-designed animal study that supports the epidemiological findings of Masters and Coplan[15] and Masters et al.[16]

It is well established that even very low levels of lead exposure can compromise the intellectual development and behavior of young children. If, as this experiment shows in animals and Masters and Coplan may have found in epidemiological studies, lead exposure is increased by the presence of hexafluorosilicic acid (or possibly even free fluoride ions) in drinking water, this should result in the end of fluoridation in any rational world.

---

* $p<0.001$ means less than one chance in a thousand that this finding is a random result.

Fluoridating Chemicals from China

As a result of the decreased availability of fluoridating chemicals in the United States, some communities have been using fluoridating agents imported from China: either sodium fluoride or sodium silicofluoride (i.e., sodium hexafluorosilicate). Both of these can be shipped as solids, but, according to recent press reports, some water departments have been unable to completely dissolve the sodium fluoride received from China. They are left with an unidentified sludge. Even though the substance has not been identified, a CDC engineer has said that it is safe.[17] In one case this problem has forced a town to stop fluoridating.[18]

Summary

Promoters of fluoridation claim that they are simply topping off the existing natural concentration of fluoride in the water supply to a supposed optimal level of around 1 ppm. However, it is not quite so simple as that. The chemicals used in most fluoridation programs—silicon fluorides obtained from the phosphate fertilizer industry—are not naturally occurring fluoride compounds or the pharmaceutical-grade substances used in dental products. They are derived from wet-scrubbing systems, contain other contaminants, and are officially characterized as hazardous waste by the U.S. EPA. Over 90 percent of the chemicals used in the U.S. fluoridation programs are silicon fluorides. A bit less than 10 percent are industrial-grade sodium fluoride, the only fluoride compound that has received extensive toxicological testing. Several potential problems with the silicon fluorides exist, including (1) reassociation of silicon and fluoride in the acidic environment of the stomach to form silicofluorides with unknown biological properties; (2) leaching of lead from brass fittings; and (3) increased uptake of lead into children's blood. Moreover, the addition of industrial-grade fluorides to the public water supply inevitably leads to exceeding the EPA's MCLG for arsenic, a known human carcinogen, which is set at zero.

• 4 •

Who Is in Charge?

One of the most puzzling aspects of the American fluoridation program is just who is in charge of it. Neither the American Dental Association (ADA) nor any of the many endorsing agencies listed by the ADA accept any liability for the practice. Historically, the agency that preceded today's Office of Public Health and Science (OPHS), the U.S. Public Health Service (PHS), endorsed fluoridation in 1950. Various other government agencies followed suit, but of today's U.S. Department of Health and Human Services (DHHS) (the ultimate parent body for all the federal health agencies in the US), no agencies, divisions or institutes that help to promote or defend this practice appear to accept any legal liability should individuals be harmed.

The DHHS agency most identified with the program today is the Centers for Disease Control and Prevention (CDC). We will discuss its role as well as that of the Food and Drug Administration (FDA) and the Environmental Protection Agency (EPA). These are the three obvious candidates for ownership of this program at the US federal level.

The Centers for Disease Control and Prevention
We begin with the CDC because there is no question that this federal agency is an avid and aggressive promoter of fluoridation, although its involvement stops short of the following:

- Overseeing the safety of the program
- Vouching for the safety of the chemicals used
- Accepting any other liability in the matter

In fact, only one division at the CDC is involved with fluoridation, and that is the Oral Health Division (OHD). This division is largely staffed by personnel with dental rather than medical qualifications. In a 2008 listing of twenty-nine employees in that division, ten had an advanced dental degree, two had a PhD (one of those was in economics), eleven had an MPH (Masters of Public Health) or other master's degree, one was a professional engineer, and five others were listed without academic or professional qualification.[1]

While academic degrees may not tell the whole story about a person's specialized knowledge, on the face of it there seems to be little evidence to suggest that the OHD personnel have the appropriate educational background to properly evaluate toxicological studies or conduct health-risk assessments.

Even though the CDC has experts in other divisions with the appropriate credentials to review health studies and conduct risk assessments, they have not been given any formal oversight or advisory role on the safety issues pertaining to fluoridation. It is true that a division of the CDC called the Agency for Toxic Substances and Disease Registry (ATSDR) updates toxicological profiles of substances found at hazardous waste sites, including fluoride; however, the profiles are prepared by outside contractors, and the 2003 update had little to say about the risks posed by fluoridation.[2]

The only apparent role that the CDC is prepared to play in the matter of fluoridation is that of the OHD's aggressive promotion of fluoridation throughout the United States. Its stated goal has been for fluoridation to reach 75 percent of the population by 2010. The OHD supports mandatory fluoridation on a statewide basis. With such a commitment to the promotion of fluoridation, it is difficult to see how the OHD could pass an objective judgment on health concerns, even if its personnel had the capacity to do so properly.

The result is that the OHD's promotion of fluoridation is not tempered by any firsthand knowledge of the safety of the program. For example, neither OHD personnel nor anyone else at the CDC investigates reports that some people may be sensitive to fluoride, even though many people claim to be in this position (see chapter 13). Nor do CDC personnel ensure that fluoride levels in the urine, blood, or bones are monitored in fluoridating communities to gauge the effects of short- and long-term exposures. There is also no evidence that the CDC is involved in any research program to investigate the toxicology of the fluoridating chemicals used.

We cannot look to the CDC to take any responsibility for the safety of water fluoridation. We return to a discussion of the role of the CDC in promoting fluoridation in chapter 23.

The Environmental Protection Agency
The EPA in the United States has no direct role in the water fluoridation program per se, but it does have an indirect role that might ultimately prove decisive. This is because, while the EPA Office of Drinking Water (ODW) does not regulate "additives" to water, it does regulate "contaminants." The EPA is required by the Safe Drinking Water Act to determine safe standards for all the contaminants that might enter the water supply from either natural

or industrial sources. Currently, the safe drinking water standard, otherwise known as the maximum contaminant level (MCL), for fluoride is 4 ppm. Above that level, water utilities are required by federal law to remove the excess fluoride.

In 2002, the ODW asked the National Research Council of the National Academies (NRC) to review that standard and the related goal (maximum contaminant level goal, or MCLG), which is also set at 4 ppm. In 2003, the NRC appointed a twelve-member panel to investigate the issue, and on March 22, 2006, the panel produced the 507-page report *Fluoride in Drinking Water: A Scientific Review of EPA's Standards* [3] (see chapter 14).

The NRC panel concluded that the 4 ppm standard was not protective of health and recommended that the EPA perform a risk assessment to determine a new MCLG. After over four years (as of April 2010), the ODW has failed to produce a new risk assessment or a new MCLG or MCL. Were the agency to produce an MCLG of 0 ppm, as some experts recommend,[4] it would force an end to the fluoridation program. This is the EPA's indirect involvement with the fluoridation program. It has the power to end fluoridation in the United States, but the issue is such a hot political potato that the agency seems unwilling to act.

The ODW takes no responsibility for the safety of the water fluoridation program itself and seems reluctant even to exercise the influence it could have on the practice by scientifically determining a protective MCLG. Thus, another federal agency is failing to protect the American people.

The Food and Drug Administration
Incredibly, even though fluoride is the most prescribed medicine in U.S. history—now given to over 180 million Americans in their drinking water every day—the FDA has never taken any responsibility for the safety of the water fluoridation program or for the safety of the chemicals used. It has not even tested or regulated the use of fluoride in prescriptions or over-the-counter supplements. As a result, fluoride has never been treated to the clinical trials required by the FDA for other drugs. There has never been a double-blind randomized clinical trial (RCT) for fluoridation's effectiveness. Nor have there been any well-conducted large-cohort studies in which all the possible confounding variables are controlled.

The FDA does, however, recognize that fluoride is a drug; its official designation is "unapproved new drug" (see chapter 1).

The FDA also regulates fluoride's use in toothpaste. If readers check the back of a tube of fluoridated toothpaste, they will find this FDA-required warning: "Keep out of the reach of children under 6 years of age. If you swallow more than used for brushing, get medical help or contact a poison control center right away." The recommended quantity for brushing is a "pea-size" dab. Such a dab contains about one-quarter of a milligram of fluoride, about the same amount as in one glass of fluoridated water. The FDA puts warnings on the former but remains silent on the latter.

So if none among the FDA, EPA, and CDC accepts responsibility for regulating the practice or fluoridation, or the fluoridating chemicals used, who does? Here the story gets even more bizarre.

The National Sanitation Foundation International

As we have seen, no federal agency regulates either the practice of water fluoridation or the chemicals used. There is plenty of advice but no responsibility. By default, regulation has been left to a private entity in the United States called the National Sanitation Foundation (NSF) International. This self-regulating, private consortium certifies water-fluoridation chemicals.

NSF Standard 60 established a standard for pollutants that is 10 percent of the maximum contaminant level. Unfortunately, NSF ignores this requirement for the chemicals used in water fluoridation. The MCL for fluoride is 4 ppm, but the NSF allows additions of fluoride between 0.7 and 1.2 ppm. Moreover, it ignores the fact that fluoridating chemicals contain arsenic, for which the EPA has assigned an MCLG of zero (see chapter 3). Thus the use of industrial-grade fluoridating agents is increasing the cancer risk for those drinking fluoridated tap water. This is in addition to any cancer risks posed by fluoride itself (see chapter 18).

In an affidavit obtained during preparation for a court case in California, the following exchange took place between Kyle Nordrehaug, lawyer for the plaintiffs, and Stan Hazan, the general manager for the NSF's Drinking Water Additives Certification Program:

> Lawyer: "Does NSF require the manufacturer to provide a list of published and unpublished toxicological studies relevant to HFSA [hydrofluorosilicic acid] and the chemical impurities present in HFSA?"
>
> Hazan: "I would say that the HFSA submissions have not come with the tox studies referenced."[5]

The NSF neither provides toxicological studies supporting the safety of the chemicals used in fluoridation nor accepts liability for its standards, as is made clear in this disclaimer in "Drinking Water Treatment Chemicals—Health Effects":

> NSF International (NSF), in performing its functions in accordance with its objectives, does not assume or undertake to discharge any responsibility of the manufacturer or any other party. The opinions and findings of NSF represent its professional judgment. NSF shall not be responsible to anyone for the use of or reliance upon this Standard by anyone. NSF shall not incur any obligation or liability for damages, including consequential damages, arising out of or in connection with the use, interpretation of, or reliance upon this Standard.[6]

So while the NSF claims that "NSF Standards provide basic criteria to promote sanitation and protection of the public health,"[7] it accepts no responsibility for damage to those who rely on its standards. Nor, apparently, do any of the agencies whose representatives belong to NSF panels. Another NSF disclaimer states, "Participation in NSF Standards development activities by regulatory agency representatives (federal, local, state) shall not constitute their agency's endorsement of NSF or any of its Standards."[8]

Thus, we must now add the NSF to the list of agencies that promote or accept water fluoridation but refuse to accept liability for any damage that the program may cause. This is quite a collection of "three-lettered" liability disowners: ADA, CDC, EPA, FDA, and NSF.

Summary

Fluoride is a drug, unapproved and untested by the FDA. It has never been subjected to randomized clinical trials for effectiveness or safety, as required for other drugs. It is added to the drinking water of over 180 million Americans each day (in some cases against intense individual opposition). The virtues of this practice are extolled by the CDC, the ADA, and many other professional bodies that vigorously promote or endorse it. However, no federal agency accepts responsibility for any damages that may accrue. All pass the buck to a self-regulating, private consortium called the NSF, which in turn accepts no liability for the "safe levels" or the "safety of the chemicals" it recommends. Thus to answer the question posed by the title of this chapter (Who is in Charge?) for the American fluoridation program, the answer is *no one.* We can only assume therefore that whatever liabilities are involved in this practice are taken on by local communities or by state authorities where the practice becomes mandatory via state legislation.

An Experimental Program

It may astound our readers to learn that fluoridation of the public water system remains an experimental procedure, even though the practice has been in effect for over sixty years. However, the facts speak for themselves:

1. When the fluoridation trials began in 1945, practically no health studies had been undertaken or published (see chapter 9).
2. When the U.S. Public Health Service (PHS) endorsed fluoridation in 1950, none of the trials had been completed and still no comprehensive health studies had been published (see chapter 9).
3. When a whole series of professional organizations followed the PHS and endorsed fluoridation in 1950, and in subsequent years, those organizations still had no comprehensive health studies to refer to and no trials had been completed (see chapter 10).
4. Since 1950 no rigorous scientific studies have established safety (see chapters 11–19) or effectiveness (see chapters 6–8). Many health questions remain unasked and unanswered.
5. Since 1950 the fluoridation program has not been monitored in a scientific or comprehensive fashion. Many basic health studies have still not been performed, and no effort has been made to monitor exposure in a scientific fashion—that is, there has been no systematic collection of measurements of fluoride levels in the urine, blood, or bones of people living in communities with fluoridated water (see chapter 22).
6. Fluoridating countries have made little or no effort to replicate studies performed elsewhere that have shown associations between fluoride exposure and increased bone fractures in children (chapter 17); arthritic-like symptoms in adults (chapter 17); lowered IQ in children (chapter 15); lowered thyroid function (chapter 16); and the accumulation of fluoride in the human pineal gland, as well as lowered melatonin production and earlier onset of puberty in animals (chapter 16).
7. Fluoridating countries have made little or no attempt to use dental fluorosis, a clearly visible manifestation of early childhood overexposure

to fluoride (chapter 11), as a biomarker to investigate health concerns in children that may be related to fluoride exposure.

8. No government that has promoted fluoridation has made any effort to investigate the many anecdotal reports that a subsection of the population is highly sensitive to fluoride's toxicity and is experiencing a range of common symptoms that, they claim, clear up when the source of fluoride is removed (see chapter 13).

9. Even when independent bodies have recommended key basic research, governments practicing fluoridation have ignored the recommendations. For example, in 1991, the National Health and Medical Research Council of Australia recommended that the government investigate the claims by a number of people that they were particularly sensitive to fluoride. The NHMRC also recommended the collection of data on fluoride levels in bone, so that health agencies would be in a better position to judge whether long-term exposure to fluoride might cause bone damage.[1] Neither federal nor state health authorities in Australia have responded to either recommendation in the nineteen years since the recommendations were made.

Basic Health Questions Unanswered

Few basic health studies have been done in fluoridating countries. In 2006, the U.S. National Research Council (NRC) was forced to make many recommendations for new research to resolve unanswered health questions about the fluoridation of water.[2] The chairman of this important review panel, Dr. John Doull, was interviewed for an article that appeared in *Scientific American* in January 2008 and was quoted as follows:

> What the committee found is that we've gone with the status quo regarding fluoride for many years—for too long really—and now we need to take a fresh look . . . In the scientific community people tend to think this is settled. I mean, when the U.S. surgeon general comes out and says this is one of the top 10 greatest achievements of the 20th century, that's a hard hurdle to get over. But when we looked at the studies that have been done, we found that many of these questions are unsettled and we have much less information than we should, considering how long this [fluoridation] has been going on.[3]

In 2001, Professor Trevor Sheldon, chair of the Advisory Group for the York Review[4] and founding director of the UK National Health Service's Centre for Reviews and Dissemination at the University of York, wrote the following about the York Review in an open letter disseminated in the UK:

> The review team was surprised that in spite of the large number of studies carried out over several decades there is a dearth of reliable evidence with which to inform policy. Until high quality studies are undertaken providing more definite evidence, there will continue to be legitimate scientific controversy over the likely effects and costs of water fluoridation.[5]

Violation of the Nuremberg Code

Those who promote and sanction fluoridation in the United States and other countries lack the answers to very basic health questions, and yet they continue to impose the practice on millions of people. Without suggesting any sinister motivations—we are sure that most of the people who promote fluoridation do so with the very best of intentions—it is clear from what we have said above that fluoridation is an ongoing human experiment and thus violates the Nuremberg Code, which requires informed consent to human experimentation from each individual being exposed to the treatment involved.[6]

Fluoridation is designed to treat people, and millions of people are receiving and drinking fluoridated water without being informed about possible side effects and without being asked to give their consent for such experimentation (see chapter 1). Moreover, those with low income have little choice but to drink the treated water whether they want to or not.

Rejections of Fluoridation

With so many basic health questions unanswered, it is little wonder that many countries have not followed the American example and fluoridated their water. In fact, contrary to the impression given by many fluoridation promoters, the vast majority of countries in the world—including China, India, Japan, and nearly all European countries—do not fluoridate their water. Only about thirty countries in the world have some percentage of their populations drinking fluoridated water, and of those only eight have more than 50 percent of their population doing so: Australia, Colombia, Ireland, Israel, Malaysia, New Zealand, Singapore, and the United States.

The European Experience

The following European countries have never fluoridated their water: Austria, Belgium, Denmark, France, Greece, Iceland, Italy, Luxemburg, and Norway. Countries that started fluoridation in one or more towns but have since stopped include the Czech Republic, Finland, Germany (West and East), the Netherlands, Sweden, and Switzerland. Some of the countries—Austria, France, Germany, and Switzerland—that do not currently fluoridate their water fluoridate their salt, but those, too, are a minority in Europe. Moreover, in those four countries non-fluoridated salt is available, leaving people with freedom of choice in the matter.

Only three countries in Europe have any significant water fluoridation: Ireland, the UK, and Spain. The Republic of Ireland has had mandatory fluoridation since 1963. Currently, over 70 percent of its population drinks fluoridated water. Less than 10 percent of the population in Spain drinks fluoridated water. The UK has had some fluoridation since the 1950s, but the percentage of people drinking fluoridated water has been stable for many years at approximately 10 percent. Since the Water Act was revamped in 2003, the UK government has renewed efforts to increase that figure. The changes made allow for the indemnification of water utilities for any liability involved in the fluoridation of drinking water.[7]

Contrary to claims made by promoters of fluoridation, the rejection of fluoridation has not been based on technical difficulties. In most cases countries have rejected fluoridation largely because they considered that a number of health issues had not been resolved and because they did not want to force it on people who didn't want it. A spokesperson in the Czech Republic, Dr. B. Havlik of the Ministry of Health, gave the following assessment of stopping fluoridation in that country:

> Since 1993, drinking water has not been treated with fluoride in public water supplies throughout the Czech Republic. Although fluoridation of drinking water has not actually been proscribed it is not under consideration because this form of supplementation is considered as follows:
>
> (a) uneconomical (only 0.54 percent of water suitable for drinking is used as such; the remainder is employed for hygiene etc.). Furthermore, an increasing amount of consumers (particularly children) are using bottled

water for drinking (underground water usually with fluor [fluoride])

(b) unecological (environmental load by a foreign substance)

(c) unethical ("forced medication")

(d) toxicologically and physiologically debatable (fluoridation represents an untargeted form of supplementation which disregards actual individual intake and requirements and may lead to excessive health-threatening intake in certain population groups; [and] complexation of fluor in water into non biological active forms of fluor)[8]

European countries have not suffered more tooth decay as a result of rejecting fluoridation. In fact, according to World Health Organization (WHO) data available online,[9] rates of tooth decay in twelve-year-olds have been coming down as fast in non-fluoridated countries as in fluoridated ones. A graphical plot of these data can also be accessed online.[10] We show a simplified version of this graph in figure 6.1 in chapter 6.

Moreover, there is no evidence that where fluoridation has been started and stopped in Europe there has been a rise in tooth decay. Indeed, two studies published in 2000, from Finland and the former East Germany, show that tooth decay continued to decline after fluoridation was halted.[11, 12] There have been similar reports from Cuba[13] and Canada's British Columbia.[14] The ADA[15] claims that in cases where fluoridation has been halted and no increase in tooth decay observed, other steps have been taken to fight tooth decay. Whether or not that is the explanation, European countries have clearly demonstrated that there are other ways of reducing tooth decay without forcing everyone to take a medicine in their drinking water.

Summary

When the fluoridation of drinking water began, there was little evidence for its long-term safety, and since then little attempt has been made to monitor its health effects systematically. Because there are so many unanswered health questions, fluoridation of water must be considered an ongoing experimental procedure, and as such it is a violation of the Nuremberg Code, which forbids experimentation on humans without their informed consent. Only a minority of countries practice fluoridation. In Europe, nearly all countries either have never fluoridated their water or have ceased doing so. Yet the incidence of caries has declined just as much in those countries as in countries that practice fluoridation.

PART TWO

The Evidence That Fluoridation Is Ineffective

One of the big surprises awaiting someone who decides to review the literature on water fluoridation is that, despite the impression conveyed by its promoters for over sixty years, the evidence that swallowing fluoride actually reduces tooth decay is weak. In chapter 6, we review the many lines of evidence that fluoridation is ineffective at reducing tooth decay. In chapter 7, we examine the evidence that the famous 1942 study by Dean, Arnold, and Elvove and the early trials in the United States, Canada, and New Zealand were either seriously flawed or fraudulent.

In chapter 8, we review many of the studies published since 1980 that indicate little or no benefit from fluoridation. We also discuss two other lines of evidence that cast doubt on the effectiveness of fluoridation: (1) the impact on tooth decay when fluoridation is halted, and (2) the dental crises being reported in American cities that have been fluoridated for over thirty years.

Fluoridation and Tooth Decay

Incredibly, in the sixty years that public water systems have been fluoridated, there has never been a study of the results of fluoridation of the quality required by the Food and Drug Administration when approving new drugs for efficacy—that is, a study involving randomized clinical trials. Such trials require random selection and double-blind testing. "Double-blind" means that neither the people being tested nor the people determining the outcome know which subjects have received the drug and which have received a placebo.

The York Report, a systematic review carried out by a team from York University at the request of the UK government, adopted the following criteria for awarding Grade A status to a fluoridation study:

- The study started within one year of either initiation or discontinuation of water fluoridation and had a follow-up of at least two years for positive effects and at least five years for negative effects.
- The study either was randomized or addressed at least three possible confounding factors and adjusted for these in the analysis where appropriate.
- The fluoridation status of participants was unknown to those assessing outcomes.[1]

Even using these criteria, an exhaustive review of the literature identified no Grade A studies. Eventually, the York Review team was able to find only six longitudinal studies that met its Grades B and C classifications. Those six studies were published over a period of years from 1961 to 1990. That does not speak well of the general quality of the studies that have addressed fluoridation. The absence of Grade A studies is extremely unfortunate because there are so many aspects of tooth decay that might have been revealed if the issue were examined using stringent scientific methods.

Instead of randomized clinical trials, proponents of fluoridation have relied heavily on the famous two-part, twenty-one-city study by Dean, Arnold, and Elvove;[2, 3] trials conducted in North America between 1945 and 1955; and an early trial in New Zealand. The methodologies and legitimacy of both the

Dean study and these early trials have been challenged by fluoridation critics for many years (see chapter 7).

Proponents of fluoridation like the CDC have claimed that the incidence of tooth decay is coming down in fluoridated communities because of the introduction of water or salt fluoridation; however, we saw in chapter 5 that most industrialized countries, including most European countries, fluoridate neither their water nor their salt, yet according to World Health Organization (WHO) data available online, tooth decay in twelve-year-olds has come down as fast in non-fluoridated countries as in fluoridated countries.[4] As mentioned in chapter 5, a graphical plot of these data can also be accessed online,[5] and a similar graph is presented in an article by Cheng, Chalmers, and Sheldon in the *British Medical Journal*.[6] Because it is difficult to distinguish which country is which in the plot, especially when the image is converted into black and white, we have selected just four of the non-fluoridated countries to compare with four fluoridated countries in figure 6.1. The four non-fluoridated countries fluoridate neither their water nor their salt, yet there is little obvious difference in the rate of decline in tooth decay in these eight countries.

We invite readers to compare figures 6.1 and 6.2. Figure 6.2 appeared (as figure 1) in the CDC report that backed up its claim that fluoridation is one of the "Ten Great Public Health Achievements" in the twentieth century.[7]

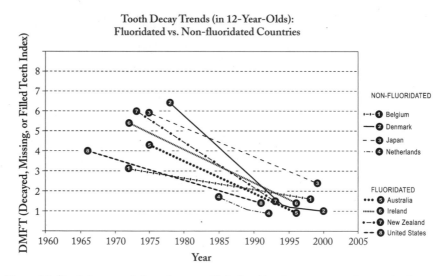

Figure 6.1. Tooth decay trends in twelve-year-olds in fluoridated vs. a representative sample of non-fluoridated countries. Graph based upon plots by Chris Neurath.[8] *Source:* World Health Organization, 2004.

In this figure, the CDC authors show the decline in tooth decay in twelve-year-olds in the United States from 1967 to 1992.[9] On the same graph the CDC authors show the percentage of the American public drinking fluoridated water increasing over the same period. The suggestion is that tooth decay has come down in the United States during this period because the number of people drinking fluoridated water has gone up. In the text the CDC authors refer to this figure in the following context: "The effectiveness of community water fluoridation in preventing dental caries prompted rapid adoption of this public health measure in cities throughout the United States. As a result, dental caries declined precipitously during the second half of the 20th century. For example, the mean DMFT among persons aged 12 years in the United States declined 68%, from 4.0 in 1996–70 . . . to 1.3 in 1988–1994."[10]

The problem with both the CDC's statement and its figure 1 (reproduced in figure 6.2) is that this agency is stating or implying a cause-and-effect relationship between increased use of fluoridation and the observed drop in tooth decay in twelve-year-olds. If the CDC authors had checked the WHO data for themselves, they would have been hard put to maintain that falling tooth decay in twelve-year-olds in the United States was simply due to the increased use of fluoridated water, as the same or greater declines have been

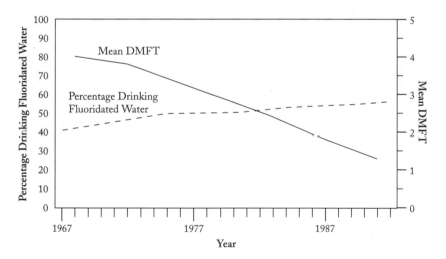

Figure 6.2. Percentage of the U.S. population in areas with fluoridated community water systems and mean number of decayed, missing (because of caries), or filled permanent teeth (DMFT) among children aged twelve years in the United States, 1967–1992. *Source:* Figure 1 in CDC (1999).[11]

40   THE EVIDENCE THAT FLUORIDATION IS INEFFECTIVE

achieved over the same time period in countries whose populations have not been drinking fluoridated water.

Journalists and officials around the world are innocently using the CDC statement that "fluoridation is one of the top public health achievements of the twentieth century" without realizing how weak the CDC's evidence for the benefits of this practice actually is.

Fluoridation vs. Income Level

One of the biggest factors that mars many studies claiming to show a benefit from fluoridated water is the failure to control for key confounding variables, and one of the most important of these is income level.

Dr. Bill Osmunson, a practicing dentist who supported fluoridation for twenty-five years before he began to research the issue for himself, has shown that, according to the results of a questionnaire administered to parents in all fifty states by the Department of Health and Human Services (DHHS),[12] there is absolutely no correlation between the percentage of parents who responded that their children had very good or excellent teeth and the percentage of the population in the state drinking fluoridated water. However, there is a very strong relation in all fifty states between the percentage of parents giving that answer and their income levels. Across the board, 80 percent of high-income parents gave that answer, but only about 60 percent of low-income parents did so (see figure 6.3).[13]

In 2002–2004 a survey of tooth decay in third graders in New York State was conducted by the pro-fluoridation New York Department of Health.[14] When Michael Connett plotted the tooth decay in New York third graders (averaged by county) against the percentage of the population of each county drinking fluoridated water, no relationship was found.[15] There was again, however, a relationship with average county income levels, though the relationship was less clear than that in the Osmunson data (see figures 6.4 and 6.5).

Other Variables

Figures 6.3–6.5 show that when comparing U.S. states or New York counties, income level is a far greater factor affecting dental decay than the percentage of the population that has fluoridated water. If this and other key variables are not carefully controlled and two towns are selected from a long list of towns (or counties or states), you can get any result you want.

Readers might not believe that promoters of fluoridation could apply such a crude means of influencing the public in these matters, but this appears to

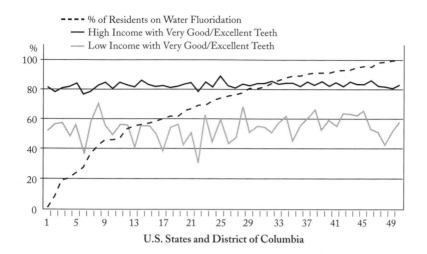

Figure 6.3. Percentage of parents (of both high and low income) who responded that their child had very good or excellent teeth compared with the percentage of the population with access to fluoridated public water in each state and the District of Columbia. *Source:* Osmunson. [16]

have been attempted in the case of the New York State survey. Before the study was published, figures for just two counties were leaked to a Syracuse, New York, newspaper.[21] Those figures purported to show that tooth decay in third graders was less in fluoridated Onondaga County than in non-fluoridated Cayuga County. However, as discussed above, the study did not take into account the key issue of income level or any other confounding variables. In 2008, Onondaga County had a median income level of $50,586 compared to a median income level of $47,308 for Cayuga County. Moreover, Onondaga County contains the large city of Syracuse whereas Cayuga County has only small towns. Larger cities tend to have more dental services than small towns and rural areas. A front-page article featuring this selective piece of information led to a push to fluoridate Cayuga County. Fortunately, the effort failed.

In the UK, promoters routinely contrast fluoridated Birmingham with non-fluoridated Manchester, with little more justification than that the two cities are comparable in size. Again, no careful account is taken of factors such as income level, ethnicity, educational level, and availability of dental services.

Non-Fluoridated vs. Fluoridated Countries

Since 1980, a number of prominent review articles and studies have found little or no significant difference in the level of tooth decay (especially of the

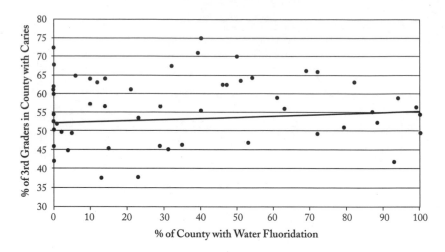

Figure 6.4. Percentage of third graders with caries (average by New York county) plotted against the percentage of the population that has fluoridated water in each county. The line drawn on the figure represents the best straight-line fit to the data, resulting from linear-regression analysis. A horizontal linear regression line means that there is no apparent statistical relationship between the two variables plotted (in this case percentage caries rate in third graders averaged by county and percentage of the population in each county with access to fluoridated water). *Source:* Figure prepared by Michael Connett for the Fluoride Action Network based on NYDOH data.[17, 18]

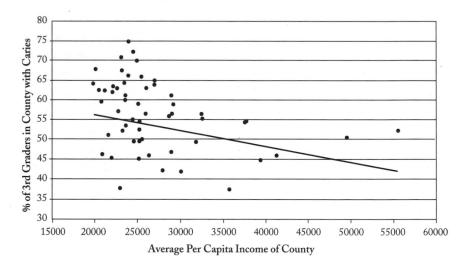

Figure 6.5. Percentage of third graders with caries (averaged by New York county) plotted against average personal per capita income in each county. The line drawn on the figure represents the best straight-line fit to the data, resulting from linear-regression analysis. The fact that this line is sloping downwards from left to right suggests that as average per capita income for each county goes up the percentage of third graders with caries goes down. *Source:* Figure prepared by Michael Connett for the Fluoride Action Network based on NYDOH data.[19, 20]

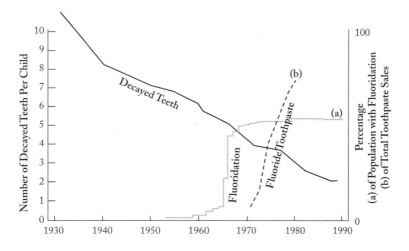

Figure 6.6. Tooth decay in five-year-olds in New Zealand plotted over the time period 1930–1990. The plot also shows the periods in which fluoridated water and fluoridated toothpaste were introduced.[22]

permanent teeth) when comparing children living in fluoridated and non-fluoridated communities. These studies also are reviewed in chapter 8.

In chapter 5, we referred to four modern studies that showed that when fluoridation was halted in communities in British Columbia (Canada), Cuba, Finland, and the former East Germany, tooth decay rates did not go up as anticipated and in some cases continued to go down. The ADA claims that that was because the communities in question took other steps to reduce tooth decay commensurate with the cessation of fluoridation.[23] Some studies have even found that tooth decay rates increase as the fluoride concentration in the water increases.[24–31]

In New Zealand one of the unique features of the dental data collected is that under the country's national health system, dental decay is measured in every five-year-old and every twelve-year-old. When John Colquhoun examined the historical data, he found that tooth decay rates in five-year-olds (1930–1990) were coming down long before fluoridation of the water began or fluoridated toothpaste was introduced (see figure 6.6).

Maximization of Fluoride Benefit

Mark Diesendorf, in his article "The Mystery of Declining Tooth Decay," published in *Nature* in 1986, showed that the rate of tooth decay was coming down before fluoridation was introduced in communities in Australia and

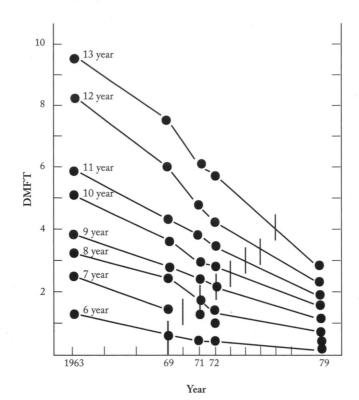

Figure 6.7. Decline in caries, measured by DMFT, in Tamworth, Australia, for children in age groups six to thirteen years. The vertical line cutting the graph line for each age group denotes the year when the maximum possible benefit from fluoridation was reached. Tamworth was fluoridated in 1963. *Source:* Figure adapted from figure 1 in Diesendorf, 1986.[32]

continued to decline after any benefits of fluoride would have been maximized (see figure 6.7).

This finding remains relevant—but often overlooked—today. For example, after twelve years of a fluoridation program, any drop in tooth decay prevalence in future generations of twelve-year-olds cannot be ascribed to fluoridation. After twelve years of the program, all subsequent generations of twelve-year-olds will have been exposed to fluoridation for their whole lives. Further declines in tooth decay can only be explained by other causes. Today, careless observers credit all further declines in successive generations to fluoridation, even after the year in which any benefit would have been maximized for each age group (shown by the short vertical lines in figure 6.7).

Factors Concealing a Lack of Benefit

A number of factors can cause an *apparent* or *real* decline in tooth decay that has nothing to do with the action of fluoride on the tooth itself. We discuss a few of these here:

- **Delayed eruption of teeth.** Until recently, few studies purporting to demonstrate fluoridation's effectiveness have controlled for a possible delayed eruption of teeth caused by fluoride, for which there is some, albeit inconsistent, evidence.[33, 34] Komárek et al. controlled for this factor and found that the apparent benefit of fluoride largely disappears.[35] We discuss the details of the Komárek article in chapter 8.

- **Primary versus secondary dentition.** Those promoting fluoridation usually use the data on primary dentition (baby teeth) rather than secondary dentition (permanent teeth). We argue that decay in the permanent teeth is more relevant, however, since those are the teeth we hope to retain for the rest of our lives. In a videotaped debate between Michael Lennon, chair of the British Fluoridation Society, and Paul Connett, director of the Fluoride Action Network, held on the Isle of Man, all the statistics Lennon cited were for primary teeth, whereas all the studies cited by Connett, showing little or no benefit of fluoride, were for secondary teeth.[36]

- **Other minerals in the water.** Many of the early trials and subsequent studies have been lax about ensuring that there are comparable levels of other minerals in the water that can affect tooth decay (e.g. calcium, magnesium, strontium) in the study and control towns. The levels of minerals in local soils might also be a factor if they enrich local food supplies with key tooth-building minerals.

Baby-Bottle Tooth Decay

Even promoters of fluoridation have conceded that it cannot prevent baby-bottle tooth decay (BBTD, also called nursing-bottle caries), a distressing example of tooth decay in infants, which often leads to extractions under anesthesia. BBTD is caused by babies sucking on sugared water, fruit juice, or carbonated beverages for hours on end.[37–44] Promoters of fluoridation are being dishonest when they use pictures of BBTD to make their case.

Explaining the Universal Decline in Decay
The Purported Halo Effect

Some promoters of fluoridation have tried to rationalize the similar rates of tooth decay in fluoridated and non-fluoridated communities by claiming a *halo effect*. They suggest that children in non-fluoridated communities are getting fluoride from food and beverages imported from fluoridated communities. However, this explanation cannot possibly explain the similar declines in rates of tooth decay in fluoridated and non-fluoridated countries in Europe (see figure 6.1), because the majority of those countries are unfluoridated; thus, there is little or no source of fluoridated beverages or foodstuffs moving into non-fluoridated countries from the fluoridated ones.

Wrong Mechanism of Benefit

A more likely explanation for the similar rates of tooth decay in fluoridated and non-fluoridated communities came in 1999 (and again in 2001) when the CDC, a longtime promoter of fluoridation, conceded that promoters had got the mechanism of fluoride's action wrong for over fifty years. The CDC admitted that the major benefits of fluoride are *topical*, not *systemic* [45, 46] (see chapter 5).

Thus, if fluoride has played any role in reducing tooth decay, it is more likely because of the universal availability of fluoridated toothpaste (which delivers fluoride topically), than because of the number of people swallowing fluoridated water. Indeed, in systematic reviews (compare Marinho[47] with McDonagh et al.[48]), the evidence that fluoridated toothpaste reduces tooth decay in children and adolescents is stronger than the evidence that swallowing fluoridated water does so. See also the review by Eaton and Carlile.[49]

High-Sugar Diets

Some opponents of water fluoridation reject even the topical benefits of fluoride. They argue that tooth decay is a result of poor diet: too much sugar and not enough minerals and vitamins. They point out that in industrialized countries where high-sugar diets are relatively common, there is a very strong correlation between poverty and tooth decay. Thus, as the standard of living increases, the incidence of tooth decay decreases. An increased standard of living allows parents more money to provide better diets (more fresh fruit and vegetables) and to pay for preventative dental care. Since World War II, we have also seen the introduction of vitamin D–fortified milk and, in some countries, school milk programs. In the United States this coincided with the introduction of fluoridation. Vitamin D, calcium, and phosphate are present in milk and are needed for the healthy development of both primary and secondary dentition. It is possible that the recent increases in tooth decay being reported in some fluoridated countries may reflect the fact that some children are drinking less milk and more soft drinks.

Antibiotics in Processed Food

Another possible explanation for the overall decline in tooth decay in industrialized countries was offered by New Zealand researcher Betty de Liefde.[50] She notes that there has been an increased consumption of processed foods containing antibiotics as preservative agents. Some of those antibiotics, she argues, would reduce the bacteria in the mouth that are responsible for converting sugars to acids, which attack the enamel and begin the decay process.

Summary

The benefits of water fluoridation have been greatly exaggerated. The early studies that served as the basis for initiating fluoridation were methodologically flawed (for further discussion, see chapter 7). Since those early studies, many studies have failed to control for confounding variables, particularly that of income level. For several decades caries rates have been declining at a comparable rate in both fluoridated and non-fluoridated countries. Together with supporting data of several kinds, this shows that factors other than fluoride ingestion have been at work. Conversely, the experience of many poor city areas has shown that fluoridation cannot compensate for the shortcomings of diet and dental care.

The Early Evidence Reexamined

Coauthored by Peter Meiers

A great deal of the conviction that fluoridation works has been derived from two sources: Dean, Arnold, and Elvove's famous two-part, twenty-one-city study in 1942[1, 2] and the early fluoridation trials in the United States, Canada, and New Zealand. Despite the weaknesses of both the Dean study and the fluoridation trials, those early studies are cited again and again to support the claim of the success of fluoridation. As Benjamin Nesin, director of the New York State Water Laboratories, stated in 1956, "It must be emphasized that the fluoridation hypothesis in its entirety rests on a very narrow base of selected experimental information. It is this very base which is vulnerable to scientific criticism. And it is upon this very narrow base that the impressive array of endorsement rests like an inverted pyramid."[3]

In actual fact, that "impressive array of endorsements" began in 1950, long before these trials, which began in 1945, were completed in 1955. Proponents really didn't need to have very much data available once the U.S. Public Health Service (PHS) endorsed fluoridation in 1950, halfway through the trials (see chapter 9).

The Dean Study

In describing Dean's early work, the Centers for Disease Control and Prevention (CDC) stated in 1999, "Dean compared the prevalence of fluorosis with data collected by others on dental caries prevalence among children in 26 states (as measured by DMFT) and noted a strong inverse relation. This cross-sectional relation was confirmed in a study of 21 cities in Colorado, Illinois, Indiana, and Ohio."[4] This raises the question, if Dean had access to data from twenty-six states, why did he use data from only twenty-one cities from four states in this critical two-part report? Did he select the cities that best supported his hypothesis? Dean's twenty-one-city plot is shown in figure 7.1.

Dean claimed that he limited the cities to those for which he had evidence that the water supply had been a constant source of natural fluoride for twenty years or more. However, according to Dr. Fred Exner, a well-known radiolo-

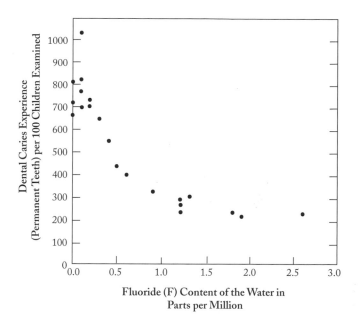

Figure 7.1. Dean's twenty-one-city graph. The original caption read, "Relation between the amount of dental caries (permanent teeth) observed in 7257 selected 12–14 year old white school children of 21 cities of 4 states and the fluoride (F) content of the public water supply." *Source:* Adapted from Dean, Arnold, and Elvove, 1942.[5]

gist and prominent critic of fluoridation, during cross-examination in court (*Schuringa v. Chicago*, 1960), Dean admitted that some of the cities did not meet that criterion.[6]

The late Rudolf Ziegelbecker, an Austrian statistician, pursued this issue. When he added in all the data he could find from the United States and Europe that compared prevalence of tooth decay with natural fluoride levels in the water, the inverse relationship reported by Dean was absent (see figure 7.2). However, when he examined the same data for dental fluorosis, he found a robust direct relationship—that is, as the level of fluoride in the water increased, so did the prevalence of dental fluorosis (see figure 7.3). One relationship (between fluoride levels and dental fluorosis) holds up over the "background noise"; the other (between fluoride levels and dental decay) does not.[7]

In a subsequent study Ziegelbecker and his son examined tooth decay data collected by the World Health Organization (WHO) in several individual countries, and again they found no relationship between tooth decay and levels

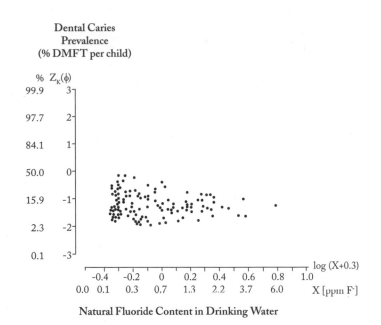

Figure 7.2. Ziegelbecker's plot of prevalence of tooth decay versus water fluoride levels. Tooth decay is plotted as the probit values of the percentages of the average DMFT in each community (the Z scale). The probit transformation is a standard procedure for making percentage data linear and more amenable to statistical analysis. The fluoride water levels (X ppm) in each community are plotted on a logarithmic scale as log (X + 0.3). The addition of 0.3 is Ziegelbecker's adjustment for other sources of fluoride in addition to water. *Source:* Reproduced from Ziegelbecker, 1981.[8]

of natural fluoride in drinking water.[9] Ziegelbecker Senior further elaborated on his critique of Dean's twenty-one-city study and the practice of fluoridation in general in a submission he made to *Codex Alimentarius* in 2003."[10]

The Early Trials

The trials conducted between 1945 and 1955 in the United States and Canada and a little later in New Zealand, which helped to consolidate the argument that fluoridation reduces tooth decay, have been heavily criticized. In those trials, pairs of cities were chosen; in one city of each pair sodium fluoride was added to the water to a level of 1 ppm, and in the other city (the control city) no addition was made. In one trial (in Brantford, Ontario) two controls were used: One control city (Sarnia, Ontario) had no fluoride added, and the other (Stratford, Ontario) had natural levels of fluoride at 1.3 ppm. In two of the trials (those in Grand Rapids, Michigan, and Hastings, New Zealand) the control cities (Muskegon and Napier, respectively) were dropped long

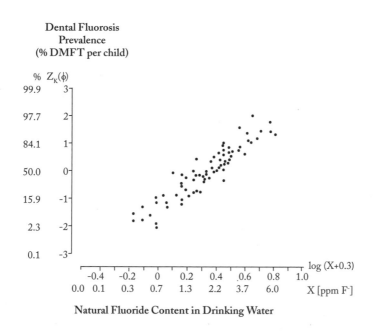

Figure 7.3. Ziegelbecker's plot of the prevalence of dental fluorosis versus water fluoride levels. Dental fluorosis is plotted as the probit values of the percentages of the children in each community with this condition (the Z scale). The scale used in the horizontal axis is explained in the legend to Figure 7.2. *Source:* Reproduced from Ziegelbecker, 1981.[11]

before the trials were due to end. The authors of this book have not studied in depth all the many reports published during those trials, but people who have done so have found many weaknesses in the methodologies used and the poor choice of control communities.[12–16] According to Dr. Hubert Arnold, a statistician from the University of California at Davis, the early fluoridation trials "are especially rich in fallacies, improper design, invalid use of statistical methods, omissions of contrary data, and just plain muddleheadedness and hebetude."[17]

In chapter 8 we discuss many factors that affect tooth decay. These include income level, ethnicity, diet, other minerals in the water, local soil and food, dental education level, and the quality of dental services available. Further complicating the issue is maintaining a consistent diagnosis of tooth decay over time and between the exposed and control communities. Many of these factors were not controlled very carefully, if at all, in the early trials, and that led to exaggerated claims of reduction in tooth decay in the conclusions of those trials.

Examples of Poor Methodology

As mentioned previously, in two trials, the control communities (Muskegon, Michigan, and Napier, New Zealand) were fluoridated before the trial was completed, so the reductions in tooth decay claimed were based on a before-and-after assessment of the fluoridated community and not a comparison with the non-fluoridated community. The reductions in the prevalence of tooth decay ascribed to fluoridation would have been negated if there had been comparable reductions in the non-fluoridating community over the same period of time.

Furthermore, when the Grand Rapids–Muskegon trial began in Michigan in 1945, children from all seventy-nine schools in Grand Rapids (the fluoridated city) were examined. By 1949, however, examiners were observing children from only twenty-five of those schools. Meanwhile, in Muskegon (the non-fluoridated control city), children from *all* the schools were still being examined.

Another example of inconsistency in sampling size is provided by the fact that when the Grand Rapids study commenced, the number of twelve- to sixteen-year-olds examined was 7,661, but by the final year of the study, the number being studied had dropped to 1,031.[18]

Along with these changes in sampling methods, the Grand Rapids study employed multiple examiners to assess the children's teeth. But at the time, studies had already shown that there is considerable variability among dentists' assessments of tooth decay.[19, 20] Dr. Philip Sutton, who authored two monographs on this subject,[21, 22] was senior research fellow in the Department of Oral Medicine and Surgery at the Dental School of the University of Melbourne, Australia. His criticisms of these early trials have never been successfully refuted by proponents, even though they have tried. Some of the efforts to critique his work, and Sutton's responses, were published in a book titled *The Greatest Fraud: Fluoridation* shortly before he died, in 1996.[23]

The Newburgh-Kingston Trial

There are three very interesting extra pieces of information about the Newburgh versus Kingston trial. The first is that even while the original researchers were claiming the benefits of fluoridation, a report emerged that far more tooth defects were being observed in fluoridated Newburgh than in unfluoridated Kingston. In a letter dated October 26, 1954 (over nine years into the trial), John Forst, MD, of the New York State Education Department, reported to Dr. James Kerwin, of the New Jersey Department of Health, that in unfluoridated Kingston 41.6 percent (2,209 out of 5,303 pupils) had defects, with 29.2 percent receiving treatment, compared with 63.2 percent (3,139 out of 4,959) that had defects, with 41.7 percent receiving treatment, in fluoridated Newburgh.[24]

The second interesting piece of information is that in the intervening years since 1955 the control community of Kingston has never been fluoridated. This has allowed researchers to continue to compare tooth decay in the two communities over a period of fifty years. Over this period the purported difference in tooth decay reported in 1955 between the fluoridated and non-

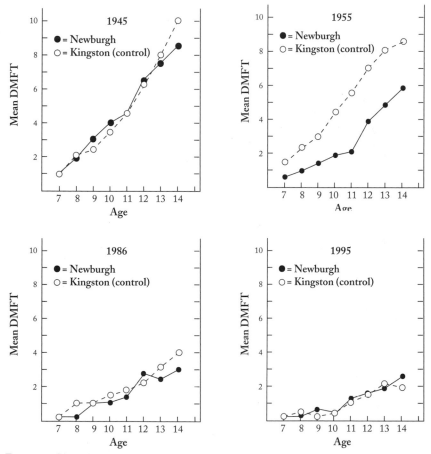

Figure 7.4. Plots of tooth decay (measured as DMFT = decayed, missing, and filled permanent teeth) of seven- to fourteen-year-old lifelong residents in Newburgh (fluoridated) and Kingston (unfluoridated), New York, published in 1945, 1955, 1986, and 1995, respectively. *Source:* Plots derived from figure 1 in Kumar and Green, 1998.[25]

fluoridated communities has disappeared. The latest study, giving rise to two separate papers (published in 1998), indicates that the teeth of the children in unfluoridated Kingston are slightly better than those in fluoridated Newburgh.[26, 27] In figure 7.4 we have plotted the reported tooth decay for children ages seven to fourteen, comparing children in fluoridated Newburgh and unfluoridated Kingston, in the comparisons conducted in 1945, 1955, 1986, and 1995, as graphically summarized by Kumar and Green.[28]

The third interesting piece of information is that the Newburgh-Kingston trial was closely monitored by Dr. Harold Hodge, chief toxicologist for the Manhattan Project.[29] Apparently, the team that was developing the atomic bomb was very interested in monitoring fluoride's low-level toxic effects on children. We discuss some of the health effects observed in this trial, including the earlier onset of menstruation in young girls in fluoridated Newburgh, in chapter 10, and we say more about Harold Hodge's long history of involvement in the promotion of fluoridation in chapters 9 and 10.

The Hastings-Napier Trial

The Hastings-Napier trial was begun in 1954 and was used to promote fluoridation successfully throughout New Zealand. However, this trial has since been shown to be fraudulent.[30–32] The control community (Napier) was dropped two years after the trial began, and the huge drop in tooth decay found in Hastings was found to be due to a change in the methodology used to determine what constituted tooth decay between when the study started and when it ended. The change in methodology was not acknowledged by the authors when they published their reports.[33–38]

Summary

There are several reasons to doubt the validity of the Dean et al. study on the relationship between caries incidence and the fluoride content of water. Subsequently, Ziegelbacker found no relationship, such as claimed by Dean, although there was a strong relationship between fluoride concentration and the incidence of fluorosis. Many serious flaws have been identified in the early trials of fluoridation, on which the modern dogma of fluoridation's safety and effectiveness is built. Subsequent developments in tooth decay in the towns of Newburgh and Kingston, New York, in the years since 1955 (the year when the study there concluded) put into question the benefits claimed in 1955.

Key Modern Studies

In the history of fluoridation a major development occurred in 1980. This was the year when Dr. John Colquhoun was sent by his superiors in New Zealand on a four-month world tour to investigate tooth decay on several continents. He expected to bring back with him evidence that would prove, once and for all, that fluoridation worked. He failed to do so.

Colquhoun's Fluoridation Activities

In the 1960s and 1970s John Colquhoun was the principal dental officer for Auckland, New Zealand's largest city. Both as a dental officer and as a city councilor, he enthusiastically and successfully promoted fluoridation throughout the country. He poured scorn on one particular councilor who opposed the measure—for which Colquhoun later apologized.

On his 1980 world tour, which took him to Australia, Asia, North America, and Europe, pro-fluoridation dental researchers told Colquhoun in private that they were not finding the difference in tooth decay between fluoridated and non-fluoridated communities that they had expected; in fact, they were finding very little difference at all.

When Colquhoun returned to New Zealand, he looked at the complete record of tooth decay in the country. At that time, under the New Zealand National Health Service, all five-year-olds and twelve-year-olds had their teeth examined. He found no difference in tooth decay between the fluoridated and non-fluoridated cities. If anything, the teeth were slightly better in the non-fluoridated communities.

After Colquhoun's assistants reported to him the extensive amount of dental fluorosis occurring in fluoridated Auckland, he made fluoridation's ineffectiveness public. To his enormous credit he spent the rest of his life trying to undo the damage he had done promoting fluoridation, by reversing his position and opposing the practice in any scientific way he could. Author Paul Connett interviewed Colquhoun on videotape in Auckland in 1997, shortly before Colquhoun died, and found that interviewing this soft-spoken but courageous man was a humbling experience.[1] Colquhoun wrote up his findings in several published papers.[2-7] After he retired he obtained a PhD, and his research thesis examined the history of fluoridation in New Zealand.[8] He argued that

New Zealand's dental education program to reduce tooth decay was superior to the use of water fluoridation for the same purpose. He offered Thomas Kuhn's famous analysis, *The Structure of Scientific Revolutions*,[9] to explain the reluctance of the New Zealand dental community to change its outlook on fluoridation's safety and effectiveness. In his thesis, Colquhoun also exposed the rigged nature of the Hastings-Napier fluoridation trial (discussed in chapter 7).

Colquhoun summarized his evolution on this issue in a journal article published in 1997 titled "Why I Changed My Mind about Fluoridation."[10] Two fluoridation proponents responded to Colquhoun's arguments in a later issue of the same journal, with an article titled "Why We Have Not Changed Our Minds about the Safety and Efficacy of Water Fluoridation: A Response to John Colquhoun." They wrote, "Colquhoun, like many opponents of fluoridation, subscribes to the conspiracy theory, according to which the government, health authorities, and the dental profession are trying to foist water fluoridation on an unsuspecting public."[11]

Leverett 1982

In the 1980s, articles began to appear in major publications like *Science* and *Nature* confirming what Colquhoun had found out privately. These articles pointed out that the prevalence of tooth decay was falling as fast in non-fluoridated communities as in fluoridated ones. Dennis Leverett reviewed many of these studies in *Science* in 1982. He noted:

> Within the past 2 or 3 years there has been increasing evidence from several developed nations of a drop in the prevalence of dental caries which cannot be attributed directly to intentional fluoride use. The data are becoming available as epidemiologists and clinical researchers review the patterns of dental caries prevalence in communities that do not have fluoridated water. The data cover children from the ages of 5 to 17 for various periods of up to 30 years; caries reductions as high as 60 per cent have been observed.[12]

Leverett cited at least nine studies that showed a decline in caries prevalence in communities without fluoridated water and speculated that the reductions were due to "an increase in fluoride in the food chain, especially from the use of fluoridated water in food processing, increased use of infant formulas with measurable fluoride content, and even unintentional ingestion of fluoride dentifrices."[13]

Diesendorf 1986

Mark Diesendorf published "The Mystery of Declining Tooth Decay" in *Nature* in 1986.[14] As did Leverett, Diesendorf reported little difference in tooth decay between fluoridated and non-fluoridated communities. He rejected Leverett's hypothesis that the drop in tooth decay in non-fluoridated areas was due to the ingestion of fluoride from other sources, because, he said, "the food processing pathway is unlikely to be significant in Western Europe where there is hardly any fluoridation."[15] He suggested, "The main causes of the observed reductions in caries are changes in dietary patterns, possible changes in the immune status of populations and, under some circumstances, the use of topical fluorides."[16]

Diesendorf concluded his article with this comment: "Perhaps the real mystery of declining tooth decay is why so much effort has gone into poor quality research on fluoridation, instead of on more fundamental questions of diet and immunity."[17]

It is worth noting that Diesendorf's background was not in dentistry but in theoretical physics. Indeed, he had previously published in *Nature* on that subject. Today he is better known in Australia for his work on alternative energy sources.[18]

Gray 1987

Another dental professional who questioned fluoridation's effectiveness was A. S. Gray, who reviewed the tooth-decay figures in British Columbia and other parts of Canada. According to Gray, those figures indicated the following:

> DMF rates in children are falling drastically in non-fluoridated areas as well as fluoridated areas. The current statements of our profession in support of fluoridation do not appear to take these changes into account. It is timely for the profession to take the lead in deciding what is scientifically appropriate to tell communities that may consider installing fluoridation equipment and holding fluoridation referendums in the late 1980s.[19]

Gray cited the following figures to support his conclusion: "Survey results in British Columbia, with only 11 per cent of the population using fluoridated water, show lower average DMFT rates than provinces with 40–70 per cent of the population drinking fluoridated water. How does one explain this? . . . School districts recently reporting the highest caries-free rates were totally unfluoridated."[20]

NIDR 1986–1987

In 1986, the National Institute of Dental Research (NIDR) stepped in and organized—at great expense to the U.S. taxpayer—the largest survey of tooth decay ever undertaken in the United States. It examined the teeth of nearly forty thousand children in eighty-four communities. Findings were published in two papers, one by Yiamouyiannis[21] and the other by Brunelle and Carlos.[22]

Yiamouyiannis 1990

When Dr. John Yiamouyiannis (a well-known opponent of fluoridation and author of the book *Fluoride: The Aging Factor*[23]) obtained the raw data from this NIDR study, he found that there was no statistical difference in the DMFTs among children who had lived all their lives in a fluoridated community (F), children who had lived their whole lives in a non-fluoridated community (NF), and children who had lived their lives part of the time in a fluoridated community and part of the time in a non-fluoridated community (PF). In figure 8.1, the three curves for DMFT across the age range from five to seventeen years are plotted for the F, NF, and PF children; the lines are essentially superimposed.

Brunelle and Carlos 1990

Subsequently, Brunelle and Carlos, who worked for the NIDR, published their own analysis of the data.[24] However, they increased the sensitivity of the study by analyzing tooth decay using DMFS (decayed, missing, and filled permanent *surfaces*) as a measure of decay. All teeth except the cutting teeth have five surfaces per tooth, so this increased the sensitivity by a factor of nearly five over a measure of DMFT (decayed, missing, and filled permanent *teeth*). Even so, they found very little difference in tooth decay in the permanent teeth of children who had lived all their lives in a fluoridated community compared to those who had always lived in a non-fluoridated community.

In the abstract of their article, the authors reported the average difference in tooth decay for five- to seventeen-year-olds as 18 percent. However, table 6 in their paper shows that this reported saving amounts to an average of

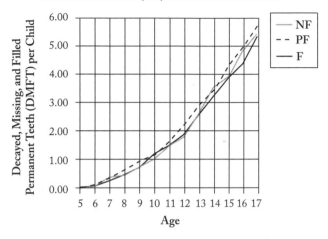

Tooth Decay in Fluoridated (F), Partially Fluoridated (PF),
and Nonfluoridated (NF) Areas: Permanent Teeth

Figure 8.1. Yiamouyiannis's plot of DMFT for children living all their lives in a fluoridated community (F), children living all their lives in a non-fluoridated community (NF), and children living part of their lives in both (PF).[25]

just six-tenths of a single tooth surface, and that is out of approximately one hundred tooth surfaces in a child's mouth. Nor did the authors subject this to any analysis to see if the result was statistically significant. What we may be looking at here are the arithmetical vagaries of comparing two small numbers. Reporting that small difference as a percentage can be very misleading. For an unsuspecting citizen or official, an 18 percent difference in tooth decay sounds a lot better than the saving of 0.6 of one tooth surface. Even so, 18 percent is a lot less than the figure of 60 percent that was being used by promoters of fluoridation at that time.

Even if we take the best figure in table 6 of their paper, an absolute saving of 1.58 surfaces for seventeen-year-olds (8.59 DMFS in non-fluoridated and 7.01 DMFS in fluoridated), this represents only an absolute saving of approximately 1.2 percent of the 128 tooth surfaces in the seventeen-year-old's mouth ($1.58 / 128 \times 100$).

Despite that very unimpressive saving in tooth decay, this is what the authors stated in their abstract: "The results suggest that water fluoridation has played a dominant role in the decline in caries and must continue to be a major prevention methodology."[26]

For most people, an average saving (averaged for five- to seventeen-year-olds) of just 0.6 of one tooth *surface*, or even 1.58 tooth surfaces for seventeen-year-olds, would hardly seem to justify the time, money, and angst involved in imposing this practice on reluctant individuals and communities. Nor would it justify taking any of the health risks outlined in chapters 11–19.

It is not unusual for dental researchers who report either meager or no savings to claim in the abstract of their paper that the results support water fluoridation (e.g., Spencer, Slade, and Davies[27]). Cynics might suggest that this is the price that has to be paid to ensure future funding for their dental research from pro-fluoridation sources. Whatever the truth of that, the claim has often proved effective for those decision makers who read only the abstract and not the details in the results section.

Spencer, Slade, and Davies 1996

Subsequently, a large survey conducted in two states in Australia found an even smaller difference in tooth decay in the permanent teeth than did the NIDR authors. Spencer et al.[28] found an *average* difference in tooth decay in the permanent teeth—again measured as DMFS—between children who had lived all their lives in fluoridated versus non-fluoridated communities of between 0.12 and 0.3 tooth surfaces per child. This is one-fifth to one-half of the meager finding of 0.6 DMFS found by Brunelle and Carlos.[29] Even if these differences are real, they represent a very small fraction of the tooth surfaces in a child's mouth. The figure of 0.3 of one tooth surface out of 128 tooth surfaces represents an absolute saving of just 0.23 percent.

de Liefde 1998

In 1998, Dr. Betty de Liefde, in a survey of tooth decay in New Zealand, confirmed what John Colquhoun had been saying for nearly twenty years. She found very little difference in permanent-tooth decay between fluoridated and non-fluoridated communities. She described the difference as "clinically meaningless."[30]

Locker 1999

In a report prepared for the Ontario Ministry of Health and Long-Term Care, Dr. David Locker of the University of Toronto reported, "The magnitude of [fluoridation's] effect is not large in absolute terms, is often not statistically significant, and may not be of clinical significance."[31]

Two years later Locker coauthored an article on the science and ethics of fluoridation with Howard Cohen, in which they state the following:

Over the past 25 years there has been a marked reduction in rates of dental caries among children, such that the benefits of water fluoridation are no longer so clear. Although current studies indicate that water fluoridation continues to be beneficial, recent reviews have shown that the quality of the evidence provided by these studies is poor . . . In addition, studies that are more methodologically sound indicate that differences in rates of dental decay between optimally fluoridated and nonfluoridated child populations are small in absolute terms . . . Canadian studies of fluoridated and nonfluoridated communities provide little systematic evidence regarding the benefits to children of water fluoridation.[32]

Cohen and Locker concluded,

Ethically, it cannot be argued that past benefits, by themselves, justify continuing the practice of fluoridation. This position presumes the constancy of the environment in which policy decisions are made. Questions of public health policy are relative, not absolute, and different stages of human progress not only will have, but ought to have, different needs and different means of meeting those needs. Standards regarding the optimal level of fluoride in the water supply were developed on the basis of epidemiological data collected more than 50 years ago. There is a need for new guidelines for water fluoridation that are based on sound, up-to-date science and sound ethics. In this context, we would argue that sound ethics presupposes sound science.[33]

Armfield and Spencer 2004

In 2004, Armfield and Spencer published a study of tooth decay in ten thousand children in South Australia.[34] While they found a small difference in the primary teeth, they found no statistically significant difference in tooth decay in the permanent teeth between those children who had drunk tank water (rainwater) or bottled water all their lives and those who drank fluoridated water.

Despite the fact that these authors clearly stated in their abstract, "The effect of consumption of nonpublic water on permanent caries experience was not significant," Spencer has responded angrily when opponents of fluoridation, including Mark Diesendorf, have reported their finding, claiming that their work is being misrepresented.[35, 36] Armfield and Spencer have also publicly advocated the fluoridation of bottled water in Australia.

Komárek et al. 2005

In a study published in the January 2005 issue of the journal *Biostatistics,* a European research team of scientists from Belgium and Finland sought to answer the question of whether fluoride intake at a young age has a protective effect on caries in permanent teeth.[37] For their response, they utilized data from the Signal Tandmobiel trial,[38] which, according to Komárek et al., "is possibly the largest longitudinal study executed with such great detail on dental aspects."[39]

In their analysis (a "Bayesian survival analysis"), the authors used dental fluorosis as the measure of the children's fluoride ingestion. The authors explained why they did that as follows: "Unfortunately, fluoride-intake in children cannot be measured accurately. Indeed, fluoride-intake can come from: (1) fluoride supplements (systemic), (2) accidental ingestion of toothpaste or (3) tap water. Further, the intake from these sources can be recorded only crudely. Therefore, it was decided to measure fluoride-intake by the degree of fluorosis on some reference teeth."[40]

The authors also took into account something that most dental studies ignore: a possible fluoride-induced delay in tooth eruption. Again, the authors explained their reasoning: "Since the emergence of permanent teeth might be delayed by fluoride-intake, evaluating the impact of fluoride-intake should take into account the time at risk for caries. Hence, in our analysis, the response will be the time between emergence and the onset of caries development."[41]

Whereas in an earlier analysis (Vanobbergen et al.[42]) the authors found a positive effect of fluoride on primary teeth, in this analysis by Komárek et al. the authors failed to find a significant effect on three of the four groupings of permanent teeth they analyzed. They reported, "Our analysis shows no convincing effect of fluoride-intake on caries development . . . This agrees with current guidelines for the use of fluoride in caries prevention, where only the topical application (e.g. fluoride in toothpaste) is considered to be essential."[43]

Pizzo et al. 2007

In 2007, a team of Italian researchers from the University of Palermo concluded the following from their review of the literature: "It is now accepted that systemic fluoride plays a limited role in caries prevention. Several epidemiological studies conducted in fluoridated and non-fluoridated communities clearly indicate that CWF [community water fluoridation] may be unnecessary for caries prevention, particularly in the industrialized countries where the caries level has become low."[44]

Waren et al. 2009.

The study by Warren et al., otherwise referred to as the "Iowa Study," is the only study that has examined tooth decay in children as a function of *individual* exposure to fluoride. All the other studies discussed above have been *population* studies, with only the Komárek study giving any indication of individual exposure to fluoride. The authors of the Iowa study found no relationship between caries experience and individual fluoride intakes at various ages during childhood. Caries rates at ages five and nine were similar for all levels of fluoride intake. The authors state that "the benefits of fluoride are mostly topical" and that their "findings suggest that achieving a caries-free status may have relatively little to do with fluoride *intake*" [emphasis in the original]. The authors' main conclusion: "Given the overlap among caries/fluorosis groups in mean fluoride intake and extreme variability in individual fluoride intakes, firmly recommending an 'optimal' fluoride intake is problematic."[45]

Dental Crises

There have been numerous press reports over the last few years of dental crises in U.S. cities that have been fluoridated for over twenty years. The fact that these crises are occurring in low-income areas again demonstrates that there is a far greater (inverse) relationship between tooth decay and family income levels than between tooth decay and water fluoride levels (see chapter 6). It also demonstrates that the tooth decay associated with low family income levels is not being eliminated by fluoridation programs.

The following excerpt from the *Cincinnati Enquirer* is fairly typical of many other press reports. Cincinnati has been fluoridated since 1979.

> City and regional medical officials say tooth decay is the city's No. 1 unmet health-care need. "We cannot meet the demand," says Dr. Larry Hill, Cincinnati Health Department dental director. "It's absolutely heartbreaking and a travesty. We have kids in this community with severe untreated dental infections. We have kids with self-esteem problems, and we have kids in severe pain and we have no place to send them in Cincinnati. People would be shocked to learn how bad the problem has become."[46]

Similar reports have appeared in the papers of other fluoridated cities, including the *Boston Globe*,[47] *New Haven Register*,[48] *Pittsburgh Tribune-Review*,[49] *Washington Post*,[50] *Lexington Herald-Leader*,[51] and *Fosters Daily Democrat* (Connecticut).[52]

In addition to these newspaper reports, formal studies have also found high levels of tooth decay in communities that have been fluoridated for several decades. For example, Burt et al. reported in a 2006 study of tooth decay in Detroit that "83 percent of low income African-American adults, 14-years-old and over, had severe tooth decay and . . . almost all of five-year-olds have cavities and most of them go unfilled."[53]

In his book *Savage Inequalities: Children in America's Schools*, Jonathan Kozol writes, "As in New York City's poorest neighborhoods, dental problems also plague the children here [in East St. Louis] . . . Bleeding gums, impacted teeth and rotting teeth are routine matters for the children I have interviewed in the South Bronx . . . I have seen children in New York with teeth that look like brownish, broken sticks. I have also seen teen-agers who were missing half their teeth."[54] The book was published in 1991; New York City's water has been fluoridated since 1965, and East St. Louis has received fluoridated water since 1968.

Almost all U.S. states produce regular oral health reports. The majority of these indicate high levels of tooth decay in low-income families, even in states with a high percentage of the water fluoridated.[55] Clearly, fluoridation is not addressing the impacts of income disparities as far as tooth decay is concerned.

Summary

Several studies and reviews published since the 1980s have confirmed that any protective effect of fluoridation is extremely small, amounting on average to only a fraction of a tooth surface for the permanent teeth and not much more for the baby teeth. Several modern studies have shown that if fluoridation is stopped, decay rates do not increase. The dental crises reported in cities across the United States and elsewhere that have long been fluoridated show that fluoridation is insufficient to combat dental caries, especially in children from low-income families.

PART THREE

The Great Fluoridation Gamble

In chapter 9, we examine the events that led up to the U.S. Public Health Service (PHS) endorsement of fluoridation in 1950 from a dental perspective, a health perspective, and an industrial perspective. We address two key questions:

1. How much of fluoride's dangers were known to the PHS in 1950?
2. What other pressures were acting on the PHS in the years leading up to this crucial event?

In chapter 10, we continue with the history of what we call the Great Fluoridation Gamble from 1950 to the present.

The Great Fluoridation Gamble, 1930–1950

Coauthored by Peter Meiers

In this chapter we look at the historical events leading up to the decision by the U.S. Public Health Service (PHS) to endorse fluoridation in 1950. Several texts have been most helpful in writing this chapter. In *The Fight for Fluoridation*, Donald McNeil gives an intriguing view of the history of the period from the dental and pro-fluoridation perspective.[1] Ruth Roy Harris gives a slightly less slanted view of that history in her book *Dental Science in a New Age: A History of the National Institute of Dental Research*.[2] In their book *The American Fluoridation Experiment*, published in 1957, the same year as McNeil's book, Exner and Waldbott give us the view of scientists who were opposed to fluoridation and were highly critical of the evidence offered for both its safety and effectiveness.[3] Finally, Chris Bryson's *The Fluoride Deception*, published in 2004, with a revised paperback edition published in 2006, discusses the industrial interests that either were directly involved in the early promotion of fluoridation or were beneficiaries of it.[4]

The Great Fluoridation Gamble Defined

As far back as the 1930s, two facts were well established. First, adding fluoride to the water would increase the number of children with dental fluorosis (see chapter 11), and, second, fluoride caused this condition by some *systemic* (internal) mechanism. What was not known was whether other developing tissues in the child's body would be affected by a mechanism similar to that which was damaging the growing tooth cells. Dental fluorosis is obvious. It is visible to the naked eye, and, as such, it cannot be denied. On the other hand, systemic effects on other tissues would not be so obvious or easy to detect without careful study.

"The Great Fluoridation Gamble" was founded on the blind trust that drinking water containing 1 ppm fluoride could damage growing tooth cells without harming any other tissues in a child's developing body and without causing any injury to adults after a lifetime of exposure.

A key question overhanging this discussion is the following: Did the U.S. Public Health Service in 1950 have enough information about the safety of ingesting fluoride at levels of 1 ppm in the water to confidently recommend that communities across the United States fluoridate their water? In this chapter we examine the evidence of harm that was available to decision makers prior to the approval of fluoridation, including the research they ignored.

This period essentially begins in 1931 with the discovery that fluoride causes mottling of tooth enamel (dental fluorosis)[5][7] and ends with the U.S. PHS endorsement in 1950. The PHS endorsement was crucial: Not only did it trigger further endorsements from most American dental, medical, and public health associations, but it was also the starting point for the massive support that the governments of the United States and a few other countries have given to fluoridation ever since.

Enthusiasm vs. Caution

Once it had been assumed (with only a modicum of scientific evidence; see chapter 7) that fluoride might reduce tooth decay, we see a battle developing between those who were enthusiastic to get water fluoridation launched, such as Gerald Cox,[8] and those who were cautious about (1) the acceptability of increasing the incidence of dental fluorosis and (2) the possibility that other conditions might be triggered by ingesting fluoride. We examine the evidence for the latter and how eventually doubts about safety were submerged.

In the history of the rhetorical support given to fluoridation we see several transitions:

- Fluoride is bad for teeth becomes fluoride is good for teeth (at low levels).
- Fluoride is bad for bones becomes fluoride is good for bones (at low levels).
- Fluoride is a toxic substance becomes fluoride is a nutrient.

These transitions, all made in the interest of promoting fluoridation, presage similar transitions we examine in later chapters.

A Short Chronology

The chronology of events leading up to the crucial year of 1950 can take on very different complexions depending on one's perspective, whether it be dental, medical, or industrial. We have tried to distinguish these various perspectives by providing a chronology using three different typefaces. We show the dental events in normal type, **the medical in bold,** and *the industrial in italics.*

1800s–1950s—*From the late nineteenth century on, there are many lawsuits pertaining to emissions near phosphate fertilizer plants and aluminum and other metal smelters. From about 1930, the cause of harm is suspected to be fluoride.*[9]

1902–1931—Mottling of tooth enamel is observed and studied.

1916—Classic study on dental mottling is conducted by Black and McKay.[10]

1920s–1950s—Doctors are using sodium fluoride to lower thyroid activity in patients with hyperthyroidism.

1928—McKay observes that tooth decay appears to be less prevalent in communities with dental mottling.[11]

1930—While studying industrial fluoride pollution in Europe, Cristiani suggests that fluoride makes bones more brittle and reports marked lesions in the thyroids of guinea pigs dying from chronic fluorine intoxication.[12, 13]

1931—Three separate research teams identify fluoride in drinking water as the cause of dental mottling, which is renamed dental fluorosis.[14–16]

1931—Alcoa scientists privately confirm dental fluorosis cases near Alcoa's aluminum smelter in Massena, New York, where the fluoride levels in drinking water are very low.[17]

1932—H. Trendley Dean of the U.S. PHS begins his studies on the incidence of dental fluorosis in the United States and also classifies its various levels of severity. Dean publishes his first paper on dental fluorosis in 1933.[18]

1932—Moeller and Gudjonsson report damage to bone caused by fluoride in Denmark.[19]

1933—DeEds (U.S. Department of Agriculture) reviews fluoride's toxicity.[20]

1933—Frank McClure publishes "A Review of Fluorine and Its Physiological Effects."[21]

1937—Roholm publishes his famous treatise *Fluorine Intoxication*. He bases his massive work on studies of animals and workers from the cryolite industry.[22]

1937—Shortt et al. publish the first study on skeletal fluorosis in India.[23]

1938—Dean reviews Roholm's study.[24]

1939—Steyn first reports an association between high fluoride levels and goiter in South Africa.[25]

1939—Gerald Cox, an industry-financed researcher, first recommends fluoridation of the water.[26]

1940—Greenwood publishes a review, "Fluoride Intoxication."[27]

1940—Pandit et al. discover skeletal fluorosis cases at levels as low as 1–3 ppm F in drinking water and find that poor nutrition exacerbates the problem.[28]

1942—Dean et al. publish their famous two-part, twenty-one-city study claiming to demonstrate an inverse relationship between levels of fluoride in the water and tooth decay. Dean's hypothesis: 1 ppm fluoride lowers tooth decay without causing dental fluorosis in its mildest form in more than 10 percent of children.[29, 30]

1944—McClure claims that boys and young adult men exposed to fluoride up to 5.2 ppm in water show no increased bone fractures, no difference in height or weight, and no indication of renal injury.[31, 32]

1945—McClure claims that all fluoride ingested up to 4–5 mg per day is excreted in the urine, that none is retained in the bones, and that only higher levels of fluoride ingestion would lead to accumulation in bones.[33]

1945—Ten- to fifteen-year trials of artificial fluoridation begin.

1948—In Donora, Pennsylvania, during a three-day air inversion, pollution from local factories in a valley kills over twenty people and makes many others sick. Scientific evidence points to fluoride as the culprit, but the U.S. Public Health Service denies this.[34]

1949—The Sugar Research Foundation (representing 130 sugar interests) declares that it needs to find a way to reduce dental caries without reducing sugar consumption.[35] *It funds researchers at universities, most notably Dr. Frederick Stare at Harvard, to investigate fluoridation, as well as sugar's role in nutrition (see chapter 26).*

1950—Cox and Hodge publish an article stating, "There is no other known toxic effect of drinking water containing 1 ppm fluorine than the 'very mild' mottling of the teeth."[36]

1950—The U.S. Public Health Service endorses fluoridation. The American Dental Association and other professional organizations quickly follow suit.

The Events in More Detail

We now review this history with the object of examining how much the promoters knew or suspected about fluoride's other health effects in addition to dental fluorosis (see chapter 11 for more about dental fluorosis).

1931: Dental Research Begins at PHS

The history of dental research within the U.S. Public Health Service started in 1931, when one dental officer, Henry Trendley Dean, DDS, was detailed to the Division of Pathology and Bacteriology with the (preliminary) assignment of investigating the occurrence of dental fluorosis throughout the United States.[37] The condition had just been ascribed to fluoride by several groups of researchers.[38–40]

It was to be expected that mottling and staining of the teeth would not be the only toxic effect of fluoride, though this was apparently the only one within the scope of dentistry. After the examination, in February 1932, of a group of children in Minonk, Illinois (where naturally occurring fluoride in the public water system was 2.8 ppm), Dean wrote in his report to the surgeon general:

> Following the Minonk examination, a new phase of this question seems ripe for further study. Is mottled enamel merely an oral manifestation of a general toxicity, or something similar? The hair of some of these mottled enamel cases is unusually coarse, almost like horse hair. Finger nails are apparently not normal. Two of the three local physicians state that there is apparently an unusually large amount of skin disorders among those using the city water supply. Future surveys will attempt to obtain this additional dermatological data in order to determine whether it correlates with the mottled enamel.[41]

There was no follow-up, however.

Texas Observations Begin

According to Dean, in 1934 a pediatrician (Lemmon) from Amarillo, Texas, reported "defective development of the long bones in babies whose diet includes water with fluorides in toxic amount . . . Some of these babies have more tendency to bowing of the legs, even in the face of constant anti-rachitic therapy, thus supporting the theory that the toxic fluorides interfere with bone and dental metabolism."[42]

In 1936, Dean made two references to the possibility that fluoride might damage the skeleton. In one paper, after discussing the period when children were vulnerable to fluoride's damage to the enamel, he cited Boissevain and Drea (1933)[43] and stated, "There is some indication that the skeletal system might likewise be affected; if this is true, it would be necessary to extend the time range [of the study] to include adults."[44] Dean also acknowledged that fluoride might make bones more fragile. He gave the following citation to Cristiani's work: "Cristiani working with guinea pigs found that the fragility of the bones was increased about 20 per cent in the fluorized animals."[45, 46]

In 1936, even though the PHS felt a need to conduct a "chronic disease survey" in several Texas cities, no mention of bone was made in a memo Dean sent to the assistant surgeon general.[47]

Fluoride's Toxic Effects

A number of studies and reviews of fluoride's toxic effects were published between 1930 and 1940. These included reviews by Floyd DeEds (1933, 1936),[48, 49] Frank McClure (1933),[50] and D. A. Greenwood (1940).[51] DeEds worked for the U.S. Department of Agriculture, which appeared to be far more concerned about the ramifications of fluoride pollution than the U.S. Public Health Service. In addition to DeEds's work, reports appeared on fluoride's impact on non-dental tissues, including studies on the bone.[52–56] In 1939, George Abbott published a short communication describing fluoride's impact on blood structure.[57] Several animal studies were published in Europe, as well as by Phillips et al. in the United States, on fluoride's possible interaction with the thyroid and parathyroid glands.[58–67] There were also numerous reports from around the world that doctors were using fluorides to lower thyroid function in patients with hyperthyroidism.[68–73]

In 1939, Steyn published the first in a series of studies from South Africa in which he reported the incidence of goiter, an enlargement of the thyroid gland that leads to a gross swelling of the neck and is normally associated with a deficiency of iodine. However, Steyn found goiter occurring in areas that were not deficient in iodine but had high levels of fluoride in the water.[74–76] In 1940, Wilson and DeEds reported dental fluorosis in rats as a result of a synergistic action of fluoride and thyroid hormones.[77]

Dean's Review of Roholm

In a very short review of Roholm's treatise in 1938, Dean was highly respectful but drew no major conclusions about any risks that might be anticipated from people drinking fluoridated water, based on either the osteosclerosis (bone hardening) observed in cryolite workers or the osteomalacia-like disease (bone-softening disease) observed in animals grazing near certain factories in Europe. In his final remarks he merely indicated that the doses that caused skeletal fluorosis appeared to be higher than those that caused dental fluorosis.[78] So it is clear that Dean, as early as 1938, was well aware of serious side effects of fluoride, even though he may have contented himself with the idea that they were occurring at higher doses than those causing dental fluorosis in the communities he was studying.

Hodges et al. 1941

Inspired by reports by Roholm and others, and considering that fluoride contamination of food was increasing in this period, Paul C. Hodges and colleagues at the University of Chicago examined people in Kempton, Illinois, where the water contained 1.2–3 ppm fluoride, and Bureau, Illinois, where the water contained 2.5 ppm fluoride. They found no *radiologically demonstrable* sclerosis of the skeleton but suggested that they continue the search for skeletal sclerosis in American communities where the fluoride content of drinking water exceeded 3 ppm.[79] Hodges should not be confused with Harold Hodge, who was to play a very important role in the promotion and defense of the safety of fluoridation (see "Cox and Hodge 1950" below).

In April 1944, during a meeting of the Technical Advisory Committee for the Newburgh (New York) Fluoridation Study, Dean questioned the validity of the results of the Illinois study because there was no statement as to how long the corresponding water supplies had been in use. There could have been several changes in the water supplies for the study areas, he said, and, further, "we really do not know what the exposure was previous to 20 years ago." Dean was of the opinion "that it was necessary to begin with a water supply of a specified number of years of continuous use, such as 30, 40 or 50 years, without any physical changes in the communal water supply involving the installment of new wells or the abandonment of old ones."[80]

Editorial in *JAMA* (1943)

On September 18, 1943, an editorial, "Chronic Fluorine Intoxication," appeared in the *Journal of the American Medical Association*. It stated, "Fluorides are general protoplasmic poisons, probably because of their capacity to modify the metabolism of cells by changing the permeability of the cell membrane and by inhibiting certain enzyme systems."

Most important, the editorial reviewed or referenced some of the key studies on fluoride's effect on bone and drew special attention to the finding of Pandit et al.,[81] who showed that fluoride's impacts on bone are made worse by a poor diet, particularly when it is low in vitamin C. Among the symptoms of chronic intoxication by fluoride listed by *JAMA* were "loss of weight, impairment of growth in young persons, loss of appetite, anemia and cachexia [wasting and weakness]."[82]

Texas Communities

At the April 1944 meeting of the Technical Advisory Committee for the Newburgh Fluoridation Study, Dean gave details of still unpublished recent findings from examinations made by the PHS in 1943 at Bartlett and Cameron, Texas, and Britton, South Dakota. Bartlett had 8 ppm fluoride in its water supply; Cameron, 0.4 ppm; and Britton, about 7 ppm. Dean explained to the committee the following:

> At 8.0 ppm F some bony changes were found although they did not result in functional impairment. These changes start in the lumbar region and the pelvis. Increased density was found in 13 of the 111 persons with over 20 years' exposure that were found by house to house enumeration in a population of 1700 to 1800. No changes were found in the controls who were using a water supply with 0.4 ppm F. In those persons who had osteosclerosis hemoglobin values averaged 2 grams less per person than in those with no evidence of osteosclerosis. It appeared that if fluorine affects the hemoglobin it does so indirectly by producing accretional bony changes which encroach on the bone marrow cavity rather than by direct toxic effect of the hemoglobin producing system.
>
> No evidence of impaired hearing was reported.
>
> There were indications of increased incidence of cataract among those 50 years of age or older in the fluoride areas . . .
>
> Another change was noted in the nails. From 10–20 percent of the younger individuals examined had a rather unusual type of nail structure, the most characteristic aspect being transverse white blotches often completely across the nail, usually symmetrical, and on all the nails, there very frequently being from three to five of these per nail. The incidence of these finally decreased with age, the oldest patient being 57. In the control area with 139 high school students examined, none showed transverse striations.[83]

The 1943 U.S. PHS findings referred to above had *not* been published. Parts appeared in the famous Bartlett-Cameron study reports that came out in

1954, 1955, and 1957,[84–87] but none of those findings were published before the PHS endorsed fluoridation in 1950.

Dean's report of these early Bartlett-Cameron findings at the April 1944 meeting nearly ended the Newburgh fluoridation "demonstration" even before it was begun, as Dean "could not agree that the proposed program could be considered a perfectly safe procedure from a public health point of view."[88] There is a hint, however, that he was raising these concerns to delay the beginning of the Newburgh-Kingston study so that "his" study in Grand Rapids would be the first fluoridation trial. This idea was articulated many years later by David Bernard Ast, dental director of the New York State Health Department, who alluded to Dean's behavior at that 1944 meeting as follows: "Territorial prerogative has always existed and continues to exist not only in the animal kingdom, but in the areas of scientific research as well. It is the kind of hide-and-seek play which frequently goes on among research people who have an overriding urge to be on record as the first to discover or the first to publish."[89]

Despite Dean's apparent opposition, members of the Newburgh Fluoridation Study group argued in support of the Newburgh-Kingston experiment. Minutes of this meeting indicate that Edward Rogers, assistant commissioner of the Medical Administration, said:

> The proposed demonstration has had much publicity. The cities of Newburgh and Kingston are ready to give enthusiastic cooperation. The setup and authorizations are complete but to date no fluorine has been added. The project can be dropped with no more serious result than embarrassment to the Department. However, committees are getting ready to do this sort of thing and it is much better that it be done under controlled conditions. Cumulative effects, if any, will not appear for a number of years. If Dr. Dean's studies produce evidence that the cumulative effects may be serious the demonstration can be discontinued. In the past the efficacy of new public health procedures has been difficult to measure because control periods were not set up clearly enough. With the exception of cataract the untoward effects presented here by Dr. Dean can be offset against the advantages which it is hoped will be obtained.[90]

Dr. Rogers also pointed out that further studies might not supply the data necessary to show whether or not there might be any untoward effects.[91]

Others at the meeting concurred that the trial should go ahead. No one mentioned the fact that this ten-year trial would not be giving any information on lifelong exposure to fluoride.[92] The meeting was chaired by Harold Hodge, the chief toxicologist of the Manhattan Project.

Editorial in *JADA* (1944)

Clearly, some of the information about fluoride's side effects was reaching the editors of the *Journal of the American Dental Association (JADA)*. In a 1944 editorial describing the history of research on dental fluorosis and indicating that fluoride might lower dental caries rates, the editors stated:

> While these data [studies on the fluoride–caries relationship] are certainly speculatively attractive as leading to possible mass treatment of caries, our knowledge of the subject certainly does not warrant the introduction of fluorine in community water supplies generally.
>
> Sodium fluoride is a highly toxic substance, and while its application in safe concentrations, and under strict control by competent personnel, may prove to be useful therapeutically, under other circumstances it may be definitely harmful.
>
> To be effective, fluoride must be ingested into the system during the years of tooth development, and we do not yet know enough about the chemistry involved to anticipate what other conditions may be produced in the structure of the bone and other tissues of the body generally.
>
> We do know that the use of drinking water containing as little as 1.2 to 3.0 parts per million fluorine will cause such developmental disturbances in bones as osteosclerosis, spondylosis and osteoporosis, as well as goiter, and we cannot afford to run the risk of producing such serious disturbances in applying what is at present a doubtful procedure intended to prevent development of dental disfigurements among children.
>
> With regard to the safety margin in the fluoride content of drinking water, the reported amount of fluorine in the water cannot be taken as the criterion for the amount taken in the system, as in an intensely hot climate much larger quantities of water would be imbibed and hence a much larger quantity of fluorine would be taken into the body. Another feature of the complex problem that demands consideration, in attempting to take advantage of

the therapeutic value of fluorine, is the quantity absorbed by the system at various age periods of life . . .

Because of our anxiety to find some therapeutic procedure that will promote mass prevention of caries, the seeming potentialities of fluoride appear speculatively attractive, but, in the light of our present knowledge of the chemistry of the subject, the potentialities for harm outweigh those for good.[93]

These comments were made just a few months before the first trials of fluoridation were to begin.

A few weeks after the *JADA* editorial, on October 30, 1944, David Ast acknowledged in a paper he gave at the meeting of the New York Institute of Clinical Oral Pathology that there were unresolved health questions about the addition of fluoride to the public water system when he asked, "Are there any cumulative effects—beneficial or otherwise, on tissues and organs other than the teeth—of long continued ingestion of such small concentrations as 1.0 part per million of fluorine in water? Again, there is much presumptive evidence that there are no such effects: but, until that is demonstrated, the procedure outlined in this paper must be regarded as an investigation."[94]

Reassuring the New York Health Commissioner

A letter from Dean's boss, Rolla E. Dyer, director of the National Institutes of Health, reached the desk of New York State's health commissioner, Edward S. Godfrey, in November 1944.[95] In an attempt to downplay the unpublished Bartlett-Cameron findings, this letter referred to some "selective service" data acquired in the meantime by biochemist Frank James McClure (see the following section), who claimed an equilibrium between the fluoride content of water and fluoride excretion in the urine. Furthermore, in Colorado Springs, where the water supply contains about 2.5 ppm fluoride naturally, three of five physicians interviewed by Dean were of the opinion that there was nothing unusual in respect to the prevalence of cataracts. Evidently, Dyer's letter did not wholly clarify some of the issues raised earlier.

McClure's 1944 and 1945 Papers

In 1944, Frank McClure published a paper on the relation of fluoride levels in water to the height, weight, and bone-fracture experience of 1,458 high school boys and 2,529 young men taking a physical examination during army recruitment. He concluded that "there was no relation of fracture experience to fluoride exposure. The average height and body weight of all the boys compared favorably with other height-weight data and accepted standards. The height-weight data were not related to fluoride exposure."[96]

In 1955, Dr. Fred Exner, in a report prepared for the City of New York, pointed out several problems with the McClure and Kinser study:

> The data for about one-fourth of the subjects were copied from army records which had nothing to do with either bone fragility or fluorides. The other subjects were asked by McClure where they lived and how many broken bones they had had. *That* was the examination . . . In some cases he measured the height and weight himself. In other cases, they measured each other . . . He took urine samples which he pooled . . . Two of the *fluoride* localities had only 0.2 ppm of fluoride in the water; while one of the *non-fluoride* places had 1.8 ppm . . . McClure, in his introduction, observes that sometimes fluorine makes bones fragile, and sometimes it makes them stronger. This would invalidate his statistical study in advance.[97] [emphasis added]

In 1945, on the basis of a study of five young men aged nineteen to twenty-four, Frank McClure published an article stating that all the fluoride ingested, up to 4–5 mg per day, was excreted in the urine; none was retained in the bones. Only higher levels of fluoride ingestion, he claimed, would lead to accumulation in bones.[98]

A subsequent study by Patricia Wallace-Durbin in 1954 using radioactively labeled fluoride showed that this was not correct (at least not in rats),[99] and today most scientists accept that approximately 50 percent of ingested fluoride is excreted in the urine and most of the rest is stored in the bone.[100] However, at the time, McClure's erroneous finding was very influential in diminishing concerns about fluoride's impact on bone.

Exner explained why he spent so much time critiquing McClure's work: "There are quite reliable reports, over a period of more than 40 years and from all over the world, of serious cumulative, chronic fluoride poisoning, especially of the teeth and skeletal structures. All these are lightly brushed aside on the basis of McClure's work, as having no applicability where there is only one part per million of fluoride in the water."[101]

The AAAS Conference 1944

The American Association for the Advancement of Science (AAAS) held its first conference on fluoride in Dallas in December 1941. Its second conference, at which McClure presented a summary of his 1944 article, was held in Cleveland in September 1944. The proceedings, titled *Dental Caries and Fluorine*, were published in 1946,[102] which allowed McClure to update his paper to include his 1945 findings.[103] Most of the other papers concerned only dental effects, but several statements indicated that some of the other authors were aware that not everything was known about the long-term health effects of fluoridation. Thus the timing of the conference (1944) and the publication (1946) is interesting because one came before the fluoridation trials began and the other came after.

In the foreword, for example, Kitchin and Moulton opined that the belief that fluoride might reduce tooth decay "does not imply that the cities and villages in this country should precipitately begin to introduce fluoride into water supplies. Science is too cautious and thorough-going for such actions. But the evidence is now sufficient to raise high hopes for the future."[104]

H. Trendley Dean, while noting that "the question of low fluoridation of the domestic water supply for the control of caries appears sound," provided a note of caution when he said, "Much investigative work, however, is necessary before a recommendation can be given for its general application . . . specifically planned, epidemiological studies should clearly demonstrate the safety of low fluoridation as it might relate to other aspects of the community's general health."[105]

Robert Weaver, in discussing studies conducted in the British Isles and India, stated, "In Somerset, Dagmar Wilson (1941) examined a number of children in two areas where the incidence of goiter was high, and found that about 15 percent of the children had some degree of dental fluorosis. She considers that fluorine may be one factor, though possibly only of subsidiary importance, in the causation of endemic goiter." This should have been another warning signal to look for changes in thyroid function in the upcoming fluoridation trials.[106, 107]

Weaver also discussed Marshall Day's studies of fluorosis in India.[108] In Kasur, a village in the Punjab with nine water supplies, of which one had a fluoride level of less than 1 ppm, five had levels between 1 and 2 ppm, and three contained 2.2, 4.2, and 6.2 ppm, respectively, Day reported that 96 percent of 203 children had dental fluorosis, according to Weaver.[109] Summing up Day's work, Weaver says he found that "the children of Kasur showed no signs of fluorosis other than the characteristic dental condition and, though rheumatoid and other arthritic conditions have been observed in old people in the endemic area, there was no convincing evidence that these conditions had anything to do with fluorosis."[110] This not only should have been a warning signal to look for early signs of arthritic symptoms in naturally fluoridated areas, but also should have drawn further attention to the problems of looking only at children, not at adults, in the upcoming fluoridation trials.

Preliminary Report from Newburgh-Kingston Study

The Newburgh-Kingston fluoridation experiment started in 1945 and was closely tracked, as mentioned previously, by Harold Hodge of the Manhattan Project.[111] A preliminary report, presented on October 25, 1949, before the Dental Health Section of the American Public Health Association, "failed to disclose any significant deviation in any of the factors studied."[112] However, only children—no adults—were examined in Newburgh and Kingston. The preliminary report was not published until June 1950—that is, after the Public Health Service had endorsed fluoridation. In the meantime, according to McNeil, certain fluoridation "zealots," especially in Wisconsin, where the state dental director, Frank Bull, was leading the charge, were making huge efforts to install fluoridation in as many cities in that state as possible.[113]

Cox and Hodge 1950

Before we examine the important research paper published by Cox and Hodge in 1950,[114] let us remind ourselves who Cox and Hodge were. Gerald Judy Cox was a researcher at the Mellon Institute whose research in the 1930s was funded by the Aluminum Company of America (Alcoa). According to Bryson, it was Alcoa's director of research who suggested to Cox that fluoride might make strong teeth.[115] Cox soon reported that fluoride gave rats cavity-resistant teeth and in 1939 made the first public proposal to add fluoride to public water supplies. Shortly after there were rumblings at the American Water Works Association that the safe level of fluoride in water should be lowered to 0.1 ppm to protect against dental fluorosis, Cox wrote, "The present trend toward complete removal of fluorine from water and food may need some reversal."[116]

Harold Carpenter Hodge, from the University of Rochester, was the chief toxicologist for the U.S. Army's Manhattan Project. In her book *The Plutonium Files*, Eileen Welsome documents that during that project Hodge supervised experiments in which unsuspecting hospital patients were injected with uranium and plutonium.[117] After the war Hodge chaired the National Research Council's Committee on Toxicology and became the leading scientific promoter of water fluoridation in the United States.[118] We return to Hodge's important role in promoting fluoridation in chapter 10.

In an article titled "The Toxicity of Fluorides in Relation to Their Use in Dentistry," which appeared in the April 1950 issue of *The Journal of the American Dental Association*, Cox and Hodge reviewed some of the literature on fluoride's health effects and in their eight-point summary concluded the following: "3. Chronic, crippling fluorosis will never appear as a result of dental uses of fluorides . . . 6. There is no other known toxic effect of drinking water containing 1 ppm fluorine than the 'very mild' mottling of the teeth."[119]

In order to dismiss concerns about fluoride's effects on bone, Cox and Hodge relied entirely on the studies of McClure discussed previously.[120] To dismiss the possibility that fluoride might interfere with thyroid function, they cited only one study, by Evans and Phillips.[121] Cox and Hodge wrote, "Evans and Phillips reviewed the evidence of fluorides as influencing the course of hyperthyroidism. They analyzed thyroids of forty thyroidectomy cases for fluorine and iodine and compared the findings with the basal metabolic rates. They concluded: 'The data obtained gave no definite evidence that fluorine in any way played a part in human hyperthyroidism by its action on the thyroid gland.'"[122]

There are several problems with Cox and Hodge using this single citation to dismiss concerns about this important issue:

1. The article by Evans and Phillips they referenced was actually an article by Evans, Phillips, and Hart that appeared in the *Journal of Dairy Science* and was titled "Fluoride Storage in Cattle Bones," which seems a long way from the subject matter quoted by Cox and Hodge. In addition, the quote cited by Cox and Hodge does not appear in that article. Cox and Hodge probably meant to reference another article by Evans and Phillips titled "The Fluorine Content of the Thyroid Gland in Cases of Hyperthyroidism,"[123] which does contain the quote.

2. While citing this single paper coauthored by Phillips, Cox and Hodge ignored the series of experiments that this same author and his coworkers performed with a number of animals (e.g., rats and chicks), in which fluoride did show interactions with the thyroid.[124–127]

3. They failed to mention other animal studies indicating fluoride's interaction with the thyroid and parathyroid glands.[128–133]

4. They ignored all the clinical evidence provided by doctors in Argentina and Germany who were using fluorides to lower thyroid function in patients with hyperthyroidism, cited previously in this chapter.[134–139]

5. They ignored Steyn's work in South Africa, in which he reported cases of goiter occurring in areas that were not deficient in iodine but had high levels of fluoride in the water.[140, 141]

6. They ignored the evidence from U.S. Department of Agriculture scientists Wilson and DeEds, who reported dental fluorosis in rats as a result of the synergistic action of fluoride and thyroid hormones.[142]

Cox and Hodge thus used one paper from McClure to dismiss all concerns about fluoride in bone and one paper from Evans et al. (with the wrong citation) to dismiss all concerns about fluoride and the thyroid.

As far as the agenda of those promoting fluoridation was concerned, this Cox and Hodge article came at a propitious time—about a month before the PHS endorsed fluoridation.

A Key Year in the History of Fluoridation

As far as the dental-medical perspective was concerned, 1950 was the key year in the history of water fluoridation in the United States. We will step back and summarize the forces at play. At that time there was a clash between two groups. On the one hand, now that the fluoridation trials were under way and the early results looked promising, dentists and dental researchers had moved from the hope that ingesting fluoride would reduce tooth decay with minimal side effects to a wild enthusiasm for a simple way of fighting tooth decay with no downside. On the other hand, a few skeptics were concerned that the rush to fluoridate was premature and that not enough was known about its long-term impacts on other tissues.

On the side of the skeptics was a considerable amount of scientific literature, particularly from Europe and from the U.S. Department of Agriculture, that fluoride posed problems to the bone and the thyroid. Some skeptics had gone as far as to write editorials on the matter in the journals of both the AMA[143] and the ADA.[144]

Those who argued that fluoridation was safe—safe enough to warrant fluoridating any community in the United States—countered the health concerns with just five studies:

1. McClure's 1944 study claiming no increased bone fractures, or changes in weight or height, in young boys and army recruits from areas with fluoridation levels as high as 5.2 ppm[145]
2. McClure's 1945 study claiming that no fluoride below an input of 5 mg a day accumulated in the bone[146]
3. A short review of health concerns in an article by Cox and Hodge[147]
4. Dean's report on the unpublished 1943 findings from the ongoing studies in Bartlett (8 ppm) and Cameron (0.4 ppm), Texas[148]
5. Preliminary unpublished findings from the Newburgh, New York, trial, which had been in progress for only a few years (those preliminary findings did not appear in print[149] until after the PHS endorsement)

On that basis, without any of the trials completed, the fluoridation enthusiasts won the day and the U.S. Public Health Service endorsed fluoridation in 1950.[150]

Donald McNeil's account of these events would lead the reader to believe that this was merely a battle between cautious and overzealous dental researchers.[151] Three other things occurred, however, that may have helped put pressure on the PHS to endorse fluoridation.

The Donora Accident

In October 1948, in Donora, Pennsylvania, an air inversion in the valley trapped the air pollution from a steel works and a zinc smelter for three days, killing at least twenty people and making hundreds of others sick. The most likely culprit, from a scientific point of view, was fluoride, but a report from the PHS denied it. This raises a serious question: Why would the PHS rush to aid the U.S. steel industry on this matter? A full answer to this question can be obtained by reading Chris Bryson's thoroughly documented book *The Fluoride Deception*.[152]

Suffice it to say here that this incident must have caused great fear among the industries producing fluoride emissions. First of all, fluoride emissions were produced in large quantities by many industries in the United States, especially the metal industries. Second, with post–World War II expansion those emissions were expected to rise considerably. Third, they left a unique telltale biomarker in children (dental fluorosis) that was visible to the naked eye. By this time it was known that children living near aluminum smelters were showing signs of dental fluorosis even when there was little or no naturally occurring fluoride in their water supply.[153] Fourth, the Donora incident made it clear that this pollutant could kill people. There could no longer be any question that, in addition to lawsuits from farmers complaining of damage to their crops and cattle (relatively small settlements), there would be complaints from people that their health—and even their lives—had been compromised by fluoride emissions downwind of those plants. That could have led to far more costly settlements. Then there was the even more costly threat that workers in the plants themselves (particularly workers in the aluminum smelter pot rooms) might sue for damages to their health.

Bryson suggests that it is these concerns about industrial liabilities that drove the U.S. PHS to endorse fluoridation. He carefully documents meetings between industry, dental interests, and PHS representatives long before the PHS endorsement. For example, he describes a meeting in April 1936 between Charles Kettering, vice president and director of research at General Motors, a delegation from the American Dental Association, and Captain C. T. Messner of the PHS.[154] Bryson also documents the aggressive role that Robert Kehoe, the director of the Kettering Laboratory, played in protecting industries involved in fluoride use, and his close ties with officials in the PHS, matters we explore further in chapter 10.[155]

Big Sugar's Influence

In 1949, in an issue of *Sugar Molecule,* the scientific director for the Sugar Research Foundation (a lobby for about 130 sugar interests) was quoted as saying that the purpose of the foundation's research was "to find how tooth decay may be controlled effectively without restriction of sugar intake."[156]

There is no question that the sugar lobby had a huge interest in distracting attention from sugar as a major contributing cause of tooth decay. Whether the lobby had a *direct* influence on the U.S. PHS's decision we leave to others to explore.

One thing we know is that the Sugar Research Foundation put a lot of money into the work of Dr. Frederick Stare, chair of the Nutrition Department at Harvard. From the 1940s through the early 1990s, Dr. Stare was one of the most prominent spokespeople on behalf of both sugar interests *and* water fluoridation (see chapter 26).

Development of the Atomic Bomb

The development of the atomic bomb in the 1940s coincided with the development of fluoridation. Production of the bomb required huge quantities of fluoride to produce the uranium hexafluoride used to separate the fissionable isotope of uranium from the nonfissionable isotope. As indicated above, the chief toxicologist of the Manhattan Project was Harold Hodge. Not only was Hodge involved in studies of fluoride's toxicity for the Manhattan Project, he was also chair of the committee set up to oversee the important Newburgh-Kingston trial of fluoridation (1945–1955) and tracked the results of medical examinations conducted in that trial.[157]

Proponents of fluoridation like to make fun of those who suggest that there might have been ulterior motives behind the rush to instigate fluoridation and often use the word "conspiracy theorist" to conjure up the notion that such people are simply exhibiting paranoia. However, Bryson's suggestion that industrial and government scientists conspired to put fluoride into the drinking water—(1) to collect low-dose data to be used to combat potential lawsuits brought by farmers and workers on the atomic bomb production line, and (2) to change the image of fluoride from a nasty air pollutant to something so harmless that children could drink it—pales beside the known fact that Hodge and his fellow Manhattan Project researchers, working for the U.S. government, actually did conspire to expose patients to injections of plutonium without their knowledge or permission.[158, 159]

The U.S. PHS Endorsement of Fluoridation

The June 1950 issue of the *Journal of the American Dental Association* was a special issue devoted to the progress of dentistry in "this first half century." Under "Advances in Research," the epidemiological studies of Henry Trendley Dean were singled out as work that "epidemiologists all over the country know and are proud of."[160] However, those studies were still missing the crowning finale.

That crowning finale came in the same month of June, but it did not arrive with much fanfare outside the dental community. There were no press conferences, no press releases, or any media coverage. The announcement of the U.S. PHS endorsement of fluoridation was printed as a small item in the ADA newsletter of June 1, 1950. The following statement appeared, referring to a report of "today" by Assistant Surgeon General Bruce D. Forsyth: "As a result of new evidence from its Grand Rapids project, where community water has been fluoridated since January 25, 1945, the Public Health Service, Dr. Forsyth said, has now altered its basic policy regarding fluoridation to read: 'Using scientific methods and procedures, communities desiring to fluoridate their communal water supplies should be strongly encouraged to do so.'"[161]

A few days later the state and territorial dental directors also endorsed water fluoridation. They did this at their annual meeting in Washington, D.C., June 7–9, 1950.

On the last day of this meeting, the PHS released a renewed statement of its position on fluoridation, which was published in the *Journal of the American Dental Association*.[162] The American Dental Association and the American Association of Public Health Dentists followed suit at their respective annual meetings a few months later.[163]

In this grand finale for dentistry in public health one can find few, if any, words of doubt about possible dangers of fluoridation. Any qualms were forgotten once the U.S. Public Health Service took the ultimate gamble and recommended fluoridation for the whole country—or at least any community that wanted it. We shall see in the next chapter that there was to be no turning back from that position. The die had been cast for the next sixty years.

Summary

As a result of studies on dental mottling, now called dental fluorosis, in the early part of the twentieth century, researchers in 1931 found that the cause of the condition was naturally occurring fluoride in the drinking water. From the outset it was established that this was a systemic effect. We define the Great Fluoridation Gamble as the notion that fluoride could cause that condition without having any other systemic effect on the body.

Whatever the reasons that led the U.S. PHS to endorse fluoridation in 1950, researchers did not have solid evidence to demonstrate either the short-term or the long-term safety of this practice. Not only was safety not demonstrated in anything approaching a comprehensive and scientific study, but also a large number of studies implicating fluoride's impact on both the bones and the thyroid gland were ignored or downplayed.

It remains an open question whether this was simply a case of zealous dentists winning out over more cautious public health officials, as McNeil suggests, or there were sugar or other industrial or nuclear interests at play, as other commentators have suggested. Either way, the PHS decision was a serious blow to the notion that public health policies should be based on the very best science available and contradicted the Hippocratic admonition "First do no harm."

We return to this matter in the next chapter, where we discuss the next phase of the Great Fluoridation Gamble, exploring the investigations of fluoride's impact on health that took place or were published *after* the all-important PHS endorsement.

• 10 •

The Great Fluoridation Gamble, 1950–

Coauthored by Peter Meiers

As we explained in chapter 9, the Great Fluoridation Gamble was the blind trust that drinking water containing 1 ppm fluoride could damage growing tooth cells without damaging any other tissue in a child's developing body or causing any damage to adults after a lifetime of exposure to uncontrolled doses. The gamble began tentatively in 1945 with the fluoridation trials and continued with a vengeance in 1950 when the U.S. Public Health Service (PHS) endorsed fluoridation with no trials completed and no comprehensive health studies published. We now examine how the gamble has continued right up to the present day.

PHS Gamble Cemented into Place

The crucial PHS endorsement of the fluoridation of public water systems on June 1, 1950, was swiftly followed by endorsements from many other distinguished authorities and professional bodies, including the American Association of Public Health Dentists (October 29, 1950), the American Dental Association (ADA; October 30–November 2, 1950), the American Public Health Association (APHA; November 1950), and state and territorial health officers (November 1950).

According to Exner and Waldbott,[1] most of those endorsements were orchestrated by a few individuals who held leading positions in several of the organizations. None of the endorsements came with a scientific review to justify them. They simply represented a follow-the-leader approach to public health and dentistry. What is surprising about the activities of the key players we examine in this chapter was their expressed *certainty* in the *absolute safety* of this measure

Prior to 1950, at least lip service was paid to the need to investigate the side effects and possible dangers of drinking fluoridated water. After 1950 even the lip service seems to have evaporated. Very quickly investigation changed to promotion.

Thus, this chapter is more about political science than physical science. We start with Dr. Frank Bull, a fluoridation zealot, and toward the end we discuss the role of Edward Bernays, the father of both public relations and propaganda in the United States.

Frank Bull and the 1951 D.C. Conference

The transcript of the remarkably candid Conference of State Dental Directors in Washington, D.C., in 1951 (whose participants apparently did not know that a transcript was being made, or suspect that the document would eventually pass into public hands) clearly shows a preoccupation with the promotion of the fluoridation program rather than a discussion of dealing with any doubts about its safety or effectiveness. The following excerpts give an idea of just how candid the comments of Dr. Frank Bull, the Wisconsin state dental director, were.

In response to his own question, "Why should we do a pre-fluoridation survey?" Dr. Bull replied, "Is it to find out if fluoridation works? No. We have already told the public that it works, we can't go back on that."[2]

Among a few dos and don'ts, Bull tells the U.S. state dental directors, "Don't use the word 'artificial' . . . and certainly don't use the word 'experimental.'"[3]

On toxicity, Bull says, "The question of toxicity . . . Lay off it altogether. Just pass it over, 'We know there is absolutely no effect other than reducing tooth decay,' you say and go on."[4]

On liability, Bull says, "The water department will say, 'What is our liability in fluoridation?' Well, we say 'You are going to look bad if they start suing you because you are not doing it.' (Laughter). You pretty nearly have to turn the thing around. If they get you answering questions for them, then they have you on the defensive, and you are like any salesman, you are sort of up against it."[5]

John Knutson and the PHS, 1952

On January 17, 1952, John Knutson, chief of the Dental Health Division for the PHS, gave a presentation to the North Shore District Dental Society in Salem, Massachusetts, which was later reprinted as "The Case for Water Fluoridation" in the May 8, 1952, issue of the *New England Journal of Medicine*.[6]

The rhetoric and argumentation used by Knutson give us a preview of the formula that was to be used again and again over the next fifty-plus years. For example, note his use of endorsements when he said, "It is now more than a year since the American Dental Association put its stamp of approval on water fluoridation as a mass method of reducing the incidence of tooth decay . . ." and:

Similar endorsements have come from all the other national groups concerned with promoting dental health—the American Public Health Association, the American Association of Public Health Dentists, the American Medical Association, the U.S. Public Health Service and many others. These highly reputable organizations did not give their blessing lightly. They approved fluoridation only after careful study by competent members and consultants, experts with broad scientific knowledge in every phase of fluoride chemistry and toxicology.[7]

This is utter nonsense. With the possible exception of the AMA, organizations rushed to endorse fluoridation within weeks or months of the PHS endorsement in 1950. We are not aware of any evidence that any of these bodies reviewed the literature for themselves after the key endorsement by the PHS.

Knutson complained that the fluoridation program in Massachusetts was "moving ahead with the speed of the proverbial snail" and asked, "Why [are] we . . . quibbling, delaying, pigeon holing—in the face of exhaustive research and overwhelming proof?"[8]

In chapter 9 we illustrate how little research had been done on safety, and what was done hardly constituted "overwhelming proof." As far as benefits were concerned, none of the trials had been completed in 1952 at the time Knutson gave this presentation.

Knutson presented the following "facts" on the matter: "An infinitesimal quantity of fluoride compound added to the water supply will reduce tooth decay by as much as two-thirds . . . this protection will . . . carry over to future generations of adults . . . save many millions of dollars in dental bills . . . does not change the color, taste or odor of the water . . . will not harm any living thing or interfere with any industrial process." He continued by asserting that behind these facts "lies a mass of proof based on years of painstaking scientific research—because fluoridation is no magic formula concocted overnight."[9] In chapter 9 we saw that most of these claims were simply not scientifically based.

Referring to the fluoridation trials still in progress, Knutson went on to say, "The purpose of these studies was not to determine whether or not 1.0 ppm of fluoride in water is a safe amount. We already knew that, simply because millions of Americans have been drinking water containing this amount of natural fluoride all their lives without ill effect."[10]

Acknowledging that fluoride was toxic in excessive amounts, Knutson introduced a calculation that he attributed to McClure: "You would have to drink over 400 gallons of water containing 1.0 ppm at one sitting to receive a toxic dose. Such a large drink of water might kill you, of course, but water alone would do the job without any help from fluoride."[11]

What Knutson and McClure were doing—and many promoters have done since—was obfuscating the crucial difference between an acute lethal dose and a chronic toxic dose. Knutson also cited a 1951 report from an ad hoc committee of the National Research Council report[12] as stating, "The margin between the optimal quantity of fluoride in drinking water which is required for maximal benefit in tooth development, and the amount which produces undesirable physiological effects is sufficiently wide to cause no concern."[13] But in 1951 there was little science on which to base such a confident statement. In the Great Fluoridation Gamble, Dr. Knutson, as chief dental officer of the PHS, perhaps qualifies as gambler-in-chief.

Nicholas Leone and Bartlett-Cameron, 1954

The first formal U.S. health study—the famous Bartlett-Cameron study—did not appear until two years after Knutson's comments above and four years after the PHS had endorsed fluoridation. This was perhaps the ultimate example of "locking the barn door after the horse escaped" and, to continue our farmyard metaphors, represented a fairly clear case of the fox guarding the chicken coop.

The name most associated with the Bartlett-Cameron study is that of Nicholas Leone, MD, the director of medical research at the NIDR. However, Leone's name was not on the study when it was first cited by the Committee on Dental Health of the National Research Council's Food and Nutrition Board.[14] The committee cited the study as follows:

> MB Shimkin, FA Arnold, JW Hawkins, HT Dean: Medical aspects of fluorosis: a survey of 114 individuals using water with 8 parts per million fluoride and of 131 individuals using water with 0.4 parts per million fluoride. Am. Assoc. Advancement Sci. 1953 (in press).

However, when the study appeared in the 1954 AAAS symposium report,[15] as well as in a *Public Health Report*,[16] some of the key authors had changed. Dean's and Hawkins's names had been dropped, and previously unlisted Nicholas Leone appeared as the lead author. It's puzzling how the authorship of this crucially important study could have changed within the space of one year. Moreover, Leone seems to have taken on this leading position with practically no background in the matter. From 1951 to 1953 he was working at the National Microbiological Institute. He did not become the chief of medical investigations at the NIDR until March 1, 1953.[17] He really did not have a lot of time to work on this study. The report *without his name on it* was in press in November 1953, and the report *with his name on it* appeared in October 1954.

Bartlett-Cameron Study Details

For a study that was destined to become the core of the argument for fluoridation's safety, the Bartlett-Cameron study was remarkably small and limited. According to Leone et al., the study began in 1943 when a team from the PHS examined 116 residents in Bartlett (where the water contained 8 ppm fluoride) and 121 residents in Cameron (where the water contained 0.4 ppm fluoride), both in Texas. The participants were all white and ranged in age from fifteen to sixty-eight. The basic requirement for inclusion in the study was having fifteen years or more of continuous residence prior to 1943.[18]

The 1953 investigation—by an entirely different team—involved tracing as many members of the group studied in 1943 as possible. According to Leone et al., 71 percent of the 237 participants still resided in Bartlett or Cameron in 1953. Eight percent of the participants had died, and the forty-seven who had moved were traced; thirty-seven of those were reexamined in 1953, and the other ten were interviewed by telephone or mail and their ten-year medical histories obtained.[19]

Each participant received a physical examination, blood and urine tests, and X-rays. Leone et al. tabulated the abnormalities in various characteristics observed in Bartlett and Cameron in 1943 and 1953, including dental fluorosis, arthritic changes, blood pressure, bone changes (density, coarse trabeculation, hypertrophy, spurs, osteoporosis), cataracts or lens opacity, thyroid function, cardiovascular system function, hearing (decreased acuity), tumors or cysts, fractures, urinary tract calculi, and gallstones. Their overall conclusion was that "no significant differences between the findings in the two towns were observed, except for a slightly higher rate of cardiovascular abnormalities in Cameron [0.4 ppm F] and a marked predominance of dental fluorosis in Bartlett [8 ppm F]."[20]

That conclusion contradicted the conclusion from the earlier NRC report (1953) of the same study, which stated, "A greater incidence in the high fluoride group of a certain brittleness and blotching of the fingernails, of hypertrophic changes in the spine and pelvis, and of lenticular opacities of the eye

requires further epidemiologic investigation."[21] Are we seeing here the beginning of the PHS spin placed on negative findings, which has been a hallmark
of fluoridation promotion to this day?

The Bartlett-Cameron Study Critiqued

If we forget for the moment that the Bartlett-Cameron study was carried
out by an agency that had already declared its support for the policy it was
investigating, to a casual observer in 1954 the study must have looked fairly
convincing, except for the glaringly obvious fact of having so few people in the
study group. However, the study had many other weaknesses, and one of the
first to spot them was Dr. Frederick Exner in 1957.

Some of Exner's criticisms of the report were:

- Both cities had fluoride in their water, Bartlett at 8 ppm and Cameron at
  0.4 ppm. Both were located in Texas, where a lot of water is drunk because
  of the very hot weather. There, 0.4 ppm is not a low concentration. (In
  fact, it is over half the level—0.7 ppm—recommended by the CDC today
  for communities in hot climates.) So it was very unfortunate that the
  study did not include a genuine control community with little fluoride
  in its water. Moreover, the 8 ppm figure for Bartlett may not have been
  accurate. The Texas Health Department listed the value as 6.6 ppm.[22]
- Although all subjects had lived in their respective communities at least
  fifteen years, only eleven (14.5 percent) of those studied in Bartlett had
  been born there, or had lived there during the period of tooth and bone
  development. Consequently, the statement that 11 or 12 percent of
  those studied in Bartlett showed evidence of osteosclerosis was misleading; actually, at least 82 percent of those exposed to Bartlett water during
  the bone-forming period showed evidence of osteosclerosis.[23]
- The actual data published were insufficient to allow any independent
  evaluation. For example, two enzymes important for bone development,
  called acid phosphatase and alkaline phosphatase, with which fluoride
  was known to interfere, were tested for "when indicated."[24] With no
  information about what the *indications* were, how many people were so
  tested, or what was found, the reader was told merely that "when the
  data are reviewed critically, it is clear that the medical characteristics of
  the two groups, with the exception of dental fluorosis, do not differ more
  than would be expected of two comparable towns with or without an
  excess of fluoride in the water supply."[25] The trouble with that was that

there were no data to review. Instead of recording what was found, the authors simply scored how many people were classified as abnormal in various respects in the two communities. Neither quantitative nor qualitative criteria of normality were given; and there was no possible basis for correlating actual findings with probable fluoride intake or other pertinent factors such as duration of intake or age of exposure.[26]

- Both in 1943 and in 1953, "significantly" more abnormalities of the neutrophilic white cells were reported at Bartlett than at Cameron. The figures given indicated that the differences were in morphology rather than in relative number. Yet for unstated reasons the authors downplayed the observation, simply claiming that "when viewed in the light of clinical experience, this finding does not suggest an association with fluoride intake."[27]

To Exner's criticisms we would add some of our own. Although the authors looked at thyroid function, they did not give any meaningful details of how thyroid function was assessed. As we document in chapter 9, a lot of information about fluoride's possible interaction with the thyroid was published between the late 1920s and the 1950s. This included animal studies, case studies of doctors treating hyperthyroid patients with sodium fluoride, and cases of fluoride-induced goiter in communities with an adequate iodine intake. So it is most unfortunate that the examiners were not more meticulous in recording their findings on the thyroid.

We also note that the examiners recorded "arthritic change" but did not give any details. There are different forms of arthritis. It would have been more helpful if we had been told how many people complained of backache and aching joints. This reveals an attitude among promoters of fluoridation that has been retained right up to the present time. Promoters have been forced to acknowledge through the work of Kaj Roholm[28] and researchers in India[29, 30] that excessive exposure to fluoride can lead to serious bone problems, ultimately leading to crippling skeletal fluorosis, in which the whole backbone is essentially frozen into one curved block. The tendency of promoters for many years has been to take seriously only the latter stages of this problem instead of the earliest manifestations, which are similar to the symptoms of arthritis (see chapter 17). We now know that the first indications of fluoride poisoning of the bone do not show up on X-rays (see chapters 13 and 17), so the emphasis placed on X-rays in the Bartlett-Cameron study, with no discussion of any evidence of pains in the joints and bones, was misplaced. Today, it is well established that there are several distinct stages of skeletal fluorosis,[31] but even in the 1950s researchers should have been aware of more subtle effects on the bones and ligaments than those that showed up on X-ray plates.

When exposing the whole population to a pharmacologically active substance, it is the earliest effects one should be concerned about. The subtle shifts are of critical importance in whole-population exposures; in a very small study like the Bartlett-Cameron study, even the gross effects are difficult to find, let alone more subtle changes. If researchers today suggested that a population of 180 million be exposed to a toxic substance based on studies done on approximately one hundred people, they would be laughed out of court.

An important point was raised by Dr. George Waldbott in *The American Fluoridation Experiment* when he stated, "Another reason why fluorosis is not recognized is that physicians, like other people, are inclined to accept as normal the things seen frequently." Referring to the Bartlett-Cameron study, Waldbott explained, "X-rays were made of Bartlett residents, and read by a competent radiologist at the Scott White Clinic in Texas. He called them all normal. They were then sent to a radiologist in New England. He found abnormal bone density in 11 percent of the people. The findings were normal for Texas, where fluoride waters are common, and quite abnormal in New England, where they are rare."[32]

There are so many weaknesses in this study that one is forced to question the objectivity of the observers. Were they really looking for all indications of harm or were they merely producing a study to vindicate the 1950 PHS decision to go ahead with fluoridation? We know little about the lead author Nicholas Leone's involvement with fluoridation prior to this report, but we know more about his activities shortly after it was published.

Leone and Industry

Chris Bryson wrote, "In August 1955, during the Martin trial [farmer Paul Martin was suing the Reynolds Metal Company for damage caused to his farm and his family from fluoride emissions], the public servant Leone spoke with a senior attorney for Reynolds, Tobin Lennon, who was also a member of the Fluorine Lawyers Association, directing Lennon to a federal safety study on fluoride that Leone had recently concluded in Texas [the Bartlett-Cameron study]." Bryson continues, "As the Martin trial hung in the balance, the government's Dr. Leone burned up the long distance telephone lines to Oregon answering questions from Reynolds' attorney."[33]

According to Bryson, Leone was also on friendly terms with Alcoa's fluoride doctor, Dr. Dudley Irwin, and wrote to Irwin after a meeting, "We are all very enthused about a group presentation at some carefully selected meeting in the near future . . . I hope that you have had the opportunity to give further thought to the type of meeting that would best suit our purpose."[34]

Thus it is not clear whether Nicholas Leone was working in the corporate or the public interest as far as fluoridation's safety was concerned. For another major player, Dr. Robert Kehoe, there is absolutely no doubt in whose interest he was working.

Robert A. Kehoe and the Kettering Laboratory

Kehoe was a key figure in the development of the fluoride story from 1930 onward. As detailed by Bryson, Kehoe came to prominence in the 1920s by successfully "sanitizing" the images of two industrial chemicals developed in the laboratory of Charles Kettering, vice president and director of research at General Motors—the gasoline additive tetraethyl lead (TEL) and the refrigerant gas Freon (Dupont's trade name for various chlorofluorocarbons that were eventually to become notorious as depleters of the ozone layer). Both of these raised safety concerns at the time, TEL because of its toxicity and Freon because of its lethal decomposition, when heated, into the nerve gas phosgene and the toxic and corrosive gas hydrogen fluoride. Thanks largely to Kehoe's research, both TEL and Freon enjoyed several decades of profitable existence in automobile fuel tanks and refrigeration units. Kehoe was rewarded in 1930 with the directorship of a new laboratory at the University of Cincinnati, named after Charles Kettering and funded initially by the Ethyl Corporation, DuPont, and the Frigidaire Division of General Motors. The Kettering laboratory under Kehoe became a bastion for industries threatened by numerous lawsuits claiming damage or injury from fluoride and other industrial pollutants. The fluoride-producing industries included aluminum smelting, Freon manufacture, and later the Manhattan Project's uranium enrichment plants, which exposed workers to high concentrations of fluoride or released large quantities in to the atmosphere. One element in deflecting such lawsuits was to establish in the public mind that fluoride was safe by promoting its addition to the public water supply.[35] In the words of Herbert Needleman, referring to Kehoe's role in protecting tetraethyl lead, he "was not burdened with a hypertrophied sense of modesty."[36] His personality enabled him to deal persuasively with lawyers, captains of industry, and senior politicians alike.

Kehoe's assistant, Edward Largent, devoted much of his time to attempting to disprove the conclusions of Kaj Roholm, whose work implicated fluoride in the production of skeletal deformities (see chapter 9) and provided a basis for compensation claims from workers affected by industrial exposure to fluoride.[37] Whatever it may have admitted in private, the Kettering Laboratory's public stance was to exonerate fluoride from causing harm in whatever context was under discussion. This was a valuable service to its industrial sponsors and to the Fluorine Lawyers Association (a group of individuals who specialized in defending corporations against fluoride-related litigation).

Although having relatively little overt involvement in the water fluoridation effort, the Kettering Laboratory did publish a PHS-funded booklet in 1963 titled *The Role of Fluoride in Public Health: The Soundness of Fluoridation of Communal Water Supplies. A Selected Bibliography.*[38] There is no doubt that Kehoe supported water fluoridation or that successful fluoridation campaigns provided a powerful boost to the Kettering Laboratory's agenda.

Edward Schlesinger and the Newburgh-Kingston Trial

In 1956, the report on the Newburgh-Kingston trial was published. David Ast and others summarized the dental findings[39] and Edward Schlesinger, MD, a pediatrician who worked for the New York State Department of Health, was the lead author in the summary of the health findings.[40] It is the latter we examine here. Three very interesting findings pertaining to health emerged, but they were apparent only to those who carefully read the study. First, a greater number of cortical bone defects were found in the fluoridated community compared with the non-fluoridated one. The ratio was about 2:1, and the finding was statistically significant. Second, young girls in the fluoridated community, on average, reached menstruation approximately five months earlier than those in the non-fluoridated community (see chapters 16 and 17). Third, some blood abnormalities were observed. None of these observations were thought to be significant at the time. Schlesinger et al. concluded, "No differences of medical significance could be found between the two groups of children [Newburgh versus Kingston]; thus further evidence was added to that already available on the safety of water fluoridation."[41]

It should also be noted that no studies on adults had been attempted up to that point in the Newburgh trial or any of the other early trials. As far as adults were concerned, the confidence that there would be no long-term effects rested almost entirely on the limited Bartlett-Cameron study discussed above.[42]

Edward Schlesinger: A Quick Convert

It is fascinating to see how quickly the lead author of the Newburgh-Kingston trial, Dr. Edward Schlesinger, cast off the mantle of "objective observer" to become an unapologetic promoter of fluoridation. In a presentation given to the annual meeting of the Academy of Pediatrics in October 1956, just six months after publication of the final report of the Newburgh-Kingston study, he produces many examples of the standard rhetoric that have become familiar hallmarks of fluoridation promotion ever since.[43]

First, he uses the authority of endorsements. He tells his audience that "the leading medical, dental and related scientific organizations have expressed a *belief* in the safety of fluoridation of water" and that "water fluoridation is universally accepted among *reputable* professional groups." The opposition, on the other hand, "is based, with rare exceptions, on *emotional* grounds." [44] [all emphasis added]

He argues that the claim "that fluoridation is mass medication" is invalid, since "fluoridation is simply a preventive measure and no different in principle from the legal requirement in some states that all bread and flour sold in these states be enriched to meet established minimal nutritional levels."[45] He, like promoters who still use that kind of argument today (see chapter 25), fails to note that fluoride is not an essential nutrient like the enrichments added to flour and bread.

As far as the safety of fluoridation is concerned, he uses the typical high-dose versus low-dose claim that "most of the voluminous literature on the toxicology of fluorides is irrelevant to the present discussion because the quantities of fluoride involved are usually the equivalent of drinking water with concentrations at least 100 to 200 times higher than the levels recommended for prevention of dental caries."[46] No citation is given to support such a blatantly false claim. Schlesinger should have known that researchers in India had found bone problems at levels of fluoride in water much lower than this. For example, Pandit had observed bone problems at levels between 1 and 3 ppm.[47]

Schlesinger adds that "the margin of safety for non-dental effects is far greater than any possible increase in intake of fluid for short or long periods of time"[48] but fails to reference any margin-of-safety analysis that would support such a claim.

As far as the Newburgh-Kingston trial is concerned, he states that the study "failed to show any non-dental differences that could be ascribed *even remotely* to the ingestion of fluoridated water" [emphasis added].[49] He makes no mention of the significant difference in cortical bone defects in boys, the earlier onset of menstruation in young girls, or the blood abnormalities mentioned above. It is one thing to dismiss the relevance or significance of those findings, but to say that there were no differences that were "even remotely" related "to the ingestion of fluoridated water" is a huge stretch.

It is highly likely that Schlesinger inherited this dismissive attitude about fluoridation's risks from Harold Hodge. Although Hodge's name does not appear in the list of authors of this final report, he was, according to Bryson, heavily involved in the Newburgh-Kingston study. Reputedly, the officials involved in the Manhattan Project were keen to have low-dose data for fluoride's impact on humans, for possible use in lawsuits that the nuclear industry might face for fluoride damage to the workers on the production lines or to farms in the localities of their plants.[50]

We discuss the important role of Harold Hodge in the promotion of fluoridation in "The False Claims of Harold Hodge" below.

The Push to Fluoridate New York City

The missionary zeal of fluoridation proponents reached its full expression in the effort that was deployed to introduce fluoridation in the city of New York. By 1956, thirty million U.S. citizens and ten major cities had fluoridated water. New York would be the jewel in the crown and pave the way for further successes. In 1957 a propaganda campaign was launched with the publication and distribution of a booklet titled *Our Children's Teeth*.[51] The sponsor was a body called the Committee to Protect Our Children's Teeth, Inc., a group of luminaries that included the celebrated pediatrician and parental guidance guru Benjamin Spock. It was funded by the W.K. Kellog Foundation, famous for both its good works and protecting sugar interests.[52] The booklet included statements from several of fluoridation's big guns whom we have already met—Dean, Ast, McClure, Schlesinger, Leone, and Kehoe—and some others, including Thomas Parran, a former surgeon general, and Herman E. Hilleboe, the commissioner of health for New York State. The booklet merits attention since it provides a blueprint for the tone, content, and even actual wording of many fluoridation promotion documents that were to follow.

There was a little more reason behind the contributors' missionary zeal than may be apparent today. For one thing, dental caries were much more prevalent then than now. However, Hilleboe could not be accused of understating the problem in his contribution, describing the "progressive accumulation of dental disease" as a "national calamity" that was beyond the muscle of the dental profession to control.[53] In that context, it is understandable that a measure apparently offering some degree of protection was seen by many as a godsend. That said, the booklet is awash with errors, evasions, and half-truths, particularly where it is attempting to sow the idea of fluoridation's safety. Hilleboe himself set the ball rolling by stating that "no satisfactory explanation has been advanced for the great prevalence of dental decay in our population;"[54] he avoided mentioning diet, especially sugar consumption, and microbial activity, although a connection had long been recognized.[55] Hilleboe also adopted the tactic, repeated many times since (see chapter 23), of denigrating opponents, describing them as "food faddists, cultists, chiropractors, and misguided and misinformed people who are ignorant of the scientific facts involved."[56]

Most of the following dubious or incorrect statements were highlighted in the booklet as being representative of the contributors' views.

Dean: "Fluoridation is a proven effective, cheap and safe method." Dean goes on to make the remarkable claim that "the literature about the relation of fluorine to health is now so voluminous that the Kettering Laboratory has developed a complete bibliography of over 8,500 references." **Our comment:** The reports in this bibliography deal with a whole variety of papers on fluoride stretching back to the nineteenth century. However, very few of them deal with either the safety or effectiveness of water fluoridation per se. Moreover, some of the papers cited underline the *dangers* posed by fluoride, so to use this bibliography, put together by the industry-funded Kettering Laboratory, as evidence that fluoridation is safe was preposterous. This 8,500 figure is possibly the origin of the claim sometimes made by proponents that "thousands of publications support fluoridation."

Kehoe: "The question of the public safety of fluoridation is non-existent from the viewpoint of medical science." **Our comment:** Here is a precursor for the self-serving statement that there is "no valid debate" on the safety and efficacy of fluoride to which we refer in the introduction and chapter 23.

Leone: "We know without question or doubt, that one part per million fluoride in a water supply is absolutely safe, is beneficial, and is not productive of any undesirable systemic effect in man."

Parran: Discussing the "wide" margin of safety between optimal and deleterious levels of fluoride, he states: "Less than 20
pounds of sodium fluoride added to one million gallons of water
provides one part per million of fluoride ion. In order to produce
the first mild symptoms of toxic fluorosis, more than two tons of
sodium fluoride would be required." **Our comment:** To support
this patently ludicrous 200-fold margin of safety Parran cites
a paper by A. P. Black, head of the department of chemistry,
University of Florida.[57] Parran did not mention that members of
Black's family were involved in a company that was selling fluoridation equipment to municipalities and that he might have a
conflict of interest in his pronouncements on this subject.[58]

Despite this veritable barrage of authority, certainty, and respectability,
NYC was not fluoridated until 1965—some nine years after this brochure
was issued—and even then not by a process that could well be described as
democratic.[59]

One notable absentee from the roster of leading fluoridation promoters
who contributed to the booklet, displaying such unanimous confidence in the
safety of fluoride, was Harold C. Hodge. Yet it was Hodge who probably
played the most decisive role in assuring the public and decision makers that
fluoridation posed no harm. We return to him after a brief consideration of
the influence that Edward L. Bernays had on the fluoridation effort.

The Spin Doctors

If Frank Bull, whose antics we described earlier in the chapter, was a clown
of spin, spin's Machiavelli was surely Edward Bernays, master of the science
and art of what he called "engineering consent."[60] Bernays was undoubtedly one of the most influential propagandists and PR men of the twentieth
century. He admitted to Chris Bryson, who interviewed him in 1991 and
1993, that he had played a part in promoting fluoridation, explaining that
selling fluoridation was child's play because of people's inclination to trust
doctors and believe what they were told by them. The full extent of his
influence is not clear, but most probably it was pervasive. As Bryson relates,
he was certainly in touch with Dr. Leona Baumgartner, health commissioner for New York City, who was steering the fluoridation effort there,
and advised her how to approach the media to sow the idea that there was
no room for controversy over fluoride and that debate on the issue was inap-

propriate. Bernays's suggestion was that it would be like "presenting two sides for anti-Catholicism or anti-Semitism and therefore not in the public interest."[61]

The False Claims of Harold Hodge

We saw in chapter 9 that Cox and Hodge produced an article—at a crucial time—exonerating fluoride of any harm other than dental fluorosis.[62] That article was published in the *Journal of the American Dental Association* in May 1950, just before the critical U.S. PHS endorsement on June 6, 1950. We note above ("Edward Schlesinger and the Newburgh-Kingston Trial") Harold Hodge's intimate involvement in the Newburgh-Kingston trial and also Chris Bryson's revelations about Hodge's role as chief toxicologist for the Manhattan Project. We should add that in the years after the PHS endorsement Hodge was the most influential voice on behalf of the safety of the fluoridation program. In government and toxicological circles he was the "guru" as far as toxicology and the safety of fluoridation were concerned.

Readers can get a glimpse of Harold Hodge in action by watching the opening sequence of a video ("Professional Perspectives on Water Fluoridation") produced by the Fluoride Action Network and accessible on its Web site.[63] In this archived footage we first hear Hodge's commanding voice saying, "There is no health hazard that justifies postponing fluoridation." When Hodge comes into view, we see a handsome man wearing a white lab coat standing in front of a blackboard. When he next appears in this film, he is saying and writing on the blackboard that "fluoridation is safe at 1 ppm." His impressive appearance and strong delivery must have inspired both contemporary viewers and his colleagues with confidence. How impressive would he have seemed if they had known what we know now, that Hodge led a team that injected plutonium into the veins of patients without their knowledge?[64]

But his contemporaries did not know that. What they did know was that Hodge repeated again and again that the science showed that "fluoridation at 1 ppm" was perfectly safe. Between 1950 and 1980 he wrote several influential articles and books or chapters of books in which he continued to exonerate fluoridation of any risks, save that of dental fluorosis.[65–74] These articles, chapters, and books appear authoritative, and his pronouncements on this matter were taken as gospel by fluoridation promoters and government officials alike. Perhaps more than any other single factor, Hodge's influence allowed the Great Fluoridation Gamble to continue for so many years after

1950. However, many of Hodge's scientific claims were blatantly false, and he should have known that. We will examine six examples of false claims from Hodge's publications.

1. *There is no extra retention of fluoride by persons with kidney disease.* In the 1960s Hodge repeatedly asserted—based on his and Frank Smith's experiments on humans and animals—that people with kidney disease would *not* retain more fluoride in their body. Hodge claimed this to be true even for animals and humans with severe kidney disease. In 1963, Hodge stated: "Serious kidney injury or disease does not interfere with fluoride excretion, e.g. in rabbits given near-fatal doses of uranium (a kidney poison), in rats poisoned with fluoride, in elderly patients and in children suffering from kidney disease."[75]

It is difficult to imagine how Hodge and Smith were unable to find increased fluoride retention with kidney disease. Today, it is generally accepted that poor kidney function increases fluoride retention.[76] The fact that Hodge and Smith did not find the effect—in repeated studies—should raise eyebrows about the quality of their research. For more on fluoride and the kidneys, see chapter 19.

2. *Fluoridation accidents cannot cause acute poisoning.* In 1956, Hodge claimed it was "impossible" for an accident with fluoridation equipment to cause acute fluoride poisoning. He further stated that a major fluoridation malfunction could occur every day for ten years and people would still not suffer "serious toxic consequences." He said the following:

> Sometimes the question is raised, What would happen if there were a mechanical breakdown at the fluoridation plant and all of one day's supply of sodium fluoride or sodium silicofluoride were suddenly dumped into the water? If this large weight of fluoride could be dissolved, mixed and distributed within an hour, there would still be a factor of safety sufficient to predict that the water could be drunk for ten years or more without serious toxic consequences . . . it is clearly impossible to produce acute fluoride poisoning by water fluoridation.[77]

It is now well known that water fluoridation accidents can, and do, result in acute poisoning—even death. A list of documented poisonings can be accessed from the Fluoride Action Network Web site.[78]

3. One hundred ppm is the threshold needed to damage kidneys. Hodge's 1963 claim that 100 ppm is the lowest concentration of fluoride that can damage kidneys is similarly flawed.[79] He made the claim based, again, on his own animal research, as well as a review of other animal studies. How could he have missed McCay et al.'s article published in 1957? In that study the authors stated the following:

> Microscopic examinations were made on the kidneys from 6 animals which had not received fluoride in the drinking water, on 3 receiving 1 ppm, on 1 receiving 5 ppm, and on 6 receiving 10 ppm. Interstitial nephritis was observed in all the animals examined histologically, and the severity increased in proportion to the level of the sodium fluoride in the drinking water. Renal tubule hypertrophy and hyperplasia were found in those animals receiving sodium fluoride in the water but not in the 6 rats which had not been given sodium fluoride supplementation.[80]

How did he overlook the 1955 Siddiqui study on humans in India, which found that people consuming water with fluoride levels between 2.5 and 12 ppm had a "marked impairment of renal function. The mean figures for the maximum and standard clearance were 26.24 and 39.67% of the normal respectively."[81]

Animal research published in the past ten years—including a long-term study by Varner et al.[82] (see chapter 15) and a study by NIH-funded toxicologists Borke and Whitford[83]—has indicated that fluoride can damage the kidneys of animals at levels as low as 1 and 10 ppm, depending on the duration of the exposure.[84, 85] According to Borke and Whitford, their study "provides the first evidence that one of the effects of long-term F exposure is a change in expression of the plasma membrane and endoplasmic reticulum Ca^{++} pumps in the kidney."[86]

4. Fifty ppm fluoride in water is the threshold needed to cause thyroid damage. Hodge claimed that fluoride can damage the thyroid in animals or humans only if the level in water consumed reaches 50 ppm.[87] His purported threshold was questionable at the time he made the claim and is even less tenable now.

As early as 1958, Galletti and Joyet published clinical evidence showing daily doses of just 2 to 10 mg fluoride could reduce the activity of the thyroid in individuals with hyperthyroidism[88] (see chapter 16). In 1985, Bachinskii showed that thyroid function in humans could be affected at levels in water as low as 2.3 ppm,[89] and in 1991 a UNICEF-funded research team in China found that humans with iodine deficiencies may be affected by fluoride levels as low as 0.9 ppm[90] (see chapters 15 and 16).

5. *Fluoride-induced bone changes (osteosclerosis) are not observed at urine levels lower than 5 ppm.* According to Hodge's 1963 review paper, bone changes do not occur in fluoride-exposed workers if their urine fluoride levels are below 5 ppm.[91] However, his source for that information is suspect. Hodge and Smith in a 1954 paper tell us that the information was derived from a "personal communication" from Dudley Irwin.[92] What they do not reveal is that Dudley Irwin was the medical director for the Aluminum Company of America (Alcoa), hardly a disinterested source of information on an issue that could cost his company millions of dollars in compensation claims.[93]

Worse, in making his claim, Hodge mischaracterizes information from India that had been published in an article in the *British Medical Journal* in 1955. To understand the mischaracterization, simply compare the following findings from A. H. Siddiqui, the author of the article, with Hodge's 1963 review of this same article:

- Siddiqui: "The urinary fluoride excretion varied between *1.2 and 5.8 ppm*"[94] [emphasis added].
- Hodge: "Crippling fluorosis has been reported from India and China in patients who apparently had ingested little fluoride . . . Fragmentary data on the urinary fluoride excretion, *13–41 ppm*, indicate that the fluoride intake may well have been within the limits known to produce osteo-sclerosis or crippling fluorosis in Western industry" [emphasis added].[95]

6. *Prolonged consumption of 20–80 mg/day is needed to produce crippling skeletal fluorosis.* For many years Hodge was cited for the claim that people would have to consume 20–80 mg of fluoride per day to develop crippling skeletal fluorosis (the terminal stage).[96, 97] Even though Hodge himself quietly changed this to 10–20 mg per day in 1979,[98] others continued to cite his higher figure. In 1993 the NRC used the lower figure,[99] and in 1997 the Institute of Medicine also used a lower figure.[100] However, as late as 1986 the U.S. EPA was relying on Hodge's higher numbers in its determination of the safe drinking water standard for fluoride of 4 ppm[101] (see chapter 20). The EPA has continued to use this standard for over twenty years, even though the basis for it had been changed by the very author most frequently cited as its source. The NRC review of March

22, 2006, called upon the EPA to determine a new standard after concluding that 4 ppm was not protective of health.[102] But, as we have pointed out, the EPA has yet to do that. So Hodge's faulty but confident assertions live on.

To his credit, in his 1963 paper, Hodge does acknowledge the cortical bone defects observed in the Newburgh-Kingston study but conveniently ignored by lead author Schlesinger in 1956 and 1957[103, 104] (see the section "Edward Schlesinger and the Newburgh-Kingston Trial" above). Hodge stated, "The higher incidence of cortical defects in the Newburgh children's long bones, although these changes are considered by the specialist in children's roentgenology to be 'normal' variants (Coffey [the correct spelling is Caffey], 1955), deserves additional study."[105]

Those cortical bone defects certainly did deserve additional study, especially in relation to a possible increase in bone fractures in children in fluoridated areas, but that extra study has not taken place in any fluoridated country in the forty-seven years since Hodge made the suggestion.

The Absence of Study

At the end of the day, this issue is not about studies but about the absence of study. Hodge's last paragraph in his 1963 paper says it all:

> What can be said of the general health of those who drink fluoridated water? A persuasive guarantee of the safety of water fluoridation lies in the fact that over 3 million people in the U.S.A. alone have for their lifetime drunk from naturally fluoridated water supplies containing 1 p.p.m. F or more, and over 7 million from supplies containing 0.7 p.p.m. F or more. Although a large scale epidemiological study is lacking, physicians and public health experts who live in these areas have not become aware of disorders peculiar to these localities or diseases more frequent, more severe, or different than elsewhere. No ill effect of drinking fluoridated water at 1 p.p.m. is known.[106]

Hodge wrote the hymnbook from which all fluoridating public health officials have sung ever since: *If there was any problem, we would have seen it by now.* However, unless you look, you will not find. There wasn't much looking before the PHS endorsement in 1950, and there has not been much more since in those countries that fluoridate their water. What studies there are have come largely from countries that do not fluoridate their water but have moderate to high levels of naturally occurring fluoride in their water and, as a result, have areas endemic for fluorosis.

The Gamble Continues

In the United States and other fluoridated countries, the Great Fluoridation Gamble has continued, virtually unaffected by genuine scientific investigation, since the 1950s. While the U.S. and other governments pour millions of dollars into endless studies on teeth, little effort has gone into tracking potential harm from fluoridation in other tissues. In fact, governments spend more time and effort trying to discredit studies done in non-fluoridated countries that have found harm from fluoride than in investigating the matter in their own countries (see chapter 22). Moreover, Waldbott[107] and Bryson[108] have documented what happens to unsuspecting researchers in the United States when they unwittingly stumble on one of fluoride's adverse effects. Whole careers have been ruined for researchers who found health problems with fluoride and dared publish their findings (see chapter 15).

Summary

The early caution about the possible side effects of fluoridation, shown by dental researchers such as Dean and Ast (see chapter 9), rapidly disappeared once the PHS had endorsed the practice in 1950. After 1950, the emphasis switched from somewhat halfhearted attempts to examine health issues to out-and-out promotion of fluoridation, which has involved downplaying and ignoring health effects. The main players set aside any doubts they may have had and embarked on what they saw as a mission, though in reality it remained a gamble. Doubts and caution were replaced with absolute certainty. The science of investigation was replaced by the politics of promotion. This situation has continued to the present day. As a result, fluoride has become a protected pollutant and fluoridation a protected practice. We examine further examples of the poor science that has protected fluoridation in chapter 22.

PART FOUR

The Evidence of Harm

As we have seen in the previous chapters, there are many arguments against the practice of water fluoridation that, in and of themselves, should persuade a conscientious decision maker not to endorse it. For some people, establishing that fluoridation is an unethical and poor medical practice is sufficient to support an end to the practice (chapters 1–2). Some are appalled that the chemicals used in fluoridation of the water are not pharmaceutical grade but a hazardous industrial waste (chapter 3). Many are further shocked that no U.S. federal agency accepts responsibility for the practice or the chemicals used (chapter 4). For others, a deciding factor is that the evidence that swallowing fluoride reduces tooth decay is weak (chapters 6–8).

In addition to all these reasons for rejecting fluoridation, perhaps the ultimate one for most opponents is that the practice may cause harm. If evidence can be found that fluoridation involves health risks, the case against it becomes overwhelming. In this respect, we would do well to remember the Hippocratic admonition, "First, do no harm."

In the following pages, we look at fluoride's potential to damage the teeth (dental fluorosis, chapter 11); the brain (chapter 15); the endocrine system, including the thyroid and pineal glands (chapter 16); bone (including fractures, arthritis, and osteosarcoma, chapters 17 and 18); and the kidney and other tissues (chapter 19). Chapter 12 summarizes the kind of information that a toxicologist would want to have before making a weight-of-evidence judgment about the safety of a chemical before exposing an individual or population. In chapter 13, we examine the evidence that a small percentage of the population may be particularly sensitive to fluoride's toxic effects, exhibiting a number of reversible symptoms that clear up when the source of fluoride is removed. Chapter 14 describes a major recent event in the science of this matter: publication of the report of the U.S. National Research Council of the National Academies, *Fluoride in Drinking Water: A Review of EPA's Standards.*

Before reviewing the evidence of health effects, however, we must stress the important difference between the possible health effects caused by *fluoride* and those caused by *fluoridation*. There is no doubt at all about the former; the debate rages over the latter.

The one area of harm even the most ardent promoter of fluoridation cannot deny is dental fluorosis, and that is where our review of fluoride's adverse health effects begins.

• 11 •

Dental Fluorosis

Coauthored with Peter Meiers

Dental fluorosis is a mottling and discoloration of the tooth enamel. Fluoride in drinking water was identified as the cause of this condition in three independently published studies in 1931.[1-3] Also in 1931, soon after these reports were published, Alcoa scientists were finding cases of dental fluorosis near the company's aluminum smelters where there was little or no fluoride in the water (e.g. Massena, New York).[4] In 1932, Dr. H. Trendley Dean, from the Dental Section of the U.S. Public Health Service, began his survey of the whole United States for this condition. In a 1934 article, he classified dental fluorosis according to the following categories: questionable, very mild, mild, moderate, moderate to severe, and severe. The article included an artist's rendition of the categories.[5] In a later article he provided black-and-white photographs.[6]

Although there have been other attempts to define the various stages of this condition, Dean's classification is still used widely, although the categories "questionable" and "moderate to severe" have tended to drop out of common use. Dean described the four main categories very precisely by the percentage of the enamel impacted:

- *Very mild* dental fluorosis involves opaque white patches or streaks ranging from small areas on the cusps of the teeth up to 25 percent of the tooth surface.
- *Mild* dental fluorosis involves an impaction of up to 50 percent of the tooth surface.
- *Moderate* dental fluorosis involves 100 percent of the tooth surface being affected, with some pitting.
- *Severe* dental fluorosis affects 100 percent of the tooth surface with more pitting and brittleness.

In time, especially with the moderate and severe categories, the white patches become progressively discolored, going from yellow to orange to brown, making the condition even more unsightly. The percentage of children affected by this condition steadily increases with the level of fluoride in the water in a very close to linear fashion (see figure 7.3).

By 1936, Dean was reporting that two hundred areas in the United States—many clustered in Arizona, Colorado, Illinois, Iowa, New Mexico, South Dakota, and Texas—had endemic mottled enamel and in another one hundred areas it had been reported but not yet confirmed by survey. These three hundred areas were distributed among twenty-three states.[7] By 1938, he was reporting that a "higher percentage of caries-free children is found in cities whose water supplies contain relatively toxic amounts of fluoride than in those communities with water supplies not so affected," but he warned that "the possibility of partially controlling dental caries through the domestic water supply warrants thorough epidemiological-chemical study."[8] His famous twenty-one-city study would not appear for another four years.[9, 10]

Percentage of Children Affected

Dean believed that with fluoride at 1 ppm in the drinking water, dental fluorosis would affect only about 10 percent of children, and then only in its *very mild* form. When it came to artificial water fluoridation, he felt that any level of fluorosis above the *very mild* level was unacceptable. In 1952, this is what Dean had to say in his testimony before the Delaney Committee of the U.S. Congress: "We don't want any 'mild' [fluorosis] when we are talking about fluoridation. We don't want to go that high and we don't have to go that high . . . I don't want to recommend any fluoridation where you get any 'mild.'"[11]

Dean's comments on the unacceptability of mild (and thus moderate and severe) dental fluorosis as a trade-off for "any advantage that might accrue from the partial control of dental caries"[12] are in sharp contrast to what fluoridation promoters say today. The latter accept both mild and moderate dental fluorosis, and become concerned only when the condition reaches the severe stage.

Modern Surveys of Dental Fluorosis

In 1997, Heller, Eklund, and Burt reported on the findings of a 1986–1987 survey conducted by the National Institute of Dental Research (NIDR) in the United States.[13] They revealed that 29.6 percent of children in artificially fluoridated areas (0.7–1.2 ppm) had dental fluorosis on at least two teeth (see table 11.1). In those communities, 22.5 percent of the children had very mild, 5.8 percent had mild, and 1.3 percent had moderate dental fluorosis.[14] This breakdown by severity level is shown in table 11.2. The figure for all levels combined (29.6 percent) is three times the rate anticipated by Dean, and, of course, not all of the fluorosis was in the very mild category.

Heller et al. also found that about 21.6 percent of children in non-fluoridated areas (0.3–0.7 ppm) had dental fluorosis, as did about 13.6 percent of children in communities with less than 0.3 ppm.[15] Tables 11.1 and 11.2 summarize Heller's findings.

The York Review panel estimated that up to 48 percent of children in "optimally" fluoridated areas worldwide have dental fluorosis in all forms, with 12.5 percent showing abnormalities of aesthetic concern.[16]

In 2005, the Centers for Disease Control (CDC) released the findings of Beltrán-Aguilar et al. of a new national survey of oral health in the United States conducted during the years 1999–2002 as part of the National Health and Nutrition Examination Survey (NHANES). The survey found an overall dental fluorosis rate of 32 percent among U.S. schoolchildren aged six to nineteen years. Incredibly, 3–4 percent of American children have dental fluorosis in the combined moderate and severe categories. These figures include children

Table 11.1 Percentage of children with dental fluorosis (DF) on at least two teeth, as a function of the level of fluoride (F) in the community's drinking water.

F (ppm)	% children with DF on at least two teeth
<0.3	13.5
0.3 – <0.7	21.7
0.7 – <1.2	29.9
>1.2	41.4

Source: Heller et al.,[17] using data from the NIDR survey of U.S. children in 1986–1987.

Table 11.2 Percentage of children with different levels of severity of dental fluorosis (based on Dean's classification) as a function of the level of fluoride (F) in the community's drinking water.

F (ppm)	Severity of dental fluorosis (%)			
	very mild	mild	moderate	severe
<0.3	10.7	2.4	0.4	0.1
0.3 – <0.7	17.3	3.1	1.2	0.0
0.7 – <1.2	22.5	5.8	1.3	0.0
>1.2	27.2	7.0	5.3	2.0

Source: Heller et al.,[18] using data from the NIDR survey of U.S. children in 1986–1987.

living in both fluoridated and non-fluoridated communities. According to the CDC, the 32 percent total represented an increase of 9 percent over the previous national survey, in 1986–1987.[19]

Black American Children Are More Vulnerable to Dental Fluorosis

The CDC survey also found that fluorosis affects more black American children than white American children. According to the CDC, "No clear explanation exists why fluorosis was more severe among non-Hispanic black children than among non-Hispanic white or Mexican-American children. This observation has been reported elsewhere, and different hypotheses have been proposed, including biologic susceptibility or greater fluoride intake."[20]

Children Are Being Overexposed to Fluoride

These surveys of dental fluorosis indicate that today, even without fluoridation, a large number of children are overexposed to fluoride from an increasing number of sources. Opponents and proponents of fluoridation offer diametrically opposed responses to this problem.

The simplest and most direct way of improving this unacceptable situation, opponents say, is to end water fluoridation. Not only would that remove a major and direct source of fluoride, but it would also eliminate an indirect source—the cumulative amounts of fluoride ending up in beverages and foods processed in fluoridated communities.

Proponents argue instead that we should go after the *discretionary* sources of fluoride (sources of fluoride over which the individual has some control) by limiting or eliminating the use of fluoride supplements and putting more effort into educating parents to stop their children from swallowing fluoridated toothpaste. While laudable, the latter recommendation is somewhat ironic, because one of the reasons for introducing fluoridation in the first place was to reduce parental responsibility in these matters.

A Cosmetic Problem?

Proponents insist that dental fluorosis is merely a cosmetic problem, not a health problem. Until the condition becomes severe, they argue, fluorosis does not interfere with the functioning of the tooth or increase susceptibility to dental decay. What this position ignores are the psychological impacts children who suffer from mild, moderate, or severe dental fluorosis undoubtedly experience. In an article published in the *New York State Dental Journal* in 2008, Elvir Dincer, DDS, concluded that children's self-esteem is harmed by even mild fluorosis.[21] As well, to claim that dental fluorosis is merely cosmetic is to ignore an indication of a *systemic* effect that has caused some alteration of the biochemistry of the growing tooth.[22]

Opponents of fluoridation are concerned that dental fluorosis in a child may signal that damage to other tissues has also occurred. That damage may be less visible and less obvious but possibly far more serious.

Possible Mechanisms of Damage
While the exact mechanism by which fluoride damages the enamel is not yet known, three possibilities have been suggested:

1. Inhibition of enzymes (proteases that remove the last traces of protein between the crystals that make up enamel) in the growing teeth[23–25]
2. Interference with G protein-signaling mechanisms[26]
3. Interference with thyroid function[27]

There is no law that says interference in biochemistry will not occur in other tissues as it does in teeth. For fluoridation promoters, it has always been an article of faith that the presence of dental fluorosis does not signal any other damage to the human body. This we have called the Great Fluoridation Gamble, the subject we address in chapters 9 and 10.

Promoters' Spin
Not surprisingly, promoters of fluoridation have always worried about how they could convince the public of the "safety" of fluoridation, while acknowledging the increase in dental fluorosis it causes. At a meeting of state dental directors held in Washington, D.C., in 1951, Dr. Frank Bull, then dental director for the state of Wisconsin and an avid and very prominent early promoter of fluoridation, gave this advice on how to handle the dilemma:

> What are some of the objections that are brought up on this fluoridation program? I think the first one that is brought up is: "Isn't fluoride the thing that causes mottled enamel or fluorosis? Are you trying to sell us on the idea of putting that sort of thing in the water?"
>
> What is your answer? You have got to have an answer, and it had better be good. You know, in all public health work it seems to be quite easy to take the negative. They have you on the defensive all

the time, and you have to be ready with answers. Now, we tell them this, that at one part per million dental fluorosis brings about the most beautiful looking teeth that anyone ever had and we show them some pictures of such teeth. We don't try to say that there is no such thing as fluorosis even at 1.2 parts per million which we are recommending. But you have got to have an answer. Maybe you have a better one.[28]

Over fifty years after Dr. Bull offered his advice to fluoridation promoters, Dr. Peter Cooney, chief dental officer of Canada, had this to say about mild dental fluorosis in a public hearing held in Thunder Bay, Ontario, on July 20, 2009:

Mild fluorosis shows teeth as being a very nice white color. It is called mild fluorosis because kids love it and adults love it. People will go to dentists to get bleaching so that they will look like this. What it does of course is to make the enamel of the teeth much harder so not only are kids happy with the color and the whiteness but it is also much more resistant to decay.[29]

We suspect very few children or adults share Dr. Cooney's enthusiasm for the appearance of mild dental fluorosis, which can affect up to 50 percent of the tooth surface (see photos at the Web site of the Fluoride Action Network, www.fluoridealert.org), especially when, with aging, the white patches slowly turn orange and brown.

Summary

The "optimal" fluoride concentration was originally defined as 1 ppm on the basis that that reduced caries but caused fluorosis in only about 10 percent of children and then only of the *very mild* type. Dean considered that even *mild* fluorosis was unacceptable aesthetically and indicative of systemic toxicity. More recent studies show that, by that criterion, many children in industrialized countries are receiving too much fluoride, even where the water is not artificially fluoridated. In fluoridated areas a substantial minority of children may have fluorosis of aesthetic concern (*mild, moderate,* or *severe*). Proponents of fluoridation admit only that this is a cosmetic problem that may call for expensive treatment. They are less ready to concede that it is in fact a manifestation of systemic fluoride poisoning.

Fluoride's Chemistry, Biochemistry, and Physiology

The standard approach used by toxicologists when assessing the potential toxicity of a substance is to investigate its properties in this sequence: its chemistry, biochemistry, and physiology; its impact on animals; and finally its impact on humans. Because of the limits on human experimentation, however, seldom do toxicologists enjoy the luxury of having numerous human studies at their fingertips. Fluoride is unusual in this respect, because millions of people worldwide have been exposed to high natural levels, with serious health consequences; these are discussed in chapters 13–19.

Chemistry
This is not the place to write a textbook on chemistry, but perhaps a brief lesson will be helpful.

Elements
Fluorine is one of approximately one hundred elements that make up our universe. Most of these elements are classified as metals (iron, copper, silver, sodium, etc.), with only a dozen or so classified as nonmetals (carbon, nitrogen, oxygen, hydrogen, fluorine, chlorine, bromine, iodine, sulfur, phosphorus, silicon, arsenic, and the noble gases—helium, neon, argon, etc.).

Fluorine forms chemical compounds with almost every other element. With sodium, for example, it forms sodium fluoride (NaF), and with calcium, calcium fluoride (CaF_2).

Compounds
When elements combine chemically, the properties of the resulting compound are completely different from those of the parent elements. For example, when sodium (a very reactive metal that has an almost explosive reaction with water) combines with chlorine (a poisonous gas used in World War I and used today to kill bacteria in water), the compound formed is sodium chloride, or the common table salt we are happy to sprinkle on our food!

There is a world of difference between the element fluorine and the fluoride compounds it forms when it combines with metals (e.g., sodium fluoride, calcium fluoride), which in turn are different from the organofluorine compounds it forms with carbon (e.g., perfluoroethylene), but commentators frequently confuse the element *fluorine* with the *metallic fluorides* and sometimes the *organofluorine compounds*. The key difference between the latter sets of compounds is that the former contain *ions* and the latter contain *molecules* (molecules are groups of atoms held together with strong linkages called covalent bonds).

Note 1: When a nonmetal element combines with another element, we change the ending of the nonmetal from *ine* to *ide*; for example, sodium and fluor*ine* combine to form sodium fluor*ide*.

Note 2: While there are only about one hundred elements, there are literally millions of compounds.

Fluorine

Fluorine—the element—is a pale yellow gas, and because it is so extremely reactive, it is never found as the free element in nature. What we find in nature are its compounds with other elements, such as calcium fluoride, which is found as the mineral fluorspar (CaF_2). Another important mineral containing fluorine is cryolite (Na_3AlF_6). This latter mineral is of critical importance in the electrolytic process used to extract the metal aluminum from bauxite.

Fluorine is the most reactive element, but the fluorides it forms with metals (such as sodium, calcium, magnesium, aluminum) are not very *chemically* reactive. On the other hand, soluble metal fluorides are very active *biologically,* as we shall see in the section on biochemistry below.

The Free Fluoride Ion (F^-)

When metal fluorides dissolve in water, their constituents separate as ions. For all intents and purposes, a solution of sodium fluoride can be treated as two separate substances—sodium ions (Na^+) and fluoride ions (F^-). You will notice that when concentrations are reported on bottled water in Canada and Europe, the concentrations of the positive ions (e.g., Na^+, Mg^{2+}, etc.) and the negative ions (e.g., Cl^-, F^-, carbonate, etc.) are reported separately.

Thus, most of the discussion on toxicology focuses on the free fluoride ion (F^-). Organofluorine compounds (certain plastics, pesticides, and pharmaceuticals) enter our fluoridation picture only if, in the human body, they are metabolized to release free fluoride ions.

This is about as much chemistry as most of us need to know to explore the issue of fluoridation's dangers.

Biochemistry

Enzymes are very large protein molecules (thousands of times larger than the simple water molecule, H_2O) that catalyze (facilitate) most of the ten thousand or so chemical reactions that occur in our bodies and other living things. Fluoride is a well-known inhibitor of enzymes in vitro (in test tube experiments). In this respect, it is interesting to note that some of the earliest opponents of fluoridation in the 1950s were biochemists who used fluoride to poison enzymes in their experiments. One of these was Dr. James Sumner, who was the director of enzyme chemistry in the department of biochemistry and nutrition at Cornell University. Sumner won the Nobel Prize for his work in enzyme chemistry. He is quoted as saying, "We ought to go slowly. Everybody knows fluorine and fluorides are very poisonous substances and we use them in enzyme chemistry to poison enzymes, those vital agents in the body. That is the reason things are poisoned, because the enzymes are poisoned and that is why animals and plants die."[1]

Even though enzyme molecules are very large, the chemical reaction they help steer is usually facilitated by a small section on the enzyme molecule called the "active center." Frequently, metal ions like Mg^{2+}, Zn^{2+}, and Cu^{2+} are located at these active sites.

Fluoride can interfere with enzyme function in two ways: either by attaching itself to a metal ion located at an enzyme's active site or by forming a competing hydrogen bond (see the next section) at this same active site. Either way, these interactions can block or interfere with the enzyme's function.

Hydrogen Bonds

The fluoride ion interferes with hydrogen bonding.[2] Hydrogen bonding occurs when a hydrogen atom in a molecule finds itself located between two atoms of either oxygen or nitrogen or one of each. These bonds (or attractions) can form within the same molecule if it is very large (e.g., a protein) or between different molecules (e.g., between water molecules). Hydrogen bonds are weaker than the *covalent* chemical bonds that link atoms together, and they can be more easily disrupted. Hydrogen bonds are of critical importance to both the structure and function of some of the most important molecules in the body. In the big polymer molecules (particularly proteins and nucleic acids), there are literally hundreds, even thousands, of these hydrogen bonds giving a stable shape to the molecules. In small molecules the shape is rigidly determined by the covalent bonds. In the larger molecules in living things the shape is much more flexible, and it is largely the hydrogen bonds that provide the final and operative shape. In biochemistry shape and function are intimately connected. Some of these hydrogen bonds can easily be pulled apart without a full chemical reaction (i.e., without breaking the covalent bonds); they are the Velcro strips of biology.

Formation of Complex Ions

Because the fluoride ion is *negatively* charged, it is attracted to *positive* ions (usually metal ions) and forms clusters with them of a fixed formula and shape called *complex ions*. (For our purposes, the only thing we need to know about the charges on ions is that opposites attract and like charges repel.) Fluoride forms these complexes with every metal ion except the alkali metals (lithium, sodium, and potassium). Two complex ions we are going to meet in these pages are silicon hexafluoride (SiF_6^{2-}) and aluminum tetrafluoride (AlF_4^-).

The fluoride ion forms complexes with metal ions that are needed in the body (e.g., calcium and magnesium) as well as with metals that are toxic to the body (e.g., lead and beryllium). This can cause a variety of problems, including the following examples:

1. Fluoride interferes with enzymes where metal ions are located at the active sites or where, as with magnesium ions, they act as an important co-factor. (A co-factor is not actually part of an enzyme's structure but expedites its action by aligning the molecules in the right position.)

2. Fluoride can form complexes with metal ions like Al^{3+} and Pb^{2+} and may facilitate their uptake into tissues where those metals might not otherwise go.[3-6]

Aluminum Fluoride Complexes

With the aluminum ion (Al^{3+}) the fluoride ion can form the ion AlF_4^-, an ion that has about the same size and shape as the phosphate ion (PO_4^{3-}), an ion of huge biological significance. Both RNA and DNA (polymers of nucleic acids) are synthesized using the triphosphates of their corresponding bases: adenosine, cytosine, guanosine, and thymine (or uracil for RNA). Phosphate is also involved in the storage and use of energy in the body; energy is stored by converting adenosine diphosphate (two phosphates on the molecule) to adenosine triphosphate (three phosphates on the molecule), and energy is released by reversing the process and converting adenosine triphosphate back to adenosine diphosphate. Some biological switching devices (e.g., see the discussion of G proteins in the next section) are controlled by substituting guanosine triphosphate for guanosine diphosphate. Any basic textbook on biochemistry goes into these processes in great detail. It is not unreasonable to think that AlF_4^- might do damage to biological systems, and much more attention needs to be paid to this possibility.

Interference with G Proteins

One of the things that the AlF_4^- ion can do, which we know most about, is to switch on G proteins in vitro and thereby disrupt the transmission of important messages across cell membranes.[7, 8]

The G protein system is located in the outer membranes of the cells in every tissue that requires external regulation. The system is needed to enable water-soluble messengers like hormones and growth factors, which cannot cross the cell membranes (membranes are made largely of fat and repel water-soluble compounds), to get their message inside the cells of the tissues they are meant to excite. The G protein system performs this function.

This is how the G protein switch works: In the off position guanosine diphosphate (two phosphates on the molecule) sits in a pocket in the G protein, but in the on position guanosine triphosphate (three phosphates on the molecule) occupies the pocket. The switch from "on" to "off" is normally triggered by a hormone or other water-soluble messenger arriving at a receptor on the cell's surface.

However, AlF_4^- has the ability to "trick" the G protein to act as if it has been switched on when it hasn't (i.e., no normal messenger has arrived). This is how that works: The AlF_4^- ion can enter the G protein in the off position and form a combination with guanosine diphosphate, which makes it look like guanosine triphosphate, thus switching the G protein to the "on" position. The result is that AlF_4^- is able to mimic the transmission of critical messages across cell membranes when no actual messenger has arrived at the receptor on the membrane surface.

Given a sufficiently high concentration (20–200 ppm F⁻), which certainly occurs in bones and teeth and possibly at the interface between calcified deposits and the soluble part of the cell in bone and other calcifying tissues, such interactions give aluminum-fluoride complexes the potential to interfere with many hormonal, some growth-factor, and some neurochemical signals.[9, 10] There are approximately three thousand reports in the scientific literature of scientists using aluminum fluoride to switch on G proteins. Researchers have suggested mechanisms involving G proteins to explain fluoride's ability to damage the growing tooth enamel (see chapter 11), as well as stimulating bone turnover. The bone, like every other tissue in the body, is continually being broken down (resorbed) and rebuilt (ossified) from its constituent materials; see chapter 17. TSH, the thyroid-stimulating hormone, is one of the hormones whose signals aluminum fluoride can mimic, at least in test tubes (see chapter 16).

An excellent summary of the biochemistry of fluoride can be found in the book by Kenneth L. Kirk titled *Biochemistry of the Elemental Halogens and Inorganic Halides.*[11]

Calcium-Fluoride Interactions

There was an old adage in the long history of lead toxicity: Lead follows calcium. The same adage also applies to fluoride: Fluoride follows calcium. In the sixty years of water fluoridation most of the attention has been focused on fluoride's interaction with the calcium in the hard tissues (the teeth and bone); however, it may well turn out that fluoride's more worrying impacts on the body will turn on its interaction with calcium ions in the soft tissues.

It is well established that fluoride interacts with the key structural material of both the tooth enamel and the bone: calcium hydroxyapatite. In this process the fluoride ion replaces a hydroxyl ion, making the enamel harder and more resistant to acid attack (which is the first step in dental decay) and also making the bone harder but possibly more brittle (see chapter 17). A great deal of research has been done on these interactions between fluoride and calcium. However, surprisingly, much less work has been done investigating fluoride's possible interaction with calcium's other functions.

Two important functions of calcium are (1) the transmission of messages across the junction between two nerve cells (the synaptic cleft) and (2) the communication between the nerve cell and muscles at the neuromuscular junction. Both of these calcium actions hinge on the remarkable fact that in our tissues the concentration of calcium ions outside the cell is about ten thousand times greater than the concentration inside. This huge difference has been exploited by nature to allow the influx of calcium ions into the cell to become a very important messenger and regulator. Equally important is to get the calcium ions out of the cell once its regulatory job has been done. This involves proteins that straddle the cellular membrane and use chemical energy to pump the calcium out of the cell (or at least away from the key action area).

So the key question to ask is whether fluoride ions can cause some kind of interference with these calcium ion movements and thereby disrupt their delicate regulatory role. The simple answer is that we don't really know because few researchers in the West have pursued the matter very closely. However, there has been a great deal of research on fluoride's impact on the brain in China, and gradually more people are hearing about these studies. For example, there are now over eighty experiments that show that fluoride interferes with animal brain, twenty-three studies that have found an association between moderate to high fluoride exposure and lowered IQ in children, three studies that have found fluoride damage to fetal brain, and one study showing altered behavior in children in areas endemic for natural fluoride exposure. All of these studies are identified, and some discussed, in chapter 15. However, there are many different ways that a toxic substance can interfere with the brain in addition to calcium-regulating mechanisms.

A very recent study (Zhang et al. 2010)[12] has found a relationship between fluoride and calcium that may explain fluoride's role in causing brain damage. However, it is not a direct interaction between fluoride and calcium ions per se; rather it appears that fluoride might be interfering with the process responsible for the production of the proteins that comprise the channels through which calcium flows or the pumps that clear it from the scene of action.

It can only be hoped that researchers will pursue this matter further and find out just what fluoride may be doing to the developing brain and determine the mechanisms involved. Hopefully, solid answers will be achieved in this before too many more children are unnecessarily exposed to excessive fluoride.

Oxidative Stress

Meanwhile, as this book goes to press, a review article by E. Gazzano et al., "Fluoride Effects: The Two Faces of Janus," has been published and summarizes much of what is known about fluoride's mechanisms of toxicity. Of particular interest is the ability of fluoride to cause oxidative stress by interfering with the body's defense mechanisms against reactive oxidative species (ROS), which can otherwise attack membranes (lipid peroxidation) and presage inflammation and a whole range of degenerative disesases.[13]

Physiology

An important starting point for a discussion of fluoride's physiology is the level of fluoride naturally present in mother's milk. This has been measured in several studies. Reported concentrations generally lie in the range of 0.004–0.04 ppm.[14-20] These concentrations are very much lower than the average level used in fluoridation programs (0.6–1.2 ppm). As discussed in chapter 1, there is little or no evidence that fluoride is an essential nutrient.

Possibly the low levels in mother's milk may tell us that there were reasons for keeping the fluoride ion away from the infant's developing tissues. Having had a glimpse of fluoride's biochemistry above, that would seem to be a fortunate result.

While there is no evidence that any mechanism has evolved for concentrating fluoride in the milk—which would be necessary if a baby were to receive anything approaching the amount of fluoride he gets from formula made with fluoridated water—there is some evidence that fluoride may be partially excluded from human milk.

Increasing daily fluoride intake does not necessarily increase the concentration of fluoride in human milk. Some studies suggest that the concentration of fluoride in milk is influenced by the amount ingested;[21, 22] others find no significant correlation.[23, 24] Overall, any correlation appears weak. One problem in interpreting these results is that they usually do not take into account the total fluoride intake from all sources. Such an accounting was, however, attempted by G. N. Opinya and colleagues, who calculated total fluoride ingestion by individual mothers living in an area with a naturally high fluoride concentration in water (9 ppm). Total daily intakes ranged between 9.5 mg and 37.2 mg, yet, despite the wide variation, there was no significant correlation with human milk fluoride, which averaged only 0.033 ppm.[25] When a single large dose of fluoride is ingested, the concentration rises sharply in the blood plasma. However, Ekstrand et al.[26, 27] found that despite the rise, the concentration in milk showed little or no change.

We can conclude from the above only that human babies are adapted to develop with very little or no fluoride in their diet. It seems reckless to imagine that we know better what is good for them. In particular, infancy is not the time when one would want exposure to a substance that can affect the brain (see chapter 15), especially at levels that are 25–250 times the concentration found naturally in mother's milk.

One of the reasons that Dr. Arvid Carlsson, a neuropharmacologist, gave in 1978 for opposing fluoridation in Sweden was the far greater exposure bottle-fed babies would get to fluoride than breast-fed babies. He wondered what this "may mean for the development of the brain and the other organs."[28] Thirty-two years later we may be beginning to find out (see chapter 15).

Circulation of Fluoride

Fluoride enters the bloodstream via the gums, the stomach, the intestinal lining, the lung (in the case of airborne fluoride), and possibly the skin during baths or showers (there seems to have been little formal study of this route of exposure). Once in the bloodstream, it circulates throughout the body and can then enter every other tissue. However, only in the calcifying tissues (which include the pineal gland; see chapter 16) will the concentration rise substantially higher than the concentration in the blood.

On average, only 50 percent of the fluoride we ingest each day is excreted through the kidneys, the remainder largely accumulating in our bones, teeth, pineal gland, and other calcifying tissues. People with poor kidney function excrete less fluoride. This affects the elderly, as kidney function decreases with age. Because the total mass of our bones is so large, 99 percent of the total fluoride accumulates there, although that does not mean concentrations reached in other tissues are not significant. This may be particularly true of the pineal gland (see chapter 16).

Inkielewicz and Krechniak showed that fluoride accumulated in rat testis in a dose- and *time*-dependent manner.[29] Others have shown that fluoride can cross the blood-brain barrier and accumulate in rat brain (see chapter 15). However, when considering the extent of accumulation in the brain, it is important to distinguish between accumulation in the brain itself and the demonstrated accumulation in the pineal gland[30, 31] (see chapter 16). The pineal gland is outside the blood-brain barrier but may have been included in some of the analyses of the whole brain.

If the kidney is damaged, more fluoride will accumulate, especially in the bone. To a certain extent, the accumulation of fluoride in the bone could be viewed as having a protective effect by keeping fluoride away from more sensitive tissues. However, it may produce two problems: First, as the fluoride accumulates in the bone over time, it may reach levels where it affects the bone itself (and connective tissue; see chapter 17), including the bone marrow, which is responsible for generating key cells and molecules involved in the immune system. Second, fluoride accumulated in the bone may cause problems for other tissues by passing into the circulation during bone turnover. Bone turnover—the dynamic process of resorption and ossification—may accelerate during fasting, ill health, and pregnancy, either by slowing down desorption or accelerating resorption, or a combination of both.

Fluoride's Slow Turnover in Bone
The time it takes a substance to go from a given concentration to half that concentration in the absence of continued input is called the substance's half-life. The half-life of fluoride in bone is thought to be about twenty years,[32]

with complete turnover occurring three or four times in a lifetime. Thus, turn-over under normal circumstances is slow; however, in times of stress, disease, or prolonged reduced diet, the turnover can increase. According to the 2006 NRC panel, twenty years may not be the true half-life. The report states, "A study of Swiss aluminum workers found that fluoride bone concentrations decreased by 50 percent after 20 years . . . Twenty years might not represent a true half-life. Recent pharmacokinetic models . . . are nonlinear, suggesting that elimination rates might be concentration dependent."[33]

Animal Studies

There are many animal studies of fluoride's impact on the bone and brain, as well as on the endocrine and reproductive systems. These are discussed in subsequent chapters along with some important human studies.

Farm and Domestic Animal Studies

Normally, when we talk about animal studies, we are thinking about animals used in lab studies, like rats, mice, and guinea pigs. However, in the history of fluoride pollution (see chapter 9) the fluoride poisoning of farmyard animals has been of great concern. Grazing cows have literally been brought to their knees by fluoride emissions from aluminum smelters.

One of the pioneers in researching the impacts of fluoride on farmyard animals was Dr. Lennart Krook, a veterinary pathologist at Cornell University. Dr. Krook passed away in April 2010. One of his last studies involved investigating the mysterious illnesses affecting a number of quarter horses on Cathy and Wayne Justus's farm in Pagosa Springs, Colorado.[34] Some of the horses died. It was only when Cathy and Wayne Justus changed the horses' water supply that the symptoms of the remaining animals began to clear up. Dr. Krook was able to show that the likely cause of the horses' ailments was fluoride. This event led to the halting of fluoridation in Pagosa Springs. A very disturbing videotape of these horses can be viewed online.[35] The Justus and Krook study was published in the journal *Fluoride* in 2006.[36]

The problem for both cows and horses is that they drink very large quantities of water, so should they be exposed to fluoridated water, their fluoride exposure can be very high indeed.

Another animal that might be very sensitive to fluoride is the dog. The dog is one of the few animals that succumbs to osteosarcoma, and larger dogs commonly lose strength in their rear legs. Fluoride is known to cause arthritic-like symptoms and is suspected of causing osteosarcoma in both rats and humans (see chapter 18). With the possibility that dogs are getting high levels of fluoride in pet food,[37] especially pet food that contains bonemeal, there is a very real chance that fluoride may be the causative agent for these conditions. These speculations need to be investigated.

Summary

The chemistry and biochemistry of fluoride, and its kinetics in the body, are such that fluoride can function as a cumulative poison when small amounts are ingested over a long period by drinking fluoridated water. Fluoride circulates in the blood and accumulates in calcifying tissues, which include the bone, the teeth, and the pineal gland. It can inhibit the function of a variety of enzymes in vitro ("in vitro" literally means "in glass" and is used to indicate an experiment performed outside the whole body). Also in vitro, in combination with traces of aluminum, fluoride can interfere with G proteins, used by many water-soluble messengers, such as hormones and growth factors, to deliver their messages to the inside of the cells of tissues they help regulate. Although more difficult to prove, it is reasonable to assume that many of the effects seen in vitro can occur in the whole body.

Fluoride Poisoning of Humans: Early Reversible Effects

Reports began to emerge soon after fluoridation of public water supplies began that some people appear to be very sensitive to fluoride, even at the supposedly low level of 1 ppm in water. Unfortunately, governments that support fluoridation have never bothered to investigate this issue in a scientific manner. In 2008, Dr. Bruce Spittle published a book, *Fluoride Fatigue*,[1] that goes into the issue of individual sensitivity to fluoride and covers many of the findings discussed in this chapter.

Dr. George Waldbott and Sensitivity to Fluoride

Dr. George Waldbott earned his medical degree at the University of Heidelberg in 1921 and emigrated to the United States shortly afterward. As a physician in clinical practice, he specialized in the treatment and study of allergic and respiratory diseases. He was the first doctor to demonstrate that some people are sensitive to penicillin and that tobacco causes lung damage. Beginning in the 1950s, he increasingly turned his attention to the adverse health effects of environmental pollutants, especially fluoride.[2] He continued that work until his death, in 1982.

H. T. Petraborg, a medical doctor practicing in the town of Aitkin, Minnesota, gave an example of Waldbott's work on sensitivity to fluoride:[3]

> In 1955 Waldbott described a case of progressive illness in a woman aged 35, characterized by weakness, severe headaches, pains in the epigastric area, diarrhea alternating with constipation, and hemorrhages of the uterus. A cardinal feature of the disease was a gradual loss of strength and increasing fatigue which led to complete disability. Waldbott attributed this disease to intolerance to fluoridated water. The patient improved promptly following elimination of fluoridated water. When the subject was given, unbeknown to herself, a test dose of fluoride the disease recurred. Subsequently, Waldbott (1956) reported a series of 52 similar cases.[4]

Later, other doctors, including Petraborg, repeated Waldbott's findings.[5, 6]

Spittle provides a long list of the symptoms that Waldbott identified and called chronic fluoride toxicity syndrome.[7] The symptoms involve various skin rashes, gastrointestinal symptoms, urinary problems, bone and joint pain, neurological symptoms (headaches, depression, etc.), and excessive tiredness not relieved by sleep.

Many of the symptoms that Waldbott reported are very common complaints and have many different causes. Some have suggested that Waldbott's patients were imagining these symptoms. That might explain some cases but certainly not all, because some patients had no prior knowledge of the issue of fluoride or water fluoridation. All that many people knew before they reported to Waldbott (and other doctors) was that they were experiencing problems, and neither they nor their doctors could explain the cause. No conventional treatment worked.

Some have pointed out that several of the symptoms described by Waldbott correspond to symptoms that appear or disappear when people are given placebos but think they are getting a particular drug—the so-called placebo effect. In *Continuing Evaluation of the Use of Fluorides*, Dr. Donald Taves cites D. M. Green[8] to explain the issue, as follows:

> A patient having gone from doctor to doctor and probably being labeled a "crock," who finds a sympathetic doctor who "knows" that fluoride is the source of his problems is going to try very hard to support his explanation. Expectation plays a very large role in what subjects experience when given placebos (such as capsules of sugar). Green reported a wide variety of symptoms (gastrointestinal, heartburn, drowsiness, blurred vision, dizziness, dry mouth, palpitation, urinary frequency and vomiting) among half of 50 professional people given placebos. The professionals, expecting that they might be getting an active drug, naturally worried about the side effects. Patients tended, on the other hand, to have a decrease in symptoms when given placebos.[9]

However, the most important and consistent finding by Waldbott and others is that these symptoms clear up within a few weeks if the source of fluoride is removed, and return when exposure recurs (often without the patient's knowledge). Where possible, Waldbott and others (e.g., Grimbergen[10]) conducted double-blind trials to demonstrate the phenomenon.

Some commentators have wondered how one substance could cause so many problems. However, since fluoride interferes with many biochemical processes (see chapter 12), we should not be surprised to see a wide range of symptoms. We should also remember that there is some indication that fluoride interferes with thyroid function, and we know that those suffering from hypothyroidism also have many symptoms that overlap with the symptoms in Waldbott's list (see chapter 16).

Moreover, many of these symptoms have also been observed in situations where people have received high doses of fluoride. We discuss some of these below. Thus, this looks like a sensitive response to a toxic substance rather than an allergic reaction mediated by the immune system (although skin reactions are somewhat reminiscent of contact allergy to nickel and other substances). Waldbott himself said, "By far the majority of my cases had no bearing on allergy (hives, asthma, allergic nasal and sinus disease and so on). They pertained to intolerance to fluoride that is true poisoning."[11]

Extreme sensitivity to any toxic substance should be expected in a small fraction of people. In any human population there is a very wide response to a toxic substance. We can expect that a small percentage will be very resistant to a particular substance, a small percentage will be very sensitive, and most of the population will be somewhere in the middle.

In 1997, Shulman and Wells analyzed reports obtained from the American Association of Poison Control Centers of suspected over-ingestion of fluoride by young children (less than six years of age). This poisoning arose from the consumption of home-use dental products, like fluoridated toothpaste. The authors made the following comment:

> Parents or caregivers may not notice the symptoms associated with mild fluoride toxicity or may attribute them to colic or gastroenteritis, particularly if they did not see the child ingest fluoride. Similarly, because of the nonspecific nature of mild to moderate symptoms, a physician's differential diagnosis is unlikely to include fluoride toxicity without a history of fluoride ingestion.[12]

These comments were made in the context of poisoning by relatively large amounts of fluoride (e.g., 50 mg in one case). If it is difficult for parents and doctors to recognize the cause of these problems at such high doses, it underlines how much more difficult it is for doctors to recognize the cause of poisoning that may accrue from very much smaller doses of fluoride among people who are particularly sensitive to fluoride.

Feltman 1956, Feltman and Kosel 1961

In the late 1940s Dr. Reuben Feltman, a researcher at the Passaic Hospital in New Jersey, started a study at his own expense to investigate the effects on pregnant women and young children of ingesting sodium fluoride tablets.[13] In 1950 he received funding from the U.S. Public Health Service (PHS) to continue the study. In the study the dose administered was 1 mg, which corresponds to 1 liter of fluoridated water at 1 ppm. The study was designed to last ten years, but when early results showed that patients were experiencing side effects, the PHS stopped funding the study. When James Rorty, the editor of Exner and Waldbott's book *The American Fluoridation Experiment*, asked about this termination in 1956, Dr. John Knutson, dental director for the PHS, stated that Feltman's "original research application proposed 'to determine the efficacy (in preventing caries) of the addition of measured doses of fluoride salts to pregnant women and children up to and through the age of eight years,'" and Knutson claimed that none of Dr. Feltman's progress reports mentioned "any ill-effects to the persons taking the fluoride pills." Knutson added, "In point of fact, there are no data based on careful scientific research to indicate that waterborne fluoride ingestion at the levels used for dental decay control has any ill effects."[14]

In 1961, Feltman, joined by a second researcher from Passaic General Hospital, George Kosel, published a final report on this work, in which they stated the following:

> One percent of our cases reacted adversely to the fluoride (1 mg/day tablets). By the use of placebos, it was definitely established that the fluoride and not the binder was the causative agent. These reactions, occurring in gravid women and in children of all ages in the study group affected the dermatologic, gastro-intestinal and neurological systems. Eczema, atopic dermatitis, urticaria, epigastric distress, emesis and headache have all occurred with the use of fluoride and disappeared upon the use of placebo tablets, only to recur when the fluoride tablet was, unknowingly to the patient, given again. When adverse reactions occur, the therapy can be readily discontinued and the patient or parent advised of the fact that sensitivity exists and the element is to be avoided as much as possible.[15]

Waldbott's Struggle to Be Heard

Waldbott summarized his work in *Fluoridation: The Great Dilemma,* a book coauthored by Albert Burgstahler and Lewis McKinney.[16] Unlike his other work, which brought him considerable fame among allergists around the world, Waldbott's work on fluoride was largely ridiculed by those who resented his opposition to fluoridation. He documented the struggle he had with the promoters of fluoridation in *A Struggle with Titans.*[17]

Moderate- to High-Dose Responses to Fluoride

Evidence that the symptoms described by Waldbott and others are real for highly sensitive persons is that they mimic the symptoms that occur at much higher doses for people who are not extremely sensitive.

In the next sections we discuss some of the skin problems, gastrointestinal symptoms, bone and joint pain, and neurological symptoms that have been described in the studies of people with moderate to high exposure to fluoride, which mirror the symptoms found by Waldbott at much lower levels.

Skin Problems

There have been many reports of skin problems (rashes, ulcers, pimples, etc., in the area of the mouth) associated with the use of fluoridated toothpaste.[18–23] As early as 1957, Thomas Douglas, MD, of Seattle, Washington, described the lesions caused by fluoridated toothpaste in 133 patients he had treated. He described the lesions as follows: "shallow superficially ulcerated areas which tend to have a whitish exudate on the surface and surrounding areas. The worst lesions and, indeed, the earliest lesions, commenced on . . . those areas which come into contact with the teeth. The tongue, hard palate, soft palate, floor of the mouth, gingival regions and oral pharynx also produced similar ulcerations." Of the 133 patients who had the lesions, 94 had gums that bled easily and 99 complained of soreness.[24]

Muscle, Joint, and Bone Pain

Sodium fluoride (as a source for fluoride) has been used in the treatment of patients with osteoporosis in an effort to increase bone mineral density and reduce fractures (see chapter 17). However, a number of side effects, including rheumatic pain, have been reported. Riggs et al. reported the following:

> Twenty-three of the fluoride-treated patients (dose = 18–27mg/day) had adverse reactions (38 per cent), which caused five of them to

discontinue therapy; 13 had rheumatic symptoms (joint pain and swelling or painful plantar fascial syndrome), nine had gastrointestinal symptoms (severe nausea and vomiting, peptic ulcer, or blood-loss anemia), and one had both rheumatic and gastrointestinal symptoms.[25]

It is also well established that the earliest symptoms of skeletal fluorosis are almost identical to the symptoms of arthritis. Here are just a few of the many reports:

> The onset was insidious, and stiffness of the back and legs was a universal complaint. Almost all the patients complained of vague fleeting pains all over the body, particularly in the spine and in the knee-joints.[26]

> The onset of chronic fluorosis is insidious and may be confused with chronic debilitating diseases such as osteoarthritis, trace-element toxicosis, and trace-element deficiencies.[27]

> In the initial stages, the complaints of the patients are not remarkable. At first they experience vague rheumatic pains, then the pains become localized in the spine.[28]

Neurological and Behavioral Problems

Headaches have also been reported as one of the early symptoms of skeletal fluorosis. For example, in a 1994 article on skeletal fluorosis in the *American Journal of Roentgenology*, Wang et al. reported, "The initial symptoms usually were headache and weakness."[29]

Waldbott wrote that as early as 1974 Russian physicians (Popov et al.[30]) had reported neurological symptoms among patients suffering from occupational fluorosis. He also noted that Polish researchers (Czechowicz, Osada, and Slesak[31]) had observed effects on brain tissue in high-dose experiments with guinea pigs. These observations prompted Waldbott to suggest, "If such a direct action of fluoride upon nerve tissue should be confirmed by further studies, it would explain some of the diverse neurological complaints in arms and legs, such as numbness, muscle spasms and pains, and the frequent headaches . . . that I and others have encountered in the early stage of fluoride poisoning before bone changes occur."[32]

To date over eighty animal and biochemical studies have indicated that fluoride damages the brain and changes behavior; twenty-three studies have indicated that fluoride at moderate doses is associated with lowered IQ; and two studies have shown behavioral changes that were associated with fluoride exposure in both children and adults (see chapter 15).

Gastrointestinal Symptoms

The excerpts in the following paragraphs illustrate numerous examples of gastrointestinal problems reported in cases where people have had moderate to high exposure to fluoride. We begin with a statement from the U.S. Environmental Protection Agency (EPA) pertaining to poisoning by fluorides in pesticides: "Ingested fluoride is transformed in the stomach to hydrofluoric acid, which has a corrosive effect on the epithelial lining of the gastrointestinal tract. Thirst, abdominal pain, vomiting, and diarrhea are usual symptoms. Hemorrhage in the gastric mucosa, ulceration, erosions, and edema are common signs."[33]

Swallowing fluoridated toothpaste.

Shulman and Wells, mentioned above, discuss parents' confusion of the symptoms associated with mild fluoride toxicity with those of "colic or gastroenteritis" when fluoridated toothpaste and other fluoridated dental products are swallowed by young children.[34]

Swallowing fluoride gels.

C.-J. Spak and his Swedish coworkers, in an investigation of the impacts of swallowing fluoride gels, demonstrated that fluoride could damage the stomach lining. They described their findings as follows: "The histopathological evaluation revealed changes in nine of ten patients, with the surface epithelium as the most affected component of the mucosa. The present study clearly shows that a treatment with a F gel of rather low F concentration may result in injuries to the gastric mucosa."[35]

Treatment of osteoporosis.

As mentioned, sodium fluoride has been used in the treatment of patients suffering with osteoporosis; this is in an effort to increase their bone mineral density and thereby reduce fractures (see chapter 17). The side effects described by those running the clinical trials studying the use of sodium fluoride to treat patients with osteoporosis included gastrointestinal damage. There are many reports; here are two:

Results from several large trials indicate that significant side effects attributable to treatment occur in about one-third to one-half of patients. Symptoms have been of two types—periarticular and gastrointestinal . . . Gastrointestinal symptoms consist of epigastric pain, nausea, vomiting, and occasionally, blood-loss anemia; these presumably result from the irritant effect of fluoride ion on gastric mucosa . . . Diarrhea occurs occasionally.[36]

Of 48 patients who began sodium fluoride therapy (dose = 9.0–27 mg/day F), 25 developed significant side-effects (10 with nausea and dyspepsia, 1 with gastrointestinal hemorrhage).[37]

Skeletal fluorosis cases in India.
Gastric problems have also been reported in studies of citizens suffering from skeletal fluorosis in areas of India with high natural levels of fluoride in the water. The following symptoms have been reported among the inhabitants consuming water with high fluoride content: "loss of appetite, nausea, abdominal pain, flatulence, constipation and intermittent diarrhoea . . . When water with negligible amounts of fluoride (safe water) is provided, the complaints disappear within a fortnight."[38]

Dr. A. K. Susheela, executive director of the Fluorosis Research and Rural Development Foundation in Delhi, India, has moved from a general description of these gastric problems to more detailed microscopic observations. In 1996, she and her colleagues reported abnormalities of the gastric mucosa in patients with outright skeletal fluorosis (osteofluorosis). They described their study as follows:

A prospective case-controlled study was performed to evaluate the gastrointestinal symptoms and mucosal abnormalities occurring in patients with osteofluorosis. Ten patients with documented osteofluorosis and ten age- and sex-matched healthy volunteers were included in the study . . . Electron microscopic abnormalities were observed in all 10 patients with osteofluorosis. These included loss of microvilli [small hairlike structures that protrude from the lining of the GI tract and facilitate the uptake of minerals and other nutrients into the blood], cracked-clay appearance, and the presence of surface abrasions on the mucosal cells. None of the control subjects had any clinical symptoms or mucosal abnormalities. It was concluded that gastrointestinal symptoms as well as mucosal abnormalities are common in patients with osteofluorosis.[39]

Dismissing Fluoride Sensitivity

In 1971, the PHS, presumably fearing that Waldbott's reports on sensitivity were threatening the fluoridation program, asked the American Academy of Allergy (AAA) to investigate the matter. Without interviewing Waldbott or any of his patients, the AAA's eleven-member executive board declared "unequivocally and unanimously" that "there is no evidence of allergy or intolerance to fluorides as used in the fluoridation of the community water supplies."[40]

However, Waldbott pointed out the following:

1. None of the board members had carried out any research into fluoride for themselves.
2. In the references, they cited Waldbott's *A Struggle with Titans*,[41] which was intended for a lay audience, and thus these board members ignored most of his published case studies.
3. The request for this statement came from the PHS, which clearly had a vested interest in the outcome.
4. At about the time the statement was released the PHS announced research grants to four of the eleven board members amounting to nearly $800,000, a huge amount of money in 1971.
5. Most of the other members of the board had previously received funding from the PHS for their work on allergies.[42]

Despite the apparent ignorance and bias in the AAA disclosed by Waldbott's criticisms, and the evidence of Waldbott's own work, this 1971 statement by the AAA has been cited again and again by fluoridation government agencies and review panels to dismiss the issue, sometimes with little further analysis. The AAA statement has been used in this way by the British Royal College of Physicians,[43] the Inquiry into the Fluoridation of Victorian Water Supplies,[44] the Australian National Health and Medical Research Council,[45, 46] the World Health Organization,[47] the U.S. Department of Health and Human Services,[48] the New Zealand Public Health Commission,[49] and the U.S. National Research Council.[50] Using this statement to negate bona fide research publications without careful scientific analysis is an evasion of responsibility.

Any criticisms of Waldbott's methodologies could have been easily resolved scientifically if the governments promoting fluoridation had been prepared to put some resources into the matter. However, they chose to resolve the issue politically, by using the authority of an expert body in the same way that they had used endorsements in the promotion of the program. The result is that health agencies in fluoridated countries have never attempted to perform systematic studies, even when it has been recommended that they do so by several independent observers.[51, 52]

Michael Prival, PhD, writing on behalf of the Center for Science in the Public Interest, made the following suggestion in 1972:

> It is important to realize that Waldbott's work constitutes a central medical core of the American anti-fluoridation movement . . . Rather than simply denying the validity of his reports, it would be to the advantage of all concerned to have them thoroughly analyzed. This could best be done if a small number of unbiased, qualified physicians, agreed upon by both "sides," would independently examine and diagnose several of the patients who are reportedly allergic to fluoride. Only when this is done will there be any possibility of resolving the long-standing controversy surrounding this issue.[53]

In 1979 Donald Taves stated, "Most of the above counter arguments [to Waldbott's findings] are based on passive observations; so while it seems unlikely to most scientists that fluoride is causing adverse effects at 1 ppm F, active study is desirable." Taves went on to recommend a study design that would take into account the criticisms leveled at Waldbott and others.[54] No such government-sponsored study has been attempted in the years since Taves's suggestions were made.

In 1991, the National Health and Medical Research Council (NHMRC), the Australian government's own research body, also recommended that the matter be put to rest with well-designed studies. The authors wrote:

> It is desirable to explore in a rigorous fashion whether the vague constellation of symptoms which are claimed to result from ingestion of fluoridated water can be shown to be reproducibly developed in these "susceptible" individuals. These claims are being made with sufficient frequency to justify well-designed studies which can properly control for subject and observer bias.[55]

Not one health agency in Australia, in the nineteen years (as of 2010) since this recommendation was made, has attempted any formal study on the matter. This, despite the fact that citizens have offered to be tested in this way.[56]

Fluoride Allergy

A very small number of people appear to be exquisitely sensitive to fluoride and have an apparent allergic reaction to it, which in some cases can be acute, even life-threatening.[57] Although a true allergy to fluoride, in the sense of an action of the immune system, initially postulated by Waldbott in some of his early cases, has generally been considered improbable, there is some experimental evidence that a response to fluoride might *mimic* a true allergy. In association with calcium, fluoride can trigger the release of histamine, a major effector substance in many allergic reactions, from mast cells in vitro.[58, 59] However, the concentrations of fluoride used in these experiments were higher than would normally be found in human plasma.

Summary

A small minority of people, perhaps 1 percent, appear to be acutely sensitive to exposure to fluoride at the concentrations present in fluoridated water. The wide range of signs and symptoms resemble those seen in poisoning with larger amounts of fluoride. These findings date from the 1950s. However, far from leading to more extensive studies, they were ridiculed when introduced and have since been largely ignored. Also, an "authoritative" statement by the board of the American Academy of Allergy has been used repeatedly for almost forty years to dismiss the issue. It is long past time that governments that promote fluoridation investigated this matter in a rigorous scientific manner, as recommended by a number of independent observers.

The 2006 National
Research Council Report

Many of the reviews of fluoride's toxicity and the risks of water fluoridation sponsored by pro-fluoridation governments have amounted to little more than self-fulfilling support for water fluoridation (see chapter 24). This support has usually been accomplished by the selection of a panel of known fluoridation promoters and/or government employees. The review by the NRC in 2006 was refreshingly different.[1]

In 2002, the Office of Drinking Water of the U.S. Environmental Protection Agency (EPA) commissioned the NRC to review the safe drinking water standards for fluoride. It did this for two reasons: (1) Such reviews are required every ten years, and (2) new scientific evidence suggested that fluoride could cause more damage than the single end point of *crippling* skeletal fluorosis that the EPA had used to determine the MCLG (maximum contaminant level goal) for fluoride in 1986.[2]

The last NRC review had been undertaken in 1993.[3] In that review, a largely pro-fluoridation panel of authors confirmed the safety of the 4 ppm MCLG but recommended that new studies should be undertaken.

In 2003, the NRC appointed a panel to undertake the review requested by the EPA. The twelve-member scientific panel was the most balanced ever appointed in the United States to do any kind of review on fluoride. It included some scientists opposed to fluoridation, others who actively promoted the practice, and still others who had never taken a position on the matter. However, the brief to the panel was to examine not the benefits of fluoridation, but the toxicology of fluoride. In fact, the name of the NRC study from its inception was *Toxicologic Risk of Fluoride in Drinking Water (BEST-K-02–05-A)* until it was published in March 2006, at which time it was changed to *Fluoride in Drinking Water: A Scientific Review of EPA's Standards*.

The task of the NRC panel was described in its report as follows:

> The committee was charged to review toxicologic, epidemio-logic, and clinical data on fluoride—particularly data published since the NRC's previous (1993) report—and exposure data on orally ingested fluoride from drinking water and other sources.

On the basis of its review, the committee was asked to evaluate independently the scientific basis of EPA's MCLG of 4 mg/L and SMCL (secondary maximum contaminant level—a concentration intended to avoid cosmetic damage) of 2 mg/L in drinking water, and the adequacy of those guidelines to protect children and others from adverse health effects. The committee was asked to consider the relative contribution of various fluoride sources (e.g., drinking water, food, dental-hygiene products) to total exposure. The committee was also asked to identify data gaps and to make recommendations for future research relevant to setting the MCLG and SMCL for fluoride. *Addressing questions of artificial fluoridation, economics, risk-benefit assessment, and water-treatment technology was not part of the committee's charge* [emphasis added].[4]

Promoters of fluoridation have claimed that the panelists looked only at studies involving exposure to fluoride at 2–4 ppm.[5–8] However, it is important to stress that no restrictions were placed on what levels of fluoride were used in the studies reviewed by the panel. In fact, the panel examined several studies that found adverse effects at levels less than 2 ppm.[9–14]

On August 12, 2003, Paul Connett was invited to give a forty-five-minute presentation to the panel. He was the only scientist known to be opposed to fluoridation who was given this formal opportunity to present his views and evidence in person.[15] The panel heard from Dr. Connett immediately after hearing from Dr. William Maas, who, at the time, was the director of the Oral Health Division at the CDC. We are happy to say that most of the concerns Dr. Connett expressed were eventually addressed in the NRC's review.

The review, which occupied the panel intensively for more than two years, was finally published in March 2006; it ran to 507 pages, including over 1,100 references.

Unlike those of the York Review[16] and the NHMRC,[17] the NRC panel members did not restrict themselves to epidemiological studies but availed themselves of all the science that might throw some light on fluoride's toxic potential. That included biochemical studies, animal studies, modeling calculations, clinical trials, and human epidemiological studies. That allowed a "weight-of-evidence" approach to assess potential harm.

The panel's exposure analysis in chapter 2 of its report indicated that certain subsets of the population consuming water fluoridated at 1 ppm were already exceeding the EPA's reference dose of 0.06 mg/kg/day (listed in the EPA's

Integrated Risk Information System[18]). These population subsets included bottle-fed infants (receiving formula reconstituted with fluoridated water); those with borderline iodine deficiency; those with impaired kidney function; and those who drank excessive amounts of water, including outdoor laborers, athletes, military personnel, and diabetics. The panel concluded that the 4 ppm standard for fluoride was not protective of health and recommended that the EPA's Office of Drinking Water perform a new health risk assessment to determine a new MCLG.

While not discounting any of the other health concerns revealed in the eleven chapters of the report, the authors singled out three clinical conditions that they believed triggered the need for a new health risk assessment:

1. Clinical stage II skeletal fluorosis: "The committee judges that stage II is also an adverse health effect, as it is associated with chronic joint pain, arthritic symptoms, slight calcification of ligaments, and osteosclerosis of cancellous [porous] bones."[19]
2. Bone fractures: "The majority of the committee concluded that the MCLG is not likely to be protective against bone fractures."[20]
3. Severe dental fluorosis: "After reviewing the collective evidence, including studies conducted since the early 1990s, the committee concluded unanimously that the present MCLG of 4 mg/L for fluoride should be lowered. Exposure at the MCLG clearly puts children at risk of developing severe enamel fluorosis."[21]

The Difference between the MCLG and MCL

The MCLG (maximum contaminant level goal) is the level of fluoride deemed safe by the U.S. EPA, based on the best science available and the application of appropriate safety factors, to protect all members of society, including vulnerable subgroups, from known, *and reasonably anticipated*, bad health effects. The MCLG is not an enforceable standard but a goal.

The MCL (maximum contaminant level) for drinking water is an enforceable federal standard. This is set by the EPA as close to the MCLG as economic considerations will allow. For example, as mentioned previously, the MCLG for arsenic is set at zero, because it is a known human carcinogen, but the MCL for arsenic is set at 10 ppb (parts per billion) because of the costs of removal of naturally occurring arsenic. Currently, both the MCLG and the MCL for fluoride are set at 4 ppm.

As of July 2010, it had been four years since the NRC recommended that the EPA produce a new MCLG, but the EPA's Office of Drinking Water has yet to produce a new health risk assessment, hence no new MCLG or MCL. Meanwhile, a former risk assessment expert at the EPA has reviewed the NRC report and concluded that if normal regulatory and toxicological procedures were followed, a new MCLG would have to be set at 0 ppm.[22] If that were to be the conclusion of the EPA, it would force an end to water fluoridation.

ADA and CDC Responses

If the EPA's response has been tardy, the response of both the American Dental Association (ADA) and the Oral Health Division at the CDC was very rapid. On the day the NRC report was released, the ADA declared that it was irrelevant to water fluoridation, erroneously claiming that the NRC panel concerned itself only with water containing 4 ppm, which the ADA said was "much higher" than the levels used in fluoridation programs (0.7–1.2 ppm).[23]

It took the CDC six days to announce the same conclusion. On March 28, 2006, the Oral Health Division of the CDC declared on its Web page, "The findings of the NRC report are consistent with CDC's assessment that water is safe and healthy at the levels used for water fluoridation (0.7–1.2 mg/L)."[24] As of July 2010 this statement still appeared on the CDC Web page.

The CDC produced no comprehensive analysis to support its claim. It is hard to believe that in six days Oral Health Division personnel could have read and digested the report, let alone its over 1,100 references. They certainly did not have time to perform a health risk assessment to determine a new MCLG to see how it would compare with the level at which communities now fluoridate their water.

It is important to put the role of the CDC in this matter in perspective. As we explained in chapter 4, there is only one division at the CDC involved with fluoridation, the Oral Health Division (OHD). This division is largely staffed with personnel with dental qualifications but very few with qualifications in general or specialized medicine. Nor do any appear to have qualifications in toxicology or risk assessment. There appears to be no individual scientist (or group of scientists), let alone a division, at the CDC with the responsibility to oversee the safety of water fluoridation. This is all left to the OHD, which has a clear conflict of interest in this matter, because it actively promotes water fluoridation.

While it is clear that political factors (i.e., doing whatever is necessary to support a long-standing policy) appear to be influencing both the ADA's and

the CDC's positions on the relevance of the NRC report to water fluoridation, it is important to stress the *scientific* flaws in their respective claims that
somehow fluoride is bad at 4 ppm but okay at 1 ppm, because the same argument is being made by several other pro-fluoridation government agencies,
spokespersons, and consultants.[25–27] We will examine the case of Bazian Ltd.

Bazian's Critique

As part of its consultation process for the proposal to fluoridate Southampton
and surrounding communities, the UK South Central Strategic Health
Authority (SHA) held three public meetings in October and November
2008. At those meetings Paul Connett and others drew attention to the NRC
report. In response, the SHA hired the consulting company Bazian Ltd. to
review the report.

Bazian's only substantive point was that the NRC panel was considering
higher concentrations of fluoride than those used for fluoridation: "The maximum levels of water-borne fluoride for cosmetic or health safety recommended
by the EPA, and examined in the book [the NRC report], are two to four times
higher than the level of water fluoridation proposed for Southampton and
higher than the 1.5ppm maximum level laid down by the European Union."[28]

Using this as a reason, SHA dismissed the NRC report without referring
to a single page, let alone a single one of the studies referenced. The following statement appeared in the final SHA report, authored by Professor John
Newton, endorsing fluoridation for Southampton: "The SHA commissioned
the . . . specialist expert organization (Bazian) to undertake a critical appraisal
of the National Research Council report. Their conclusion was that the report
is not relevant to the proposed scheme because it considers much higher levels
of fluoride (4ppm) than those envisaged in Southampton (1ppm)."[29]

Bazian's actual wording in its summary was as follows: "The question it [the
report] examines does not have *direct* relevance to the issue of fluoridation in
Southampton" [emphasis added].[30] In other words, Bazian did not deny the
obvious fact that the NRC data were relevant but found a way to imply that
the relevance was "indirect," whatever difference that may make. Although
Bazian's words were quoted in the SHA paper, the word "direct" was omitted
in Professor Newton's text. For whatever reason, Newton felt free to ignore the
NRC report when recommending fluoridation in Southampton—an action
that many may deem incautious or even reckless.

It is difficult to know just what Bazian meant to imply with the word
"direct" and what the firm's representatives would have said if asked to

explain what "indirect" evidence the NRC review had provided. Had they been challenged, they might have been forced to acknowledge the crucial difference between *concentration* and *dose* that we discuss in chapter 1 (someone drinking 2 liters of water with a *concentration* of 1 ppm would get the same *dose* of fluoride as someone drinking 1 liter of water at 2 ppm). They might have admitted that what was needed here was an analysis that would establish that there was an adequate margin of safety sufficient to protect *everyone* in the Southampton area from the adverse health effects documented in the NRC review (see chapter 20). Such an exercise would have required consideration of the *doses* at which these effects were observed, and the expected range of dose experienced by a population whose consumption of water and of fluoride obtained from other sources was uncontrolled. It would have also required choosing an adequate safety margin to account for the range of sensitivity to any toxic substance expected across a large population (see chapters 1, 13, and 20). Establishing safety under these vital requirements would have been difficult to do, especially since in chapter 2 of the NRC review, the panel established that certain subsets of the American population are exceeding the EPA's IRIS reference dose of 0.06 mg/kg/day[31] while drinking fluoridated water at 1 ppm, including infants who are fed formula made with tap water.

Here are just two of several other pieces of *indirect* evidence that needed consideration. The NRC reviewed studies that indicated an association between a tripling of hip fractures in elderly people drinking water at 4.3 ppm, and a possible doubling at 1.5 ppm, in a relatively small study population[32] (see chapter 17). It is difficult to see how Bazian or the SHA could justify exposing a much larger population to fluoride at 1 ppm over a lifetime, especially since that population would include some people with impaired kidney function. Similar considerations apply to the association between altered thyroid function and people drinking water with fluoride at 2.3 ppm.[33] Such considerations are discussed further in chapter 20.

Kathleen Thiessen, PhD, an NRC panel member, responded to the claim that the NRC report is not relevant to public water fluoridation in the course of two statements,[34, 35] of which excerpts follow:

> *Scope of the NRC report.* The National Research Council's committee on fluoride in drinking water was asked to review the adequacy of EPA's Maximum Contaminant Level Goal (MCLG) of 4 mg/L fluoride in drinking water and the corresponding Secondary

Maximum Contaminant Level (SMCL) of 2 mg/L. The committee concluded that those regulatory limits are not protective of public health. The committee was not asked to review the safety of so-called "optimal" concentrations of fluoride in drinking water (0.7–1.2 mg/L, as used in deliberate fluoridation of public drinking water supplies), although much of the report is relevant to such a review (discussed further below). In addition, the committee was not asked to review the efficacy or reported benefits of fluoridation, on the basis of which community water fluoridation was instituted. The committee also did not review in any detail either the history or the politics of water fluoridation.

Relevance of the NRC report to water fluoridation. Although the NRC report did not examine the safety, efficacy, or benefits of water fluoridation, or specifically evaluate the toxic effects of "optimal" levels of water fluoride on humans, the committee did examine a number of issues that are relevant to such evaluations. In particular, the committee did an extremely thorough review of fluoride intake in the U.S., by age group, considering all sources of fluoride intake (water, dentifrices, food, air, soil, pesticides, pharmaceuticals), including fluoridated drinking water. In addition, the committee looked specifically at population subgroups of special concern, for example, due to very high water consumption or to impaired fluoride excretion. A number of the toxicity studies that the committee reviewed involved fluoridated water or exposures equivalent to those expected with fluoridated water . . .

Hazards of fluoride exposure. The NRC report concluded that the existing MCLG of 4 mg/L is not protective of human health. This conclusion was based largely on health effects that have long been considered specific to fluoride and significant enough to warrant protection, namely dental fluorosis and skeletal fluorosis. The NRC's review differed from previous reviews of fluoride by saying that severe dental fluorosis is an adverse health effect (not merely a cosmetic effect), that stage II as well as stage III skeletal fluorosis is an adverse health effect, and that a fluoride concentration of 4 mg/L is likely not protective with respect to an increased risk of bone fracture. The NRC report indicated that at 2 or 4 mg/L, bone fluoride concentrations can reach the ranges historically associated with stage II and III skeletal fluorosis. The committee was not able to rule out a carcinogenic effect of fluoride or of "water fluoridation" (i.e., due to some substance added along with an impure fluoridating agent). Nor was the committee able to rule out the possibility that fluoridation is associated with an increased risk of Down syndrome in children of young mothers. The committee also reported that fluoride exposure is plausibly associated with a number of other health effects, including neurotoxicity, gastrointestinal problems, and endocrine problems, and that even though these effects are not necessarily specific to fluoride exposure, the associations cannot be ruled out and need further study.

With respect to dental fluorosis, skeletal fluorosis, and risk of bone fracture, the NRC committee considered primarily studies in which populations were exposed to concentrations of fluoride in drinking water of around 4 mg/L; from those studies the committee concluded that 4 mg/L is not protective of those effects. The committee did not, for any endpoint, determine a "no-effect level," an individual intake level (mg per day of fluoride intake per kg body weight) below which no adverse health effects occur. However, the ranges of intake levels, or estimated average intake levels, associated with a number of adverse effects, are in the range of intakes expected with fluoridated drinking water in the U.S. Fluoride exposures in the U.S. are driven largely by consumption of drinking water and beverages made with tap water. Water intake for a given age group varies substantially— around a factor of 100 between the highest and lowest consumption rates (discussed in the NRC report). The result of this is that for water fluoride at 1 mg/L vs. water fluoride at 4 mg/L, there will be a huge overlap between the respective populations, with apparent differences only at the very highest water intakes. In other words, any effect seen at 4 mg/L is probably going to occur in some people at 1 mg/L (e.g., in the people with highest water consumption or in people with impaired fluoride excretion), but this might easily be missed in the sample sizes typically used in studies.[36]

Carcinogenicity. Chapter 10 of the NRC report also reviewed human and animal studies of carcinogenicity, in addition to genotoxicity studies, although the NRC's review did not include a number of the older studies . . . The committee unanimously concluded that "Fluoride appears to have the potential to initiate or promote cancers," even though the overall evidence is "mixed." Referring to the animal studies, the committee also said that "the nature of uncertainties in the existing data could also be viewed as supporting a greater precaution regarding the potential risk to humans." The committee also discussed the limitations of epidemiologic studies, especially ecologic studies (those in which group, rather than individual, measures of exposure and outcome are used), in detecting small increases in risk—in other words, the studies are not sensitive enough to identify small increases in cancer risk; therefore a "negative" study does not necessarily mean that there is no risk . . .

While the NRC committee did not assign fluoride to a specific category of carcinogenicity (i.e., known, probable, or possible), the committee did not consider either "insufficient information" or "clearly not carcinogenic" to be applicable. The committee report includes a discussion of how EPA establishes drinking water standards for known, probable, or possible carcinogens; such a discussion would not have been relevant had the committee not considered fluoride to be carcinogenic. The question becomes one of how strongly carcinogenic fluoride is, and under what circumstances. As mentioned, fluoride may be a cancer promoter rather than an initiator, although the two mechanisms are not mutually exclusive.[37]

Basis for establishing fluoride concentrations in local drinking water supplies. Historically, the local temperature (the "annual average of maximum daily air temperatures" over a minimum of 5 years) has been used as the basis for recommending a given level of fluoride in the drinking water (e.g., CDC 1995). In practice (reviewed by the NRC), there seems to be little difference in water consumption for many people with temperature, season, or location. Obviously, for people with high levels of activity, water consumption can be very high. At present, basketball players or gymnasts, for example, will probably have similar rates of water consumption no matter which state they live in; however, under current guidelines, some of them will have water with 0.7 mg/L fluoride, while others will have water with 1.2 mg/L. Also, most states do not appear to account for temperature variations within a state, such that the water fluoridation levels are the same for the colder and hotter parts of the same state.

Concerns about silicofluorides. A number of issues have been raised concerning the use of silicofluorides as the fluoridating agent in most public water supplies (discussed briefly in the NRC report). These include increased lead in children's blood, increased leaching of lead into water from plumbing fixtures, and the addition of other substances to the drinking water along with the silicofluorides. For instance, the MCLGs for arsenic and lead are 0, based on health risks; however, the actual level permitted (the Maximum Contaminant Level, or MCL) is above 0 (to account for difficulty in removing it or in measuring it). However, in the addition of the impure silicofluorides to drinking water, some arsenic and lead are generally added as well, although the resulting concentration must stay below the MCL. Given that the MCLGs are 0, the obvious question is whether knowingly adding any amount, however tiny, is appropriate.[38]

Summary

The 2006 National Research Council report was the first U.S. report to look at low-level fluoride toxicity in a balanced way. The reporting panel's task was to determine whether the maximum contaminant level goal for drinking water, currently 4 ppm, was appropriate for protecting health. The report concluded that the MCLG was too high and should be reduced. The report is clearly relevant to fluoridation since, if 4 ppm is too high (by an unspecified amount) to be acceptable as a contaminant, it cannot be sensible to deliberately add 1 ppm. That implies a safety margin of less than four times, possibly much less—absurdly small by normal toxicological standards. Despite this, the major promoters of fluoridation hastened to state that the report was irrelevant to fluoridation and could be completely disregarded, on the spurious grounds that it dealt only with exposure to fluoride at more than 2 ppm. Acceptance of such a tiny margin of safety indicates a cavalier disregard for public health. The report identified three main concerns—stage II skeletal fluorosis, bone fractures, and severe dental fluorosis—but also drew attention to other potential health hazards especially to the endocrine system and the developing brain.

In the following chapters we review the impacts of fluoride on various tissues of concern and buttress our comments with citations from the NRC review, the most comprehensive text on fluoride's toxicology available to date. However, several important health studies have been published or translated into English since the NRC report was published in 2006, and they add further weight to the NRC findings. These studies include many more research papers on fluoride's impact on the brain (chapter 15) as well as Bassin et al.'s important paper on osteosarcoma[39] (chapter 18).

Fluoride and the Brain

Nowhere do the dangers of exposing a whole population to uncontrolled doses of a toxic substance become more apparent than in the possibility that they may damage brain function. It has been documented time and again that very small amounts of some chemical substances can cause subtle yet significant changes in a child's mental development and behavior. Once a small chemical change occurs over a wide and varied population, there may be unintended and unfortunate consequences, not only for the individual but for the entire population. Such changes might not be recognized until the damage becomes irreversible or irreparable. This appears to have happened in the case of the impact of airborne lead on children's IQ in the United States, when lead was present in gasoline. It doesn't take a very large downwind shift in IQ in the whole population to have a dramatic effect in decreasing the number of intellectually gifted children and increasing the number of mentally handicapped.

The story of fluoride's possible interaction with the brain began independently on at least three continents:

- The use of uranium hexafluoride to separate uranium isotopes exposed atomic bomb workers to large amounts of fluoride. In the 1940s, the late Harold Hodge, working as chief toxicologist for the Manhattan Project, asked the head of the medical section, Colonel Stafford Warren, for funding to do an animal experiment to investigate the possible impact of fluoride on the brain.[1] However, the results of such an experiment would not emerge until almost fifty years later.
- In the late 1980s, Dr. Phyllis Mullenix, a toxicologist, developed a novel technique for exploring the possible changes to animal behavior that a chemical might cause. When she was hired by Forsyth Dental Center in Boston and asked to use that technique to analyze the neurotoxicity of the chemicals used in dentistry, she had little idea of how much trouble her discoveries would provoke in her life and career.
- When, in 1994, the New Zealand doctor Bruce J. Spittle, who specialized in psychiatric medicine, published a review speculating on the potential for fluoride to damage the brain, he probably had little idea how his work would become part of the findings that would ultimately

challenge the practice in which his dental colleagues so firmly believed.[2] Spittle taught at Otago University, which housed the only dental school in the country.

- In the late 1980s, Chinese researchers found that children had lower IQs in villages in areas with high natural levels of fluoride in the water. Those researchers also probably had little notion of how their work— when it was eventually translated into English—might threaten the whole edifice of artificial water fluoridation.

Gradually, over the last twenty years or so, these strands have come together.

Hodge and Mullenix

In the late 1980s, many years after his animal experiment was turned down, Harold Hodge joined the staff of the Forsyth Dental Center and quietly watched Phyllis Mullenix as she found what he may have privately suspected to be the case. Fluoride did indeed alter animal behavior, but Hodge died before this finding was published and ruined Mullenix's career.

Chris Bryson, in his book *The Fluoride Deception*,[3] gives the sordid details of the treatment meted out to Mullenix when her 1995 paper[4] was accepted for publication. At the time, she was chairperson of the first toxicology department established in a dental school in the United States. Nevertheless, she was told that her work "was no longer relevant to dentistry,"[5] and she was fired. Contrary to previous assertions,[6] her paper showed that fluoride did accumulate in rat brains, and that the animals dosed before birth showed movement patterns associated with hyperactivity (i.e., were overactive) and the animals exposed after birth showed hypoactive patterns (i.e., were underactive).

Spittle

In the summer of 1994, a year before Mullenix's paper was published, Spittle's article "Psychopharmacology of Fluoride: A Review" appeared. In it, Spittle concluded that "chronic exposure to fluoride may be associated with cerebral impairment affecting particularly concentration and memory." While he admitted that the evidence was suggestive rather than conclusive, he listed several possible mechanisms whereby fluoride could affect brain functioning, including "influencing calcium currents, altering enzyme configurations, inhibiting adenyl cyclase activity and increasing phosphoinositide hydrolysis."[7]

When Spittle wrote his article, he was unaware of the Chinese studies (discussed next) but he had read Waldbott and colleagues' book *Fluoridation:*

The Great Dilemma[8] and was aware of their reports of cognitive impairment from those who were hypersensitive to fluoride (see chapter 13).

Chinese Studies

One year after the publication of Spittle's paper and shortly after Mullenix's paper appeared, the first articles from China on lowered IQ appeared in the journal *Fluoride*.[9, 10] There have now been twenty-three studies from four different countries (Iran, India, Mexico, and China) demonstrating a possible association between fluoride exposure and lowered IQ in children; these are listed in appendix 1. Five of the Chinese studies have yet to be translated into English.

After Mullenix

There have now been over eighty animal studies confirming what Mullenix et al. reported in the published paper that got her fired.[11] These studies demonstrate that fluoride does accumulate in animal brains, causing damage in areas of the brain involved with memory and learning, and that fluoride can alter behavior. (All of the animal studies are listed in chronological order in appendix 1, including those that are identified individually below.)

Prior to Mullenix's work, published in 1995, it was generally assumed that little fluoride entered or accumulated in the brain.[12] However, several researchers have now shown that fluoride can accumulate in the brain, some even specifying the areas of the brain where the fluoride is located.[13–19]

In a critique of Mullenix's work that was sent to an engineer at the CDC's Oral Health Division but not to Mullenix herself, Dr. Gary Whitford intimates that the fluoride levels in the water she gave to the rats were high and suggested that they were sufficient to cause behavioral problems by indirect means.[20] Mullenix responded to that claim by pointing out that the levels she used were not high because one must use about twelve times more fluoride in water to reach the same plasma levels in rats as one would get with humans. Specifically, to achieve the same range of plasma levels, rats must drink water with 75–125 ppm fluoride, while humans require 5–10 ppm fluoride.[21] In a very recent publication, Sawan et al. stated that a fluoride level of 100 ppm in water fed to rats was necessary to reach the same plasma level as humans drinking water at 8 ppm—this again is a ratio of about 12 to 1.[22]

Guan and colleagues have consistently found neurotoxic effects among rats drinking water with 30 ppm fluoride, which according to Mullenix and Sawan would be equivalent to humans drinking water with fluoride at 2.5 ppm.[23–25]

Several papers have shown that fluoride is concentrated in, or has an effect upon, the hippocampus.[26–38] Damage to the hippocampus usually results in difficulties in forming new memories and recalling events that occurred prior to the damage.

Varner et al. 1998

Julie A. Varner's study was a continuation of the work of Robert Isaacson at the State University of New York at Binghamton.[39] In the Varner study, rats were fed for one year with 1 ppm fluoride in their water (which was doubly distilled and de-ionized), using either sodium fluoride or aluminum fluoride. In the rats treated with either fluoride compound, the authors discovered the following:

- Morphological changes in the kidney and the brain
- An increased uptake of aluminum into the brain
- The formation of beta-amyloid deposits usually associated with Alzheimer's disease[40]

These findings prompted both the Environmental Protection Agency (EPA) and the National Institute of Environmental Health Sciences (NIEHS) to recommend the study of aluminum fluoride as a possible neurotoxin.

The National Research Council

In 2006, the National Research Council became the first government-appointed review body to examine the literature on fluoride's impact on the brain in any depth. In chapter 7 of its report, the panel reviewed both animal and human studies.[41] The NRC panel had this to say about the studies on the brain:

> On the basis of information largely derived from histological, chemical, and molecular studies, it is apparent that fluorides have the ability to interfere with the functions of the brain and the body by direct and indirect means . . .
>
> Fluorides also increase the production of free radicals in the brain through several different biological pathways. These changes have a bearing on the possibility that fluorides act to increase the risk of developing Alzheimer's disease.[42]

The NRC panel recommended "additional animal studies designed to evaluate reasoning."[43]

The NRC panel also recommended that studies of populations "exposed to different concentrations of fluoride" be undertaken to "evaluate neurochemical changes that may be associated with dementia," adding that "consideration should be given to assessing effects from chronic exposure, effects that might be delayed or occur late-in-life, and individual susceptibility."[44]

In 2006, the NRC panel had access to five of the twenty-three IQ studies that have been published to date and concluded:

> A few epidemiologic studies of Chinese populations have reported IQ deficits in children exposed to fluoride at 2.5 to 4 mg/L in drinking water. Although the studies lacked sufficient detail for the committee to fully assess their quality and relevance to U.S. populations, the consistency of the results appears significant enough to warrant additional research on the effects of fluoride on intelligence.[45]

The NRC panel recommended that future research "should include measurements of reasoning ability, problem solving, IQ, and short- and long-term memory."[46]

More on the IQ Studies

Contrary to fluoride proponents' claims that an association between fluoride and lowered IQ has been demonstrated only at high fluoride levels, one of the IQ studies, which the NRC authors considered to have the "strongest study design," indicated that IQ in children could be lowered by exposure to concentrations as low as 1.9 ppm.[47, 48] In the abstract of the first of two articles on that study, Xiang indicated that, from a regulatory point of view, it was significant that IQ could be affected at any level above 1 ppm. Another Chinese study indicated that even lower levels of fluoride exposure (e.g., 0.9 ppm in the water) could exacerbate the neurological effects of iodine deficiency.[49]

In a trip to China in 2006, Paul Connett was able to visit the two villages that were the focus of the Xiang study. He noted that from an epidemiological point of view, the villages appeared to present an ideal model for comparison. In both, the population was highly stable, most families having lived in the same area for many generations. Occupations, housing, diet, and education were the same. Xiang et al. controlled for both lead exposure[50] and iodine intake,[51] two factors that could also cause lowered IQ. The obvious difference was the level of fluoride in the well water used by the two villages. The well water in one village contained fluoride at levels between 2.5 and 4.5 ppm; the fluoride in the well water of the other village was less than 0.7 ppm. Across the age range of the children examined, the study showed an IQ difference between the two villages of between five to ten IQ points. There was also a clear shift in the IQ distribution curve, with more children in the mentally handicapped and fewer in the very bright category in the high-fluoride village. Howard Pollick has criticized some of the methodological aspects of the study, in a series of published exchanges of views on fluoridation with Paul Connett.[52–56] However, far more disturbing than any weakness in this study (or the other twenty-two IQ studies) is the fact that no fluoridating country (except for one small study in New Zealand[57]) has attempted to replicate this research.

Other Human Studies of Fluoride's Impact on the Brain

In addition to the studies that have shown a possible link between fluoride exposure and lowered IQ in children, there have been other studies from China adding to the weight of evidence of fluoride's ability to damage the human brain.

Three different Chinese research groups have shown that fluoride has damaged the brains of aborted fetuses in areas endemic for fluorosis.[58–60] For example, Du et al. examined the brains of fifteen aborted fetuses at five to eight months gestation from an area with endemic fluorosis and compared them with fetuses from an area where fluorosis was not endemic. Fetal brains from the endemic area revealed a significant reduction in the density of mito chondria (the parts of the cell that produce energy) and a reduction in the mean volume of neurons (brain cells).[61]

Other human studies, using a batch of standard psychological tests, have revealed behavioral differences in adults exposed to high industrial levels of fluoride[62] and behavioral differences in neonates in endemic fluorosis areas.[63]

Pro-Fluoridation Governments

Despite the cumulative evidence emerging in Western scientific literature in the mid-1990s that fluoride could damage the brain,[64–68] there has been prac-tically no research into the issue in fluoridated countries. In 2002, the UK Medical Research Council (MRC) even put a higher priority on more studies of dental fluorosis than on any investigation of fluoride's potential to affect neurodevelopment.[69]

Almost no studies have been undertaken in any fluoridated country to explore a possible relationship between fluoride exposure and lowered IQ. In the United States one small behavioral study found no apparent relationship between childhood behavior and the severity of dental fluorosis.[70] In New

Zealand one small study compared eight- and nine-year-old children who had lived up to seven years in a fluoridated community (1 ppm) or a non-fluoridated community (0.1 ppm). The authors reported no significant difference in IQ between the two communities.[71] These studies seem to represent the sum total of interest in this issue among countries practicing fluoridation.

Other Scientists' Concern

While fluoridation promoters continue to ignore—or dismiss—the studies of fluoride's impact on both animal and human brains, some scientists are taking the issue more seriously. In May 2000, Greater Boston Physicians for Social Responsibility published a report titled *In Harm's Way: Toxic Threats to Child Development*.[72] The authors included a discussion of fluoride's potential to damage the brain. After briefly reviewing two animal studies[73, 74] and two IQ studies,[75, 76] they concluded:

> Studies in animals and human populations suggest that fluoride exposure, at levels that are experienced by a significant proportion of the population whose drinking water is fluoridated, may have adverse impacts on the developing brain. Though no final conclusions may be reached from available data, the findings are provocative and of significant public health concern. Perhaps most surprising is the relative sparseness of data addressing the central question of whether or not this chemical, which is intentionally added to drinking water, may interfere with normal brain development and function. Focused research should address this important matter urgently.[77]

In 2006, Philippe Grandjean and Philip Landrigan identified fluoride as a possible neurotoxicant in an article titled "Developmental Neurotoxicity of Industrial Chemicals," published in *Lancet*. In a section titled "Emerging Neurotoxic Substances," they wrote, "Three obvious candidate substances deserve particular attention, including two that have not seemed to cause neurotoxicity in adults." Fluoride was one of those candidate substances.[78]

As discussed in chapter 3, the use of silicofluorides as water fluoridating agents has been associated with a greater uptake of lead into children's blood.[79, 80] This association received some strong biological support from an animal study by Sawan et al. published in 2010.[81] The authors found that exposure of rats to a combination of fluoride and lead in their drinking water increased the uptake of lead into blood some threefold over exposure to lead alone. There is no argument that lead causes serious mental developmental problems for children; thus, should fluoride increase the uptake of lead into the blood, as these epidemiological and animal studies suggest it may, fluoride could enhance the brain damage caused by lead exposure.

Dismissal of the IQ Studies at Southampton

At the three public meetings organized by the UK's South Central Strategic Health Authority (SHA) in Southampton in October and November 2008, mentioned earlier, Paul Connett drew attention to the IQ studies from China, India, Iran, and Mexico and provided copies of eighteen of the studies that are available in English to the SHA. This matter, too, was referred to the consultants Bazian Ltd. (see chapter 14).

By criticizing the methods used in some of the studies and claiming that the fluoride concentrations involved were generally higher than those planned for Southampton, Bazian felt able to conclude that "from these studies alone, it is *uncertain* how far fluoride is responsible for any impairment in intellectual development seen. The amount of naturally occurring fluoride in drinking water and from other sources and the socioeconomic characteristics in the areas studied is different from the UK and so these studies do not have *direct* application to the local population of Southampton"[82] [emphasis added].

These conclusions are highly equivocal and fall far short of giving fluoride a clean bill of health, emphasizing uncertainty and dismissing the studies' "direct" relevance to Southampton on relatively trivial pretexts. Anyone reading the details of Bazian's report can see that there is indeed serious cause for concern. Had Bazian done a margin-of-safety analysis (described in chapter 20), as is normal in toxicological evaluations, the high relevance of the IQ data to any fluoridation program would have been even clearer. Which brings us once again to the issue of the crucial difference between *dose* and *concentration*. A child drinking 2 liters of water at 1.0 ppm would get a higher dose of fluoride (dose = 2 mg) than a child drinking 1 liter of water at 1.9 ppm (dose = 1.9 mg), a level at which damage was estimated to occur by Xiang et al.[83]

However, Southampton SHA either failed to notice Bazian's implied reservations or chose to disregard them, stating baldly, "Their advice was that the studies are unreliable and do not constitute convincing evidence of harm."[84] On this basis, the SHA ignored the IQ studies entirely when recommending fluoridation for Southampton.

One wonders how convincing the evidence has to be. Here we have a proposal to mass-medicate 100,000 or more people. On the one hand, there is a putative modest benefit to the dental health of young children (which could be achieved by other means; see chapters 6–8). On the other hand, there are about twenty studies (albeit with questioned methodologies in some cases) suggesting potential damage to the brains of young children at levels quite close to the concentration of 1 ppm to be used in Southampton. That medication does not sound like a very good deal; it is hard to believe that many parents would choose it for their own children. The SHA's attitude is in fact a particularly glaring example of an irresponsible mind-set that seems to be common among fluoridation proponents: that it is okay to fluoridate the public water supply until incontrovertible proof is provided that it does some devastating harm. This attitude is all the more indefensible since fluoridating countries show more interest in belittling what evidence there is than in carrying out any investigations themselves.

Summary

In this chapter we have summarized the animal and human studies that show associations of fluoride with damages to the brain. Animal studies have indicated that fluoride can enter the brain and that the accumulation is dose-dependent. Animal studies have also shown biochemical changes and damage that can be viewed microscopically. Many of these studies have been carried out at relatively high doses, but one remarkable study by Varner et al. showed effects at a low level of exposure—1 ppm in rats' drinking water over one year of exposure. At this level a greater uptake of aluminum into the brain was observed, as well as beta-amyloid deposits such as have been associated with Alzheimer's disease. There have also been twenty-three studies indicating a lowered IQ in children associated with levels as low as 1.9 ppm of fluoride in drinking water. We do not claim that these IQ studies add up to conclusive evidence that water fluoridation impairs cognitive development. However, when you have twenty or more reports consistently suggesting a problem, and these have been backed up by studies indicating possible brain damage in aborted fetuses in areas endemic for fluorosis in China, as well as animal data indicating brain damage and abnormal behavior, and very little to set in the balance against them, it is wise to sit up and pay attention. The health authorities and governments of fluoridating countries show little sign of doing that. We return to this failure to pursue important health studies in chapter 22. Meanwhile, we have to ask whether the saving of any amount of tooth decay, which we believe is slight at best (see chapters 6–8), could possibly justify taking the risk of interfering with the development of a child's brain.

Fluoride and the Endocrine System

We saw in chapter 9 that prior to the start of the fluoridation program there was considerable interest in the possibility that fluoride interfered with the thyroid gland. However, the U.S. Public Health Service (PHS) paid little attention to those concerns before endorsing fluoridation in 1950. Most recent government reviews have given the matter short shrift.[1-5]

The Endocrine System

The endocrine system consists of a number of glands (e.g., thyroid, parathyroid, adrenal) that secrete hormones into the bloodstream. Hormones are responsible for regulating the chemistry of the cells in different tissues. The hormones (e.g., thyroxin, adrenaline, estrogen, testosterone, insulin) are usually secreted at precise times and circulate in the bloodstream until they reach the tissues they regulate.

Hormones can be subdivided into fat-soluble and water-soluble groups. Solubility in fat or water makes a huge difference to the way hormones interact with the cells in the target tissues. If the hormone is fat soluble, it can cross the cell membrane (which is made up largely of fats) and enter the cell. There it will find a receptor (usually a protein) with a site on its surface, into which the hormone will fit into like a hand fitting into a glove. When the hormone fits into the protein, the protein becomes "activated," meaning it is ready to start the first step in a sequence that will ultimately change the activity of the cells in the tissue. In this way, the tissue is regulated; processes inside the cells of the tissue are switched on or off, or existing processes may simply be speeded up or slowed down.

If the hormone is water soluble, it will not be able to cross the cell membrane, so the receptor protein has to be located on the *outside* surface of the membrane. In this case, once the hormone has attached to the receptor, a process is triggered by which the hormone's *message* (not the *messenger*) is carried across the membrane. The *message* triggers the production of a second messenger inside the cell that changes cellular activity, and hence the activity of the tissue involved.

A simple example may help clarify this. Most people are familiar with the adrenaline-induced "fight or flight" response. Here is how it works: When something frightens us, the adrenal glands release adrenaline into our bloodstream. This circulates in the blood until it finds the muscles. Being water soluble, it cannot cross the membranes of the cells that make up the muscles, so it finds the receptor molecule on the outside of the membranes. The message is transmitted across the membranes by the G-protein message system (described in chapter 12), producing a second messenger (cyclic AMP) inside the cell. This second messenger then activates a sequence of enzymes, which act as catalysts to break down sugar molecules more quickly—thereby releasing a lot of energy into the muscle cells so we are better equipped to fight or run away.

This is what the NRC report of 2006 had to say about fluoride's interaction with the endocrine system:

> In summary, evidence of several types indicates that fluoride affects normal endocrine function or response; the effects of the fluoride-induced changes vary in degree and kind in different individuals. Fluoride is therefore an endocrine disruptor in the broad sense of altering normal endocrine function or response, although probably not in the sense of mimicking a normal hormone. The mechanisms of action remain to be worked out and appear to include both direct and indirect mechanisms, for example, direct stimulation or inhibition of hormone secretion by interference with second messenger function, indirect stimulation or inhibition of hormone secretion by effects on things such as calcium balance, and inhibition of peripheral enzymes that are necessary for activation of the normal hormone.[6]

Fluoride and the Thyroid Gland

The thyroid gland produces two major hormones called T3 and T4, which contain three and four iodine atoms, respectively. Another hormone, the thyroid-stimulating hormone (TSH), is produced in the pituitary gland, and it regulates the production of the hormones by the thyroid gland (see the discussion below). This is a simplified picture, but it will suffice for our purposes.

The literature dealing with the interaction between fluoride and the thyroid gland has a long history stretching back to a paper written in 1854 by Maumené, who linked goiter in dogs with exposure to fluoride.[7] The group Parents of Fluoride Poisoned Children (PFPC) provides an extensive summary of that history on its Web site.[8]

There are four lines of evidence that fluoride interferes with the thyroid gland:

1. *Fluoride-induced goiter.* The condition known as goiter (also spelled "goitre"), which involves a gross swelling of the thyroid gland, in turn producing very marked swellings in the neck, is known to be induced by iodine deficiency. Significantly, the condition has also been found by some studies to occur in areas where there are adequate supplies of iodine but an excess of fluoride in the water.[9-15] Other studies have failed to find that relationship.[16]

2. *Treatment of hyperthyroid patients.* Between the 1920s and the 1950s, some doctors in Argentina and Europe treated patients suffering from hyperthyroidism with sodium fluoride.[17-23] The treatment was successful in many but not all cases. Doses as low as 0.9–4.2 mg fluoride per day were enough to reduce the basal metabolic rate (BMR) of hyperthyroid patients and alleviate their condition.[24] This corresponds to the range of fluoride ingested by many people living in fluoridated areas. The U.S. Department of Health and Human Services estimated that an adult in a fluoridated community ingests between 1.6 and 6.6 mg of fluoride a day from all sources combined.[25]

This raises an obvious question: If fluoride calms an overactive thyroid, what might it do to a normal or underactive one? Little information has been available until recently. However, a study conducted by Bachinskii et al. in the Ukraine found that prolonged consumption of water with 2.3 ppm fluoride produced changes in normal thyroid function. The authors described this as "a tension of function of the pituitary-thyroid system that was expressed in TSH [thyroid-stimulating hormone] elevated production, a decrease in the T3 concentration and more intense absorption of radioactive iodine by the thyroid as compared to healthy persons who consumed drinking water with the normal fluorine concentration" and went on to say, "The results led to a conclusion that excess of fluorine in drinking water was a risk factor of more rapid development of thyroid pathology."[26]

These responses were mirrored in a study by Mikhailets et al.[27] In that case, the authors examined the thyroid function of 165 workers in an aluminum plant. They detected thyroid abnormalities that were "characterized by a moderate reduction of iodine-absorbing function of the thyroid, low T3 with normal T4 level, and a slight increase of TSH concentration." The authors noted that these changes became more pronounced the longer the workers were exposed to these working conditions. They concluded, "The syndrome of low T3 and reduced absorption of I[131][iodine isotope 131] may be considered as diagnostic signs of fluorosis."[28] We examine the possible mechanisms whereby fluoride may exert its influence in "Possible Mechanisms of Action" below.

3. *Low iodide and brain development.* It has long been known that one of the consequences of iodine deficiency in mothers is an increased risk of developmental disabilities in their children. With the introduction of iodized salt, this is now a less frequent occurrence in industrialized countries, but the problem has not been eliminated completely. In the United States declines in iodine intake have recently been recorded, and in Australia (a fluoridating country), outright iodine deficiency is still a serious problem.[29, 30]

It is well established that the pituitary-thyroid system is important in the early mental development of children. Thus, if fluoride interfered with the thyroid, it could, among other things, result in lowered IQ in children. In this respect, the results of a UNICEF-sponsored study of "the relationship of a low-iodine and high-fluoride environment to sub-clinical cretinism" in China is particularly revealing. In the Xinjiang region of China Lin et al. found that even a modest amount of fluoride in the water (i.e., 0.88 ppm versus 0.34 ppm) led to a greater reduction in IQ and increased frequency of hypothyroidism (elevated TSH levels with normal T4 and T3 levels) than simply low iodide by itself. IQ and TSH were negatively correlated (as TSH goes up, IQ goes down).[31]

4. *The thyroid-stimulating hormone.* In conjunction with aluminum, fluoride may mimic the action of thyroid-stimulating hormone. See "Possible Mechanisms of Action" below.

NRC Report and Fluoride-Thyroid Connection

Fluoride could impact several areas of human health through the mediation of the thyroid. It is unjustifiable that almost no relevant research has been carried out in fluoridating countries. In contrast to most of the other governmental reviews of fluoride's toxicity, the 2006 NRC panel did express concern about fluoride's potential to disrupt the endocrine system in general, and about a possible fluoride-thyroid interaction in particular.[32] The authors of the report stated, "Several lines of information indicate an effect of fluoride exposure on thyroid function"[33] In terms of specific effects and the dosages at which they occur, they wrote:

> Fluoride exposure in humans is associated with elevated TSH concentrations, increased goiter prevalence, and altered T4 and T3 concentrations; similar effects on T4 and T3 are reported in experimental animals . . . In humans, effects on thyroid function were associated with fluoride exposures of 0.05–0.13 mg/kg/day when iodine intake was adequate and 0.01–0.03 mg/kg/day when iodine intake was inadequate.[34]

Such dosages are extremely low; a child would reach them by drinking one or two glasses of water fluoridated at 1 ppm.

Regarding the situation in the United States, the NRC authors showed particular concern about the impact of fluoride on people suffering from iodine deficiency or borderline iodine deficiency: "The recent decline in iodine intake in the United States could contribute to increased toxicity of fluoride for some individuals."[35–37]

In an article published in the January 2008 issue of *Scientific American*, Dan Fagin wrote the following about the 2006 NRC panel:

> The NRC committee concluded that fluoride can subtly alter endocrine function, especially in the thyroid—the gland that produces hormones regulating growth and metabolism . . . Says John Doull, professor emeritus of pharmacology and toxicology at the University of Kansas Medical Center, who chaired the NRC committee: "The thyroid changes do worry me. There are some things there that need to be explored."[38]

Possible Mechanisms of Action

There are at least two plausible mechanisms, supported by some evidence, by which fluoride may influence the activity of the thyroid and its hormones.

Inhibition of Deiodinase

Deiodinase enzymes play an important role in the functioning of the thyroid system. The thyroid hormones thyroxin (T4) and triiodothyronine (T3) contain four and three iodine atoms, respectively. Most of the molecules secreted by the thyroid are T4. A deiodinase is responsible for removing one of the iodines from T4 to form the much more active but shorter-lived T3. T3 in turn is eventually deactivated by another deiodinase. Since T3 stimulates the body's metabolic rate, its activity needs to be constantly monitored and regulated; otherwise, signs and symptoms of hyper- or hypothyroidism will appear. Deiodinases perform that function, probably at two levels: (1) in the body generally, by directly controlling the concentration of T3 in the blood and tissues (particularly the liver); and (2) by indirectly controlling the output of T4 from the thyroid.

This second control mechanism is more complicated. Briefly, thyroid activity is controlled by another hormone, thyroid-stimulating hormone (TSH), which is produced by the anterior pituitary gland in response to a signal from a part of the brain called the hypothalamus. T3 exercises negative feedback, down-regulating the production of TSH by the pituitary. It appears that deiodination of T4 to T3 within the pituitary plays an important part in that process.[39] Although there is no direct evidence that fluoride can inactivate deiodinases, it is well known as an inhibitor of many enzymes, and the hormonal derangements reported in fluoride-exposed people have been interpreted in terms of effects on deiodinases.[40, 41] According to that interpretation, there are at least three levels at which fluoride could plausibly upset regulation of the thyroid system:

1. Conversion of T4 to T3 in tissues and blood,
2. Local conversion of T4 to T3 in the pituitary gland, resulting in inappropriate continued production of TSH, and
3. Inactivation of T3.

Interpretation of events in the thyroid is further complicated by the existence of other "minor" hormones structurally related to T3 and T4 and by the varied activities and functions of the three deiodinases in different tissues.[42] Interference with deiodinases also affects the availability of free iodide, which may affect not only the brain (see chapter 15) but other tissues as well.[43]

Fluoride Mimicking TSH

As suggested in the preceding section, a possible mechanism exists whereby fluoride could bring about an excessive production of TSH from the pituitary. This may help explain why elevated TSH levels have been reported in cases of hypothyroidism with lowered T3 in aluminum workers occupationally exposed to fluoride.[44] But fluoride may itself mimic the action of TSH. TSH is water soluble and sends its message across the membrane of the thyroid via G proteins. Fluoride has a well-established ability, in the presence of a trace amount of aluminum, to switch on G proteins (see chapter 12).

Thus, a mechanism of fluoride's action here might be an activation of the G-protein messaging system, leading to excess production of the secondary messenger inside the cell (cyclic AMP). Excess production of this secondary messenger may in turn lead to desensitization of the TSH receptor, thereby reducing the stimulus by otherwise normal levels of TSH. Some evidence of this was found in a study of Chinese hamster ovary cells by Tezelman et al.[45]

We emphasize that proof that fluoride acts on the thyroid in these ways in vivo is still lacking. Further research is needed, but, meanwhile, the mechanisms are plausible and based on existing science.

Proponents' Claims

Proponents of fluoridation claim that there is no "credible" evidence that fluoridation harms the thyroid. For example, early in 2006 the British Fluoridation Society (BFS) placed a statement to that effect on the front page of its Web site:

> The available medical and scientific evidence suggests an absence of an association between water fluoridation and thyroid disorders.
> Many major reviews of the relevant scientific literature around the world support this conclusion. Of particular importance are:
>
> - an exhaustive review conducted in 1976 by an expert scientific committee of the Royal College of Physicians [RCP] of England;
> - a systematic review in 2000 by the NHS Centre for Reviews and Dissemination at the University of York; and,
> - a 2002 review by an international group of experts for the International Programme on Chemical Safety (IPCS), under the joint sponsorship of the World Health Organisation (WHO), the United Nations Environment Programme (UNEP), and the International Labour Organisation (ILO).
> - none have found any credible evidence of an association between water fluoridation and any disorder of the thyroid.[46]

This statement remained on the BFS site as of March 2010, though less prominently displayed. It sounds quite impressive, the more so since it goes on to say that the York Review "identified over three thousand references in total" and the IPCS review "included 788 original studies."[47, 48] But somehow the BFS fails to mention that only a handful (none in the IPCS review) dealt with the thyroid, and that only four short paragraphs of the thirty-year-old RCP review were relevant.[49] In fact, they are talking about a classic case of "no look, no see," but cushioning it in verbiage designed to suggest that plenty of work has been performed and reviewed to reassure the reader that fluoridation is no threat to the thyroid system. Such tactics can be persuasive even to supposedly informed and perceptive people. The British Thyroid Association (BTA), no less, was moved to endorse the BFS statement—not merely the conclusion, but the whole misleading statement. Curiously, neither organization has significantly modified its stance since publication of the 2006 NRC review, which adduced some highly relevant evidence; however, in 2007 the BTA added a rider to its endorsement, implicitly admitting that there might be a significant risk, but merely recommended that thyroid status should be monitored in any new fluoridation program. This reluctance to acknowledge risk is perhaps understandable in the case of the BFS, which exists to promote fluoridation, but one might expect the BTA to exercise more caution on behalf of its own base.

The ADA adopts a quite different approach on its Web site but one equally economical with the truth. Its *Fluoride Facts* states, "There is no scientific basis that shows that fluoridated water has an adverse effect on the thyroid gland or its function"[50] and backs this up by describing a small and, by modern standards, simplistic study by Leone et al. (a questionable source; see chapter 10) that used only very basic parameters and was published forty-five years ago.[51]

Both the BFS and the ADA are careful to talk about *fluoridated water*, perhaps believing that that absolves them from paying attention to any data relating to naturally occurring fluoride—a somewhat legalistic approach.

Our Concerns

At present there is no direct and unassailable proof that fluoridation per se harms anyone's thyroid. This may be due to the paucity of studies conducted; the 2006 NRC panel identified several areas where more research is needed. Meanwhile, although the evidence is mixed, there are clearly grounds for caution. When one considers the millions of people affected by hypothyroidism (underactive thyroid) in fluoridated countries and the millions more probably suffering from subclinical (undiagnosed) hypothyroidism, the omissions in many government-sponsored reviews are unfathomable.

With public water fluoridation, we are forcing people to drink a possible thyroid-depressing medication that could cause higher levels of both subclinical and clinical hypothyroidism in the general population, with all the attendant problems such as depression, fatigue, weight gain, muscle and joint pain, increased cholesterol levels, and heart disease, as well as cognitive dysfunction and damage to the developing brain.[52] Significantly, in the United States in 1999, the second-most prescribed drug was levothyroxine (Synthroid), a hormone-replacement drug used to treat hypothyroidism.

The interaction between fluoride and thyroid function warrants far more attention from governments promoting fluoridation than it currently receives, which is practically nil. Millions of people worldwide are affected by thyroid dysfunction, and if the condition of only a small fraction of those people is caused or worsened by fluoride, it is a very serious matter indeed. With such uncertainties in the background, continuing to press on with mass medication is inappropriate.

Fluoride and the Pineal Gland

The pineal gland is located between the two hemispheres of the brain. Its most recognized function is production of the extremely important hormone melatonin. Situated outside the blood-brain barrier, the pineal gland has the highest blood flow per unit volume of any tissue except the kidney. It is also a calcifying tissue, laying down crystals of calcium hydroxyapatite, the mineral formed in teeth and bones.

From those known facts, Dr. Jennifer Luke, a dentist in the UK, hypothesized that, like teeth and bones, this little gland would concentrate fluoride. Her theory was confirmed when she had the pineal glands from eleven corpses of elderly people extracted and analyzed. The average level of fluoride found in the crystals in those glands was 9,000 ppm, one case reaching the extremely high level of 21,000 ppm. Significantly, 9,000 ppm approaches the level of fluoride found in the bones of someone suffering from skeletal fluorosis, and 21,000 ppm is even higher than the bone levels associated with the crippling phase of skeletal fluorosis. This finding was the subject of Luke's 1997 PhD thesis[53] and was published in an article in *Caries Research* in 2001.[54]

The Hormone Melatonin

Melatonin is produced in the pineal gland in a four-step process starting with the natural amino acid tryptophan. Melatonin acts as a biological clock in many timed events in human physiology and development, including jet lag, sleep patterns, and aging. The onset of puberty is another timed event that melatonin is thought to influence. It is at its highest level in young children and decreases as they get older. At a certain point, it is believed that the low level of melatonin triggers the production of sex hormones that leads to puberty.

In her PhD thesis (available at www.FluorideAlert.org), Dr. Jennifer Luke presented evidence that animals (Mongolian gerbils) exposed to high levels of fluoride had lowered melatonin levels and reached puberty earlier than gerbils exposed to lower levels of fluoride.[55]

Health agencies in several fluoridating countries have been given copies of Luke's work, yet none has financed or requested a study to reproduce her findings. By contrast, the 2006 NRC panel acknowledged the potential seriousness of her work:

> The single animal study of pineal function indicates that fluoride exposure results in altered melatonin production and altered timing of sexual maturity . . . Whether fluoride affects pineal function in humans remains to be demonstrated. The two studies of menarcheal age in humans show the possibility of earlier menarche in some individuals exposed to fluoride, but no definitive statement can be made. Recent information on the role of the pineal organ in humans suggests that any agent that affects pineal function could affect human health in a variety of ways, including effects on sexual maturation, calcium metabolism, parathyroid function, postmenopausal osteoporosis, cancer, and psychiatric disease.[56]

One of those "earlier menarche" studies was the Newburgh-Kingston study published by Schlesinger et al. in 1956 and discussed in chapter 10.[57] The authors of that study found that, on average, girls in fluoridated Newburgh reached menarche five months earlier than girls in unfluoridated Kingston. This finding was ignored at the time and is still ignored by those promoting fluoridation more than fifty years later.

Fluoride and Diabetes
The 2006 NRC review indicated that fluoride may affect diabetics in two ways:

> The conclusion from the available studies is that sufficient fluoride exposure appears to bring about increases in blood glucose

or impaired glucose tolerance in some individuals and to increase the severity of some types of diabetes. In general, impaired glucose metabolism appears to be associated with serum or plasma fluoride concentrations of about 0.1 mg/L or greater in both animals and humans. In addition, diabetic individuals will often have higher than normal water intake, and consequently, will have higher than normal fluoride intake for a given concentration of fluoride in drinking water. An estimated 16–20 million people in the U.S. have diabetes mellitus; therefore, any role of fluoride exposure in the development of impaired glucose metabolism or diabetes is potentially significant.[58]

Plasma fluoride concentrations of 0.1 mg/L are easily achieved by people drinking water fluoridated at 1 ppm. With so many people suffering from diabetes today, it is again astonishing how little work has been done to see whether fluoride exposure is worsening their condition. This underlines an important concern: When an entire population is exposed to a toxic substance, simply setting regulatory levels to protect the average person is not enough; those levels must be set to protect the most vulnerable citizens, such as people with diabetes and those susceptible to it.

Summary

The influence of fluoride on the human thyroid gland has a long history, going back to before the days of artificial fluoridation. Until recently, however, fluoridating countries have put virtually no effort into finding out whether drinking fluoridated water might adversely affect the functioning of that gland or other components of the endocrine system. The matter has been ignored or glossed over in officially sponsored reviews. This may well appear negligent, considering the prevalence of thyroid disorders in those countries. There is evidence that consumption of naturally occurring fluoride, even in amounts comparable to the amounts in artificially fluoridated water, can affect human thyroid function, particularly when iodine intake is inadequate. Meanwhile, in vitro experiments confirm that there is cause for concern. Such experiments suggest that fluoride may inhibit the deiodinase enzymes that fine-tune thyroid function; and, in combination with traces of aluminum, fluoride can inappropriately activate intracellular signals on which much hormone function depends, including production and action of thyroid-stimulating hormone. Does fluoridation threaten the thyroid and through it many aspects of human health? We don't know, but it certainly looks more than possible, and the question should be pursued urgently, not ignored.

The pineal, another endocrine gland, is located between the two hemispheres of the brain and is responsible for the synthesis and secretion of melatonin. Research published in 2001 showed that fluoride accumulates in the human pineal and can reach very high concentrations in old age. Whether this affects pineal function is unknown. However, preliminary animal experiments indicated that fluoride reduced melatonin production and shortened the time to menarche (Luke, 1997). Thirteen years have passed, apparently without any attempt to replicate those potentially important findings.

Fluoride at doses achievable by drinking fluoridated water may impair glucose tolerance in some individuals. In view of the increasing prevalence of diabetes, this is of concern, particularly since diabetics often drink more water than non-diabetics. This requires further research and, meanwhile, underlines the inadequacy of regulatory levels for fluoride that are set merely to protect the majority of people, not the most vulnerable.

Fluoride and Bone

It has been known for many years that about 50 percent of the daily intake of fluoride is absorbed by and accumulates in the bones.[1] In this chapter, we review the evidence that this accumulation damages the bones of both children and adults.

Bone Fractures in Children

One of the earliest trials of fluoridation (Newburgh, New York, versus Kingston, New York, 1945–1955) found approximately twice as many cortical bone defects in the fluoridated city, Newburgh, compared with Kingston, the unfluoridated city.[2, 3] The fact that the defects occurred in the cortical part of the bone is significant for the potential for fractures.

The bone is in two parts: the trabecular (or cancellous) and the cortical. The *trabecular* bone is the inside meshwork that gives the bone its load-bearing ability. (It gets its name from the Latin *trabs*, which refers to the structures that hold up the roofs of barns and churches built in medieval times.) Weakness in the trabecular bone can lead to increased rates of *compression fractures* of the spine in those suffering from osteoporosis.

The *cortical* bone is the outer sheath of bone, consisting of a layered structure (the lamellae). The cortical bone is critical for protection against breakage when the bone is exposed to a heavy blow or torsional stress.

It is surprising that the finding of a higher frequency of cortical bone defects in fluoridated Newburgh did not prompt a careful investigation of the rates of bone fractures in young children exposed to fluoridated water, either after the Newburgh study or in the fifty-plus years since. This neglect may be explained by McClure's claims, mentioned previously, that he found no extra bone fractures in boys and army recruits coming from communities with up to 4.2 ppm of fluoride in the water (see chapter 9).

While very few children's bone studies have been done in fluoridated countries, an interesting study was done in Mexico in 2001. Dr. M. Teresa Alarcón-Herrera et al. investigated bone fractures in people living in a high-fluoride area (1.5–5.5 ppm fluoride in water) and reported that as the severity of dental fluorosis increased, so did the incidence of bone fractures for both children and adults. Although the validity of the scoring methods used for fractures is

acknowledged by the authors to be questionable, this is a potentially important finding, because the severity of dental fluorosis can be used as a biomarker
of the extent of overexposure to fluoride before the permanent teeth have
erupted. Simply put: As fluoride exposure went up, so did the incidence of
bone fractures.[4]

Spokespersons for governmental agencies promoting fluoridation have
contented themselves with criticizing the methodology used in this study;
not one of these fluoridated countries has sought to repeat the study since its
publication in 2001, even though dental fluorosis affects over 30 percent of
children in the United States[5, 6] (see chapter 11). This is further evidence of
the very poor monitoring of the safety of the fluoridation program, an issue
that we summarize in chapter 22.

Fluoride and Arthritis

It has been known since the 1930s that ingesting too much fluoride can cause
stiff and painful joints. Some of the early symptoms of skeletal fluorosis—
a fluoride-induced bone and joint disease that affects millions of people in
India, China, and several other countries with high natural levels of fluoride—
mimic the symptoms of arthritis, making it easy to misdiagnose, especially by
doctors who are not trained in detecting fluorosis.[7–12]

The only stage of skeletal fluorosis recognized by the U.S. EPA in determining the safe drinking water standard for fluoride in 1986 was stage III,
the crippling phase. According to a review on fluoridation published in 1988
in *Chemical & Engineering News* by senior science editor Bette Hileman,
"Because some of the clinical symptoms mimic arthritis, the first two clinical
phases of skeletal fluorosis could be easily misdiagnosed."[13]

Few, if any, studies have been done to determine the extent of misdiagnosis,
or whether the high prevalence of arthritis in America (one in five American
adults has some form of arthritis[14]) is related to lifelong and ever-growing
exposure to fluoride.

According to *American Medical News*, researchers at the U.S. National
Arthritis Data Workgroup compiled data from various large national surveys
and found that "some 46.4 million people, or 21 percent of the population,
have physician-diagnosed arthritis. Of this group, 27 million have clinical osteoarthritis, and 1.3 million have rheumatoid arthritis." The number
appears to be rising and is predicted to reach 67 million by 2030.[15]

The failure to explore the plausible connection between fluoridation and
arthritis in any fluoridating country is difficult to understand. It is particularly

surprising since the causes of most forms of arthritis (e.g., osteoarthritis) are unknown but are usually associated with the aging process. For those living in fluoridated communities the aging process will coincide with lifelong accumulation of fluoride in their bones and joints.

In 2006, the NRC report discussed the four stages of skeletal fluorosis:

> Excessive intake of fluoride will manifest itself in a musculoskeletal disease with a high morbidity. This pathology has generally been termed skeletal fluorosis. Four stages of this affliction have been defined, including a preclinical stage and three clinical stages that characterize the severity. The preclinical stage and clinical stage I are composed of two grades of increased skeletal density as judged by radiography, neither of which presents with significant clinical symptoms. Clinical stage II is associated with chronic joint pain, arthritic symptoms, calcification of ligaments, and osteosclerosis of cancellous bones. Stage III has been termed "crippling" skeletal fluorosis because mobility is significantly affected as a result of excessive calcifications in joints, ligaments, and vertebral bodies. This stage may also be associated with muscle wasting and neurological deficits due to spinal cord compression. The current MCLG is based on induction of crippling skeletal fluorosis (50 Fed. Reg. 20164 [1985]). Because the symptoms associated with stage II skeletal fluorosis could affect mobility and are precursors to more serious mobility problems, the committee judges that stage II is more appropriately characterized as the first stage at which the condition is adverse to health. Thus, this stage of the affliction should also be considered in evaluating any proposed changes in drinking-water standards for fluoride.[16]

The panel recommended more research to fill the gaps in knowledge in this area. They specifically recommended the following:

> A systematic study of stage II and stage III skeletal fluorosis should be conducted to clarify the relationship of fluoride ingestion, fluoride concentration in bone, and clinical symptoms. Such a study might be particularly valuable in populations in which predicted bone concentrations are high enough to suggest a risk of stage II

skeletal fluorosis (e.g., areas with water concentrations of fluoride above 2 mg/L).

More research is needed on bone concentrations of fluoride in people with altered renal function, as well as other potentially sensitive populations (e.g., the elderly, postmenopausal women, people with altered acid-balance), to better understand the risks of musculoskeletal effects in these populations.[17]

In a 2003 review Paul Connett and Michael Connett could find only sixteen studies published between 1941 and 1994 in which bone fluoride levels were reported.[18] Worldwide a grand total of 1,397 bones were measured for fluoride in over fifty years. This, again, despite the fact that since at least the 1960s scientists have known that approximately 50 percent of the fluoride ingested each day accumulates in bones[19]—more in the bones of people with poor kidney function.

The problem with this "research gap" on fluoride and arthritis was underscored in 2007 by three studies, one from India and two from the United States.

Gupta et al. 2007

A thirty-five-year-old woman who regularly drank water with 1.9 ppm fluoride developed a subtle form of fluorosis that doctors initially suspected to be a form of seronegative arthritis. *Seronegative arthritis* refers to a form of arthritis that mimics the symptoms of rheumatoid arthritis (RA) but lacks the auto-antibodies diagnostic of RA. In this case study, the woman "presented with joint pain involving the lower back, both heels, and the knee for the past 3 years." In addition to the joint pains, the patient suffered from "gastrointestinal disturbance," prompting the doctors to suspect "the possibility of enteropathic arthritis." *Enteropathic arthritis* is a form of arthritis associated with inflammatory bowel diseases.

The doctors finally began to suspect the role of fluoride after X-rays revealed increased bone density in the pelvic area and calcification of some ligaments. Follow-up tests revealed elevated levels of fluoride in the patient's drinking water and slightly elevated levels of fluoride in the patient's blood (0.05 ppm).[20]

Hallanger Johnson et al. 2007

A study published by doctors at the Mayo Clinic suggested that similar cases of fluorosis may be occurring in the United States among habitual tea drinkers (tea leaves often contain high levels of fluoride), especially those with weak kidney function. In this study, the Mayo doctors detailed the cases of four patients who developed bone pains, and in some cases gastrointestinal problems, from drinking large amounts of tea. As with the Indian study, at least one of these patients had previously been misdiagnosed as having arthritis. One woman, who "developed chronic pain and stiffness in her lower back that progressed to include bilateral hip and knee pain," had been treated for seven years with various drugs "but with no improvement in symptoms."

It wasn't until the Mayo Clinic doctors identified fluorosis as the cause of her pain that the woman took steps to reduce her tea intake, which led, at last, to a diminution of symptoms. According to the Mayo doctors, "Fluoride toxicity can present in an insidious manner, and clinicians may overlook its signs and symptoms. Unless recognized and the source of excessive fluoride identified and discontinued, fluoride toxicity can be both progressive and crippling."[21]

Whyte et al. 2007

In a third study, doctors reported a similar scenario. A forty-nine-year-old woman (without kidney disease) developed skeletal fluorosis by drinking large volumes of instant tea made with fluoridated water. As with the above cases, the woman "developed widespread musculoskeletal pains" and was misdiagnosed for years as having fibromyalgia and osteoarthritis. The authors stated:

> We surmise that habitual consumption of 3 quarts daily of some regular-strength preparations for more than 10 years, especially if made with fluoridated water, could cause clinically significant skeletal fluorosis . . . This fluoride exposure seems possible for many individuals who like instant or bottled teas. In fact, when a 36-year old coworker learned of our index case, she confided drinking 3–4 qts daily of what she described as a triple strength preparation of Nestea dissolved in unfiltered, municipal tap water over the past year . . . With increasing use of DXA [bone density scans], additional instances of skeletal fluorosis from instant tea will likely be revealed.[22]

Fluoride and Hip Fracture

Hip fracture is a very serious issue for the elderly. About 300,000 Americans are hospitalized for a hip fracture every year. "In the UK, the mortality following a fractured neck of femur is between 20 percent and 35 percent within one year in patients aged 82 ± 7 years."[23] Many patients never regain an independent existence.[24, 25] Thus, if fluoridation were to increase the rates of hip fracture in the elderly, it would be serious and certainly grounds in itself to eliminate water fluoridation.

In our view, the best way to resolve the issue of whether fluoridation increases hip fractures in the elderly is to use a "weight-of-evidence" approach, which avails itself of all the evidence that can be brought to bear on this matter, including clinical trials, animal studies. and epidemiological studies. The 2006 NRC review used this approach, and the majority of the panel concluded that bones are not protected at the current safe drinking water standard of 4 ppm. Lowering the MCLG (maximum contaminant level goal) would reduce the risk of fractures, especially for those with poor kidney function and others who are prone to accumulate fluoride in their bones.[26]

Neither the York Review[27] nor the 2007 review by the NHMRC[28] used a weight-of-evidence approach. Instead, both used a meta-analysis of the very limited database of epidemiological studies that examined only fracture rates with fluoride concentrations close to 1 ppm, thereby missing the significance of the trend observed by Li et al. (see "Li et al. 2001" below).

One danger of limiting an assessment of this problem to epidemiological studies is that we are always looking at the past; by the time those studies show a definitive result, it is far too late to be of help to people who have already been exposed. The use of clinical trials and animal studies, as well as epidemiological studies, allows us a better opportunity to protect future generations— that is, before exposure has taken place. Another approach would be to apply the precautionary principle when reasonable warning signals are presented of a potential problem (see chapter 21). On fluoride's impact on bone, we have an abundance of warning signals, which are largely being ignored by fluoridating governments.

Clinical Trials

High doses of fluoride (26 mg per day on average) have been used in trials to treat patients with osteoporosis in an effort to strengthen their bones and reduce fracture rates. However, the results were disappointing; while the fluoride did increase bone mineral density, the treatment frequently led to a *higher* number of fractures, particularly hip fractures. Sources for eleven trials that found an increased incidence of hip fracture are given in appendix 2.

Simple arithmetic shows that the cumulative doses used in these trials (i.e., a high dose over a short period) are exceeded by the lifetime cumulative doses (i.e., a low dose over a long time) ingested by many people living in fluoridated communities.[29]

Animal Studies

Many animal studies have found that fluoride decreases the strength of bone in several species. References to twenty-two studies that show weakening of animal bone by fluoride can be found in appendix 2. The authors of some of these studies (Turner et al.) have reported thresholds for these effects ranging from 2,500 to 4,500 ppm in bone.

In nearly all of sixteen fluoridated communities examined between 1941 and 1994, one or more individuals had bone fluoride levels within that range.[30]

Epidemiological Studies

At least nineteen studies (three unpublished, including one abstract) since 1990 have examined the possible relationship of fluoride in water and hip fractures among the elderly. Eleven of these studies found an increased hip fracture rate; eight did not. Thus, to claim, as some proponents do, that there is *no* evidence that hip fractures are increased in fluoridated communities is inaccurate and misleading. A more accurate statement is that the evidence is *mixed.* An annotated list of references to all nineteen studies is given in appendix 2.

Li et al. 2001

Li et al. 2001 (one of the nineteen hip fracture studies) has been used by both proponents and opponents of fluoridation to support their respective cases. It is a particularly strong study, because it looked at hip fractures in six villages in China that had six different levels of fluoride in their well water, ranging from 0.25 ppm to 7.97 ppm. Other than this difference, the subject populations were similar and highly homogeneous and stable, sharing similar occupations, lifestyles, and diet, as well as being free of many other possible confounding variables, such as access to other sources of fluoride and use of hormone replacement therapy. The authors controlled for a number of other factors that could influence fracture frequencies including gender, smoking, and alcohol consumption.[31]

Li et al. recorded two sets of data: (1) all fractures combined and (2) hip fractures only.

All Fractures

When the prevalence of *all fractures* was plotted for the six villages, Li et al. found what they described as a U-shaped pattern: The lowest prevalence was found in village 3 (about 3 mg/day fluoride) and the highest in villages 1 (about 0.3 mg/day) and 6 (about 14 mg/day intake), the other villages being intermediate. The statistical confidence limits shown for these data are wide,

Table 17.1 All fractures (since the age of 20 years) in six Chinese villages with average fluoride intakes varying from 0.7 to 14 mg/day

Village	Water Fluoride (ppm)	Average Daily Intake (mg/day)	Number Surveyed	Number of All Fractures	Prevalence (%)
1	0.25–0.34	0.73	1,363	101	7.41
2	0.58–0.73	1.62	1,407	90	6.40
3	1.00–1.06	3.37	1,370	70	5.11
4	1.45–2.19	6.54	1,574	95	6.04
5	2.62–3.56	7.85	1,051	64	6.09
6	4.32–7.97	14.13	1,501	111	7.40

Source: Li et al., 2001.[32]

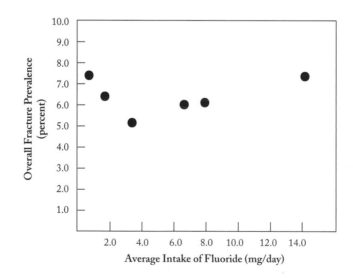

Figure 17.1. Prevalence of *all* bone fractures (since the age of twenty years) plotted against average daily fluoride intakes in six Chinese populations; data from Li et al., summarized in table 17.1.[33]

but if the U-shaped relationship is real, it suggests that intakes of fluoride of about 3 mg/day may confer some protection against fracture compared to lower and higher intakes. The water in village 3 contained 1 ppm fluoride, so some proponents of fluoridation have argued that this supports their case for artificial fluoridation at 1 ppm. That argument is fallacious, however, since it ignores the fact that, at over 3 mg/day, fracture rates increase. This is still more evident for hip fractures (see the discussion in the next section). Without the ability to control water intake and fluoride from other sources, keeping intakes at or near 3 mg/day for everyone would be impossible. There are many other sources of fluoride besides the water in fluoridating countries but no other significant sources in the rural Chinese villages studied by Li et al.

Table 17.1 summarizes Li's data for *all* fractures, and in figure 17.1 we have plotted the prevalence of all fractures in the six villages against Li's estimated daily intake for each village in mg/day.

Hip Fractures Only

When the prevalence of *hip fractures alone* was plotted for the six villages against Li's estimated daily intakes for each village (as tabulated in table 17.2), no U-shaped pattern was apparent: The prevalence was low in villages 1–3 and much higher in villages 4–6, with a possible rising trend across the whole range of fluoride intakes (see figure 17.2). Thus, there was no evidence for a protective effect of low intakes of fluoride, but daily fluoride intakes above 3 mg/day appeared harmful.

Thus, Li et al.'s results show a clear, threefold increase in hip fractures in the village with the highest fluoride concentration (village 6) and suggest that the tendency for fractures may rise progressively from an intake of about 3 mg/day (1 ppm in the water) or possibly even lower.

Returning to our discussion above about a possible benefit of protection against all fractures for villagers drinking fluoride in water at 3 mg/day, such a benefit is clearly negated by the much more pronounced and more serious problem of hip fractures increasing above 3 mg/day (or even lower). Readers should compare figures 17.1 and 17.2.

With both figures 17.1 and 17.2 in front of us, it may astonish readers to learn that a New York State Health Department official presented this study before the village board in Corning, New York, in 2007, to support his claim that water fluoridation, which Corning was considering at the time, strengthened bones.

Two WHO reports cite Li et al. as offering evidence that intakes of fluoride of 6 mg/day could damage bones.[34, 35] A review by the U.S. Department of Health and Human Services has estimated that fluoride exposure in fluoridated communities in the United States ranged from 1.6 to 6.6 mg/day, but it may be higher today and will certainly be exceeded by people who drink large amounts of water.[36]

The finding of Li et al. is buttressed by a 1999 study from Kurttio et al. in Finland that showed an increased hip fracture rate in a subset of the

Table 17.2 Hip fracture rates (since the age of 20 years) in six Chinese villages with average fluoride intakes varying from 0.7 to 14 mg/day

Village	Water Fluoride (ppm)	Average Daily Intake (mg/day)	Number Surveyed	Number of Hip Fractures	Prevalence (%)
1	0.25–0.34	0.73	1,363	5	0.37
2	0.58–0.73	1.62	1,407	6	0.43
3	1.00–1.06	3.37	1,370	5	0.37
4	1.45–2.19	6.54	1,574	14	0.89
5	2.62–3.56	7.85	1,051	8	0.76
6	4.32–7.97	14.13	1,501	18	1.20

Source: Li et al., 2001.[37]

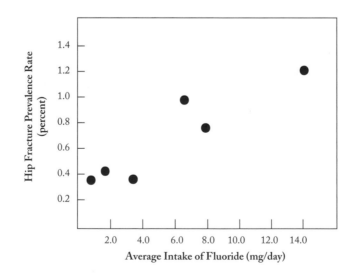

Figure 17.2. Prevalence of hip fractures (since the age of twenty years) plotted against average daily fluoride intakes in six Chinese populations; data from Li et al., summarized in table 17.2.[38]

elderly population exposed to fluoride above 1.5 ppm.[39] As mentioned above, Alarcón-Herrera et al. noted an increase in bone fractures in both children and adults associated with an increase in the severity of dental fluorosis, a biomarker of exposure to fluoride before the permanent teeth have appeared.[40] These studies require confirmation, but epidemiological findings are always greatly strengthened when, as here, there appears to be a dose-related increase in the effect being studied.

According to the 2006 NRC panel, "The combined findings of Kurttio et al. (1999), Alarcón-Herrera et al. (2001), and Li et al. (2001) lend support to gradients of exposure and fracture risk between 1 and 4 mg/L."[41] However, the panel members found it difficult to specify at what level increased fractures were likely to occur. Overall, the majority of the NRC panel members concluded that the current EPA MCLG of 4 ppm should be lowered: "Lowering the MCLG will prevent children from developing severe dental fluorosis and will reduce the lifelong accumulation of fluoride into bone that the majority of the committee believes is likely to put individuals at increased risk of bone fracture and possibly skeletal fluorosis, which are particular concerns for subpopulations that are prone to accumulating fluoride in their bones."[42]

Summary

In the sixty-year history of water fluoridation, the studies carried out on teeth in fluoridated communities vastly outnumber the studies done on bone. This reflects not the relative importance of these two systems but rather the fact that the fluoridation program has been largely driven by dental interests. It is surprising, given that 50 percent of the fluoride ingested each day accumulates in the bone, that the medical profession has not taken more interest in the matter. It does the profession little credit that bone levels of fluoride in fluoridated communities are not being monitored, an issue that we discuss further in chapter 22. Despite the paucity of study on fluoride and bone, those studies that have been carried out indicate that there is an inadequate margin of safety to protect everyone's bones from damage over a lifetime of exposure to fluoride, especially those who have impaired kidney function.

Bone damage can result in symptoms almost identical to the first symptoms of arthritis: aching bones and joints. Bearing in mind that more than 46 million American adults are currently diagnosed with some form of arthritis—and the numbers are expected to rise—the failure to pursue a possible connection with lifelong consumption of fluoridated water is inexplicable. A weight-of-evidence analysis of clinical trials, animal studies, and mixed epidemiological findings is highly suggestive that the accumulation of fluoride in bones from lifelong exposure to fluoride from fluoridated water and other sources will increase the risk of hip fractures in the elderly, especially those who have impaired kidney function. One important study from China (Li et al., 2001) indicates practically no margin of safety sufficient to protect a whole population with a lifelong consumption of water at 1 ppm from hip fracture. There is enough evidence on an increase in hip fractures to show that water fluoridation should be ended.

• 18 •

Fluoride and Osteosarcoma

Osteosarcoma is a rare but frequently fatal bone cancer found particularly in young men. With the topic of osteosarcoma and fluoride, we are talking about a possible relationship between fluoridation and deaths, few in number but nonetheless real.

The evidence that fluoride causes osteosarcoma is not clear-cut. The studies of the relationships in both animals and humans are mixed. The issue has had a long scientific and political history.

Observations in 1955

While the cortical bone defects observed in the Newburgh-Kingston study were ignored as far as bone fractures were concerned (chapter 17), they did prompt discussion on another front. This is how Donald Taves described the matter in a report published by the U.S. National Academy of Sciences (NAS) in 1977:

> There was an observation in the Kingston-Newburgh (Ast *et al.*, 1956) study that was considered spurious and has never been followed up. There was a 13.5% incidence of cortical defects in bone in the fluoridated community but only 7.5% in the non-fluoridated community. With 474 and 375 children in the respective groups, the t value was 2.85, which is statistically significant (Schlesinger, 1956). Caffey (1955) noted that the age, sex, and anatomical distribution of these bone defects are "strikingly" similar to that of osteogenic sarcoma. While progression of cortical defects to malignancies has not been observed clinically, it would be important to have direct evidence that osteogenic sarcoma rates *in males under 30* have not increased with fluoridation [emphasis added].[1]

Osteogenic sarcoma is now called osteosarcoma.

This observation by Caffey in 1955,[2] underlined by Taves in 1977, was the beginning of a long history of concern about whether fluoridation might increase the incidence of osteosarcoma in young men. Before we look further into that history, we will first consider the "biological plausibility" of a fluoride-osteosarcoma link.

Three key findings support the plausibility of such a link:

1. The bone is the principal site for fluoride accumulation within the body, and the rate of accumulation is increased during periods of rapid bone development as occurs in growth spurts during childhood. Thus, the cells in the bone are exposed to some of the highest fluoride concentrations in the body.

2. The preponderance of laboratory evidence indicates that fluoride, in sufficiently high concentrations, can cause genetic damage or genetic interference. Specifically, it can cause chromosomal damage and interfere with the enzymes involved with DNA repair, as shown in a variety of cell and tissue studies.[3–6] Recent studies have also found a correlation between fluoride exposure and chromosomal damage in humans.[7–9]

3. Fluoride is a mitogen, a substance that can stimulate cell division. It has been shown that fluoride can stimulate the proliferation of bone-forming cells (osteoblasts).[10, 11] This is important because osteosarcoma is a cancer caused by an *abnormal* proliferation of osteoblasts.

According to the authors of the 2006 NRC report, "Principles of cell biology indicate that stimuli for rapid cell division increase the risks for some of the dividing cells to become malignant, either by inducing random transforming events or by unmasking malignant cells that previously were in non-dividing states."[12]

Fluoride and Osteosarcoma, 1975–2010

Despite the recommendation by Taves that the rates of osteosarcoma in males under thirty be investigated in fluoridated communities, it took another thirteen years before that suggestion was followed. But before that, in 1975, further demands for research on cancer were stimulated by the work of Dr. John Yiamouyiannis, a biochemist, and Dr. Dean Burk, former head of the Cytochemistry Section of the U.S. National Cancer Institute. These two scientists stirred up a hornet's nest when they testified before the U.S. Congress and claimed that there was a greater rate of cancer in ten fluoridated U.S. cities compared to ten non-fluoridated ones.[13] Their findings were published in *Fluoride* in 1977.[14]

Robert Hoover and others at the National Cancer Institute attempted to rebut these findings, claiming to have looked at the same data and found no such relationship when they adjusted for age, sex, and race.[15] Several other researchers, including Sir Richard Doll in the UK, joined in what became an intense exchange of studies, with charges and countercharges flying in both directions. The ins and outs of this debate are far too complex to resolve here.

Meanwhile, Yiamouyiannis, Burk, and Doll have passed away. But two key players remain alive today. Dr. Robert Hoover, of the National Cancer Institute, continues to play a role in the cancer story and since 1991 has been involved in the osteosarcoma saga (see the section "Other Osteosarcoma Studies" below). John Remington Graham, a lawyer, worked very closely with Dr. Dean Burk for many years and published a recapitulation and reanalysis of his work in volume 61 of the *Proceedings of the Pennsylvania Academy of Science* in 1988.[16] Graham was the trial lawyer in three celebrated court cases in Pennsylvania, Illinois, and Texas from 1978 through 1984, wherein the most eminent experts in the world on both sides of this dispute testified under direct and cross-examination by seasoned trial lawyers before experienced trial judges. All three cases were settled in favor of Burk and Yiamouyiannis. With Dr. Pierre Morin, Graham has a carefully documented the legal history of this dispute for a publication of Florida State University College of Law[17] as well as fleshing out the story in the book *La fluoration: Autopsie d'une erreur scientifique*, which has recently been republished in English.[18]

Whoever was right about the effect of fluoridation on the cancer rate, the furor generated by Yiamouyiannis and Burk's work led a congressional committee to call for animal studies to determine whether fluoride caused cancer under laboratory conditions. The U.S. National Toxicology Program (NTP), a division of the U.S. Public Health Service (PHS), commissioned Battelle Memorial Institute's labs to do these studies. Oral, liver, and bone cancer received special attention. The results, which should have been completed and released in 1980, were not released until 1990. When they were released, they led to much press attention, including a cover story and commentary in *Newsweek*.[19]

It was clear that the NTP results threatened the fluoridation program. We will first examine the NTP study and then see how the PHS, now the DHHS, attempted to contain the issue, with the help of the National Cancer Institute (NCI).

NTP Animal Study

The Battelle lab researchers, contracted by the NTP to do the animal study, found a small but statistically significant dose-related increase in osteosarcoma in male (but not female) rats exposed to fluoride.[20] After a government peer review panel downgraded one of the osteosarcomas, this finding was classified as "equivocal evidence of cancer" by Bucher et al., whose study was finally published in 1991.[21, 22]

In the spring of 1990, with the NTP's findings attracting media attention, Procter & Gamble, a manufacturer of fluoridated toothpaste, released the findings of its own rat study of fluoride and cancer, which the company had conducted in 1981–1983 and which claimed not to have found this relationship in mice or rats.[23] While Procter & Gamble's study found several bone tumors in the fluoride-treated animals (versus none in the controls), the results do not achieve statistical significance and were thereby dismissed as random. According to Procter & Gamble's published report, "All bone neoplasms were considered to be incidental and spontaneous and not related to fluoride treatment, because of their low incidence and random distribution."[24]

An FDA review of this study appeared in appendix D of the Department of Health and Human Services (DHHS) report of 1991. In its analysis, the FDA identified two additional osteosarcomas in the fluoride-treated rats that were not identified in Procter & Gamble's published report. According to the FDA, "The adequacy of the gross examination at necropsy was questioned based upon the rat tumors that were not identified by the contract [Procter & Gamble] laboratory."[25]

However, even with the newly identified osteosarcomas, the FDA noted that the incidence of bone tumors in the Procter & Gamble study still did not achieve statistical significance. The FDA thereby concurred with Procter & Gamble that the bone tumors are incidental.[26]

Other Cancers in the NTP Study

As well as osteosarcoma, the original Battelle study reported an increase in liver and oral cancers and thyroid follicular cell tumors. However, the same government review panel mentioned above downgraded all the non-bone cancers to a less severe classification via a questionable rationale.[27] When, in May 1990, Dr. William Marcus, chief toxicologist of the Office of Water at the EPA, pointed this out, he was fired. (He was later reinstated, with full pay and compensation, after Labor Secretary Robert Reich ratified a December 3, 1992, ruling by administrative law judge David Clarke that the EPA "retaliated" against Marcus by firing him for scientific reports that recommended removing fluoride from drinking water.)[28]

Dr. Marcus pointed out that one of the cancers downgraded was a rare form of liver cancer called hepatocholangiocarcinoma. The peer reviewers examining the slides prepared for microscopic examination claimed that it was not a case of hepatocholangiocarcinoma. However, Dr. Melvin Reuber, an independent pathologist formerly with the National Cancer Institute and the first to describe this rare form of liver cancer, concurred with the pathologist at Battelle Memorial that the downgraded case was indeed a case of hepatocholangiocarcinoma.[29] In light of the importance of this study, in 2000 the union representing professionals working at the EPA headquarters in Washington, D.C., requested that Congress establish an independent review panel to reexamine those cancer slides.[30] That has so far not been done. The union had previously objected to the way the EPA determined the 1986 safe drinking water standard for fluoride[31, 32] (see chapter 20) and also objected to the dismissal of Dr. Marcus for raising red flags on the peer review panel's downgrading of cancer in the NTP study.[33]

The NTP findings prompted the NCI to review osteosarcoma rates in fluoridated communities in the United States (which Taves had recommended thirteen years earlier).[34] To do that, Hoover et al. used the Surveillance, Epidemiology and End Results (SEER) registries. Both the NTP results and the NCI survey were hastily published in a review by the Department of Health and Human Services titled *Review of Fluoride: Benefits and Risks.*[35] Thus, Hoover et al.'s studies were presented to the public before they had been published in a peer-reviewed journal.[36, 37] Publication in a peer-reviewed journal is widely considered by scientists to be essential to acceptance of research findings. Peer review would have been especially important in this case, as the agency publishing this report (DHHS) has a policy of promoting fluoridation.

Hoover et al. Survey of the SEER Registries

In 1991 Hoover et al. examined the nine SEER cancer registries (registries that cover about 10 percent of the U.S. population) for bone cancer and found a greater incidence of osteosarcoma in young males (not young females) in fluoridated versus non-fluoridated counties.[38] However, the same authors, using a subset of the data, claimed that the greater incidence was unrelated to duration of exposure and discounted the original finding.[39]

Today, more credence is given to Hoover et al.'s first finding than their second. This is largely because, by the time the NCI authors had used a subset of the data and divided it among four different durations of exposure, there were so few cases left in each grouping that the study lacked any statistical power.[40-43]

However, Hoover's second finding certainly helped fluoridation promoters to allay concern about this issue. Promoters included the authors of the DHHS report, who continued to argue that fluoridation was safe and effective. Here is what the DHHS authors had to say in their abstract about the animal studies (including the NTP study) as well as the human surveys on the question of a possible connection between fluoridation and cancer:

> Taken together, the only two methodologically acceptable animal studies [the NTP study and the earlier study by Procter & Gamble] available at this time fail to establish an association between fluoride and cancer. In humans, optimal fluoridation of drinking water does not pose a detectable cancer risk as evidenced by extensive human epidemiological data reported to date, including new epidemiological studies [the reviews of the SEER data by Hoover et al.] prepared for this report. No trends in cancer risk, including the risk of osteosarcoma, were attributed to the introduction and duration of water fluoridation.[44]

Somehow the osteosarcoma finding in male rats reported in the NTP study and the designation by peer reviewers of "equivocal evidence" of cancer have been lost from public view. Nor does the DHHS mention Hoover et al.'s initial finding of a greater incidence in osteosarcoma in young males in fluoridated communities compared to non-fluoridated communities, which they later discounted. Someone reading only the abstract of the DHHS report would get a very different view of the issue than someone who studied the details of both the animal and the human studies.

So to what extent was this DHHS report rushed through in an effort to protect the fluoridation program from this latest threat? An indication of the mind-set of those who set up this review is given in the last paragraph of the February 16, 1990, letter Dr. James Mason (assistant secretary for health and acting surgeon general) sent to the federal employees who made up the review panel: "Given the tangible public health benefits of fluorides in reducing tooth decay, the rarity of the tumor type in humans that is implicated by the study, and the preliminary nature of the NTP findings, our current policy supporting fluoridation must be maintained until your review is finished."[45]

McGuire et al. 1991

Two months after the DHHS review was published, a small study by S. M. McGuire et al. came out in the April 1991 issue of the *Journal of the American Dental Association* (*JADA*).[46] One of the coauthors of this study was Professor Chester Douglass, chair of the department of oral health policy and epidemiology at the Harvard School of Dental Medicine (see more below and under "Bassin 2001"). Even though this paper was a very small, preliminary study, it was given the full treatment by *JADA*. It was made the cover story, complete with a cover picture showing mountains and a lake seen through a huge glass of water.

It is clear that McGuire, Douglass, and the other authors of this study knew that a finding that fluoride might cause osteosarcoma would threaten the fluoridation program. Nor do they hide their concerns about such an eventuality, as the following quotes make clear:

> An incorrect inference implicating systemic fluoride carcinogenicity and its removal from our water systems would be detrimental to the oral health of most Americans, particularly those who cannot afford to pay for increasingly expensive restorative dental care . . .[47]
>
> Because of its strengthening action, fluoride has been widely accepted as the responsible agent for the dramatic declines in the tooth decay rates of U.S. children and adolescents . . . A disruption in the delivery of fluoride through municipal water systems would increase decay rates over time . . . Linking of fluoride ingestion and cancer initiation could result in a large-scale defluoridation of municipal water systems under the Delaney clause.[48]

Luckily for those who believed in the fluoridation program, the authors did not find that fluoridation was associated with an *increase* in osteosarcoma. In fact, they found that the very opposite might be the case, stating that "fluoridation at recommended levels *may* provide a *protective* effect against the formation of osteosarcoma" [emphasis added].[49] This speculative finding allowed the authors to reach the conclusion that they (and the *JADA* editors and the ADA) clearly wanted out of this study: "Given present knowledge, every effort should be made to continue the practice of fluoridating community water supplies."[50]

Chester Douglass, coauthor of the *JADA* article, received a sizable grant from the National Institute of Environmental Heath Sciences (NIEHS) to continue researching the fluoride-osteosarcoma issue after the article was published. It is surprising that the NIEHS would choose any dental researcher to oversee research on a life-or-death issue that might be related to the fluoridation program, let alone someone who had already expressed his understanding that a positive finding on the fluoridation-osteosarcoma connection would sabotage the practice that he favored so strongly. Douglass's further involvement in this issue is discussed under "Bassin 2001" and subsequent sections below.

Cohn 1992

In 1992, Perry Cohn, working for the New Jersey Health Department, reported a significant increase in osteosarcoma in young males in fluoridated communities in three New Jersey counties—again, not in young females.[51] Most significantly, Cohn suggested that there might be a time frame when young boys are particularly vulnerable to fluoride's carcinogenic effect:

> If rapidly growing bone in adolescent males is most susceptible to the development of osteosarcomas (Glass and Fraumeni, 1970), *it is possible that fluoride acts as a cancer promoter during a narrow window of susceptibility.* The interplay of hormonal influences and the intensity of the growth spurts may be potent influences. Since fluoride is toxic to cells and a variety of enzymes at high concentrations (reviewed by Kaminsky et al., 1990; and Department of Health and Human Services, 1991), it may exert tumor-promoting effects in the osteoblast cell microenvironment during bone deposition. Genetic predisposition may also play a role.[52-55] [emphasis added]

Other Osteosarcoma Studies

Other epidemiological studies of various sizes and quality have failed to find a relationship between fluoridation and osteosarcoma.[56-60] A full review of these and other studies on osteosarcoma is included in submissions to the National Research Council by the Fluoride Action Network (FAN).[61, 62] FAN's submissions were triggered by the discovery of a DMD thesis by Elise Bassin, discussed in the next section.

Bassin 2001

Dr. Elise Bassin investigated a possible relationship between osteosarcoma and exposure to fluoride as part of her doctorate in dental medicine thesis at the Harvard Dental School.[63] Suspecting a possible window of vulnerability for this problem, as Cohn had conjectured in 1992,[64] Bassin examined osteosarcoma rates as a function of the age at which boys were exposed to fluoride.

In a matched case-control study, Bassin reported what she described as a "robust finding" that young boys exposed to fluoride in their sixth to eighth years (which corresponds to the mid-childhood growth spurt) had a fivefold to sevenfold increased risk of contracting osteosarcoma by the age of twenty.[65]

It is extraordinary that, after Bassin's thesis was successfully defended in 2001, it was not followed up with a swift publication of her results, or any kind of statement made to warn the scientific community and the public about her findings. After all, if she was correct, a chemical that was given daily to millions of Americans in their drinking water might actually be killing people. For several years Bassin's thesis disappeared from view.

Professor Chester Douglass, coauthor of the 1991 McGuire et al. study, was Bassin's research sponsor and signed off on her thesis. Clearly, he knew the very serious implications of her findings for the future of fluoridation, as indicated in our discussion in "McGuire et al. 1991" above.[66] However, it appears that even though he was given several opportunities to do so over the next three to four years, he failed to warn his colleagues about Bassin's findings. The first opportunity occurred when he gave a presentation before the British Fluoridation Society (BFS) in 2002. He told the audience that his studies found no relationship between fluoride and osteosarcoma, but somehow he failed to mention his own graduate student's findings. This is how the BFS described his report in its piece on fluoridation titled "One in a Million," which is still posted on its Web site today: "Professor Chester Douglass of Harvard University presented preliminary results, as yet unpublished, from that and a separate National Cancer Institute study by Hoover et al., at a symposium held at the Royal College of Physicians, London, in November 2002. These two large case-control studies showed no association between fluoride exposure and osteosarcoma."[67] Eight years later (as of July 2010) these promised studies have still not been published (see the discussion in the next section) and meanwhile, in the period 2006 to 2010, the BFS has not felt the need to mention the existence of Bassin's study.

Douglass's second opportunity to mention Bassin's findings came when he was invited to send a summary of his work to the NRC panel (which published its report in March 2006).[68] He again asserted that *his* work showed no significant association between fluoride and osteosarcoma. In his short statement he did include a citation to Bassin's thesis as a footnote but did not indicate to the NRC that her findings contradicted what he had said.[69] He sent a similar statement to his funders at the NIEHS.

Bassin's Thesis Discovered

Eventually, Bassin's thesis surfaced in the Harvard Medical School Rare Books Room, where Michael Connett accessed it in January 2005. The resulting public release of this material triggered a demand by the Environmental Working Group (EWG) for an official enquiry into Douglass's behavior by the NIEHS, the body that had funded this work. This led to a great deal of press attention, including a lengthy article in the *Wall Street Journal*.[70] The NIEHS passed on the request for an enquiry to Harvard. After a year, Harvard produced a short statement declaring that Douglass did not "intentionally" hide Bassin's findings.[71] Harvard has refused to provide any arguments or explanations supporting this finding, despite repeated requests from alumni, other U.S. citizens, and even members of Congress.

Bassin's findings were published in May 2006 in the journal *Cancer Causes and Control*.[72] However, the same issue of the journal published a letter coauthored by Douglass downplaying the significance of her findings.[73] It is interesting to contrast Douglass's failure to warn the public of Bassin's findings between 2001 and 2005 with his alacrity in claiming that her findings might be "premature" on the same day that her article appeared in press.

In their letter, Douglass and Kaumudi Joshipura pointed out that Bassin's findings were based on a subset of a larger cohort and claimed that the larger cohort did not support her thesis. However, they provided no evidence that her methodology had been applied to the larger cohort, nor is it clear that it has ever been so applied. The letter further claimed that Douglass's larger study (to be coauthored by Robert Hoover, mentioned previously in connection with his critique of the Yiamouyiannis and Burk study and the NCI review of the SEER cancer registries) was "currently being prepared for publication." The NRC report had cited a January 3, 2006, communication from Douglass that their study "was expected to be reported in the Summer 2006."[74] It is now over *four years* since Douglass made that promise, and the study has not yet been published. Douglass has since retired from his position at Harvard.

Douglass's Methodology

The methodology described by Douglass et al. could not test the central thesis of Bassin's work, because the biometric of exposure those authors used—bone fluoride levels found at the time of diagnosis or autopsy—could not ascertain exposure during the years of age (six to eight) so critical to Bassin's thesis.[75, 76] Fluoride accumulates over time, so a level at, say, age twenty gives no indication of the level of exposure at six, seven, or eight years of age.

Moreover, the controls used in the *promised* Douglass-Hoover study are other bone cancers. The choice of that control makes the assumption that none of those bone cancers are caused by fluoride. The study would be invalidated if fluoride were associated with any of those cancers, like Ewing's sarcoma, which is not impossible.[77]

Despite the non-appearance of the promised Douglass-Hoover study, and the limitations in the methodology they have used to refute Bassin's work, the Douglass-Joshipura letter is being used by fluoridation proponents in several countries as if it were the final word on the issue. To use the *promise* of an unpublished study to negate Bassin's published conclusions is extraordinary. Clearly, a double standard is operating here. The same proponents who are now using the promise contained in the Douglass-Joshipura letter of 2006 to negate Bassin's findings previously used the fact that her thesis was unpublished to deflect attention from her work.

This is how the Australian National Health and Medical Research Council (NHMRC) used the Douglass-Joshipura letter in the systematic review it published in 2007:

> The attention of the reader is drawn to a Letter to the Editor that appeared in the same issue of *Cancer Causes and Controls* by co-investigators on the larger Harvard study (Douglass & Joshipura, 2006). The authors point out that they had not been able to replicate the findings of Bassin and colleagues in the larger study that included prospective cases from the same 11 hospitals. Furthermore, the bone samples that were taken in the broader study corroborate a lack of association between the fluoride content in drinking water and osteosarcoma in the new cases. As Bassin and colleagues acknowledged, the shortcomings of their study mean that their results should be interpreted with caution pending publication of the larger study results.[78]

A local health authority pushing for fluoridation in Southampton, UK, used the Douglass-Joshipura letter in its public consultation brochure in 2008. The authors do not make it clear that the reference (13) they cite is not a study or a "comprehensive review" but a letter promising a study:

Since 2006, fluoridation opponents have pointed to a study in the United States of America (12) [the Bassin study] that appears to suggest a possible increase in osteosarcoma (bone cancer) rates in young males—but not females—living in fluoridated areas. However, this was part of a larger study (13) [the Douglass letter] looking at many more osteosarcoma cases over a longer period of time and including an examination of bone samples. This more detailed and comprehensive review had found no link between water fluoride levels and osteosarcoma. The researchers therefore advised caution in selectively interpreting the results of the smaller study in isolation.[79]

This is how Dr. Peter Cooney, the chief dental officer of Canada, described the Bassin study and the Douglass-Joshipura letter in a presentation he gave in Dryden, Ontario, on April 1, 2008: "You are going to hear about osteosarcoma . . . some of the studies that did show that there may have been a concern in young males with osteosarcoma have been—in the bigger studies—completely discounted."[80]

California Proposition 65

Proposition 65 is the name given to the California Safe Drinking Water and Toxic Enforcement Act of 1986. This act requires the governor of California, at least once a year, to publish a list of chemicals known to the state to cause cancer or reproductive toxicity and to inform citizens about exposures to these chemicals. In March 2009 the California Office of Environmental Health Hazard Assessment (OEHHA) solicited public comments on thirty-eight chemicals selected for prioritization for evaluation by the state's Carcinogen Identification Committee. "Fluoride and its salts" were included, and in October the state announced that that was one of five chemicals selected for consideration.[81]

Very extensive comments were sent into the OEHHA by a number of individuals and organizations, including Paul Connett and Chris Neurath of the Fluoride Action Network;[82] the Environmental Working Group;[83] and Kathleen Thiessen, PhD, an NRC panel member.[84] There is a wealth of additional material in these submissions for those who want more details than we can provide in this chapter.

It is interesting to note on the Web site of the California Dental Association (CDA) that the organization received $200,000 from the ADA to help stop the state's investigation of the carcinogenicity of fluoride. The CDA states that "ADA granted CDA $200,000 to assist in our effort to prevent the placement of 'fluoride and its salts' on the List of Chemicals Known to the State to Cause Cancer or Reproductive Toxicity that is produced by the State of California, Environmental Protection Agency, Office of Environmental Health Hazard Assessment (OEHHA)."[85]

Here we see yet another example of how the ADA seems more determined to protect the fluoridation program than to protect the health of the American people, even on an issue that is life threatening. We look at more examples of the tactics and strategies used by proponents of fluoridation in chapter 23.

On October 15, 2009, a sixty-day comment period began on the five chemicals (including fluoride and its salts), out of thirty-eight originally nominated. This comment period ended on December 15, 2009.[86] To our knowledge, as of July 2010, the carcinogenicity of fluoride is still being considered by the California OEHHA.

Summary

The possibility that fluoridation may be associated with an increase in osteosarcoma in boys and young men was raised as long ago as 1955. The matter was raised again, in 1977, by one of the authors of an NAS panel, which recommended that osteosarcoma rates be examined in *young men* less than thirty years of age in fluoridated areas. Nothing was done about this suggestion until an NTP study in 1990 reported a dose-related association between osteosarcoma in *male* rats that were fed fluoride. In 1991 the NCI reported that there was such an association in *young males* but not females in the U.S. population but discounted it on the grounds that it appeared unrelated to the duration of exposure. From 1991 to 2001 reports on this possible association have been mixed. In 1992, in a study of fluoridated communities in New Jersey, Cohn reported an association; other studies have not. In 2001, using a different approach, Elise Bassin found that *young boys* exposed to fluoridated water in their sixth, seventh, and eighth years had a five- to sevenfold greater risk of contracting osteosarcoma by the age of twenty.

Bassin's thesis research sponsor, Chester Douglass, failed to warn the public, his peers, the NRC, or his funders about this issue for four years. Bassin's thesis did not appear in public until 2005, and her data were not published until 2006. When they were published, the same journal published a letter from Douglass in the same issue claiming that his larger study would refute Bassin's findings. That study was promised for the summer of 2006, but after four years it has not appeared. This same study had been mentioned even earlier in 2002 by Douglass at a meeting organized by the BFS in London. A possible reason that Douglass's paper has not appeared is that his methodology is seriously flawed: It cannot test the central finding of Bassin's thesis.

Meanwhile, promoters of fluoridation are using that promise of a study as a way of dispelling concern over the possibility that drinking fluoridated water may contribute to boys and young men contracting a disease that is frequently fatal. All parties agree that it is highly plausible from a biological perspective that fluoride could cause bone cancer. Fluoride reaches its highest concentration in bone and the pineal gland. Fluoride is known to increase bone turnover, and it is also established that fluoride can interfere with the genetic machinery of the cell in a variety of ways. Mutations (genetic mistakes) are most likely to occur during rapid bone turnover. Rapid bone turnover occurs during the mid-childhood growth spurt that corresponds to the window of vulnerability discussed by Cohn and identified by Bassin.

Fluoride and the Kidneys, and Other Health Issues

Two issues pertain to fluoride and the kidneys. The first is the possibility that fluoride can damage the kidneys, especially at high levels. The second is the fact that someone with poor kidney function has a limited ability to clear fluoride from the body, which would make that person more vulnerable to fluoride's other toxic effects.

Fluoride Damage to the Kidney

With the exception of the pineal gland, the kidney accumulates more fluoride than all other *soft* tissues in the body.[1-3] It is well known that high doses of fluoride can damage the kidney after short periods of exposure—for example, to an anesthetic that contains fluorinated hydrocarbons such as methoxyfluorane, which are metabolized to free fluoride ion.[4-8]

There is also evidence that low doses of fluoride, taken over longer periods of time, can damage the kidney. For example, both Varner et al.[9] and McKay, Ramseyer, and Smith[10] found kidney damage in rats drinking water with just 1 ppm of fluoride. Manocha, Warner, and Olkowski[11] found kidney damage in monkeys drinking water with 5 ppm fluoride; while Borke and Whitford found significant biochemical damage to the kidney in rats drinking water with 10 ppm fluoride. In the latter study, the average blood fluoride levels of the rats with kidney damage was 38 ppb—a concentration commonly exceeded in people living in 1 ppm areas. Borke and Whitford state:

> Our study provides the first evidence that one of the effects of long-term F exposure is a change in expression of the plasma membrane and endoplasmic reticulum Ca++ pumps in the kidney. In summary, we provided rats with fluoride in their drinking water, which produced graded, plasma fluoride concentrations that occur in humans. Our studies showed that chronic high fluoride ingestion decreases the rate of Ca++ transport across renal tubule endoplasmic reticulum and plasma membranes, and reduced the amount of ER and PM Ca++ pump protein present in the kidney membranes. We conclude that chronic high fluoride ingestion

may decrease the expression, increase the breakdown, or increase the rate of turnover of plasma membrane and endoplasmic reticulum Ca^{++} pump proteins and possibly other enzymes as well. The observed decreases in the rate of Ca^{++} transport and associated decreases in plasma membrane and endoplasmic reticulum Ca^{++} pump expression could affect in vivo Ca^{++} homeostasis.[12]

Complementing this animal research, many studies have found kidney disease to be a common feature of human skeletal fluorosis.[13-22]

Also, and perhaps most significant, a human study by Liu et al. in China has found a dose-dependent relationship between fluoride ingestion and kidney damage in children.[23] The study found evidence of kidney damage among children drinking water with as little as 2.6 ppm fluoride.

Consequences of Poor Kidney Function

Of huge concern is the impact of drinking fluoridated water on people with impaired kidney function. It is well known that in a healthy person approximately 50 percent of ingested fluoride is excreted. However, when someone has impaired kidney function, far less fluoride is excreted, leading to higher accumulations of fluoride, especially in the bones.[24] It has been reported that individuals with impaired kidney function have developed skeletal fluorosis drinking water at levels as low as 1.7 ppm.[25]

2006 NRC Report

The NRC report said the following about fluoride and the kidney:

> Human kidneys . . . concentrate fluoride as much as 50-fold from plasma to urine. Portions of the renal system may therefore be at higher risk of fluoride toxicity than most soft tissues . . . Early water fluoridation studies did not carefully assess changes in renal function . . .[26]
>
> On the basis of studies carried out on people living in regions where there is endemic fluorosis, ingestion of fluoride at 12 mg per day would increase the risk for some people to develop adverse renal effects.[27]

The NRC made these recommendations for future research on fluoride and the kidneys:

Future studies should be directed toward determining whether kidney stone formation is the most sensitive end point on which to base the MCLG . . .[28]

The effect of low doses of fluoride on kidney and liver enzyme functions in humans needs to be carefully documented in communities exposed to different concentrations of fluoride in drinking water.[29]

Kidney and Other Stones

Little investigation has taken place on the possible involvement of fluoride in the formation of kidney stones or, once stones have formed, on the possible accumulation of fluoride in or on them. Similar considerations may apply to other tissues (gallbladder, brain) where calcified deposits may occur. We agree with the NRC panel members that more research is needed on what might be a very important concern.

Other Health Issues

The 2006 NRC panel reviewed a number of other health issues, including potential fluoride interactions with the gastrointestinal, hepatic, immune, and reproductive systems.[30] Effects on the gastrointestinal system are discussed in chapter 13. Most of the concerns about the immune system are largely speculative; once again the scarcity of literature on this reflects a lack of interest by governments that promote fluoridation. The same can be said about reproductive effects; despite an extensive literature indicating that, at high levels of exposure, effects of fluoride on the reproductive system have been observed in a wide range of animals and reptiles, very few human studies on the subject have been published or even undertaken. In chapter 22 we refer to the unscientific way that the ADA dismissed a significant study on this subject by Freni.[31] For a wide-ranging review of fluoride effects on the reproductive system, see Long et al. (2009).[32]

Effects on the Cardiovascular System

There is little evidence of attention to the possibility of effects of fluoride on the cardiovascular system. The 2006 NRC report mentions cardiovascular effects only with respect to thyroid function. However, two recent studies of sixty-three adults with "endemic fluorosis" and forty-five healthy controls found that fluorotic individuals had decreased elasticity of the aorta and dysfunctions of the left ventricle.[33, 34] The papers include references to other studies on fluoride and the cardiovascular system.

Summary

Most of the possible impacts of fluoride on tissues such as the kidneys and the reproductive, hepatic, and immune systems suffer from a lack of serious study in fluoridated countries. Since the kidneys concentrate fluoride to a greater extent than any other soft tissue except the pineal gland, they may be particularly at risk. Also, if the kidneys are not functioning well to begin with, less fluoride is excreted, and more lodges in the skeleton. Moreover, because kidneys become less efficient with age, the elderly are at greater risk. The issue of a possible relationship between fluoride and kidney stones (and stones in other tissues) is potentially important but has not been explored.

Studies on the other systems mentioned do not leave much room for complacency. Some people ridicule opponents of fluoridation for the long list of health effects sometimes claimed for the simple fluoride ion. It is easy to score cheap points here, but the fact is that, as we indicated in chapter 12, fluoride has a high biological activity that is very general in nature—for example, it inhibits many enzymes, it interacts with calcium ions (either directly or indirectly), and in the presence of a trace amount of aluminum, it interferes with hormonal messaging systems. Since enzymes and hormones are essential to all physiological processes, such activities are likely to produce a wide variety of effects.

PART FIVE

Margin of Safety and the Precautionary Principle

In part 5 we address the kind of information that a thoughtful decision maker might wish to consider before endorsing or halting fluoridation.

In chapter 20, we discuss what is meant by a margin of safety. It is not disputed that, at moderate to high doses, fluoride can cause serious health problems and other adverse effects. The crucial question is whether there is a sufficient margin of safety between the doses that cause those effects and the doses experienced in fluoridated communities. We explain why this margin of safety has to be sufficiently large to protect *everyone*, including the most vulnerable, not just the *average* person. Moreover, it has to be large enough to protect the whole population over a *lifetime* of exposure.

In chapter 21, we discuss the precautionary principle. Application of this principle allows decision makers a way of resolving public health and environmental issues when the evidence of harm is mixed and has not reached the level of absolute certainty.

Margin of Safety

Proponents of fluoridation in Australia,[1] Canada,[2] the UK,[3, 4] and the U.S.[5, 6] have all dismissed the 2006 National Research Council report[7] as being irrelevant to water fluoridation, claiming that it applies only to "high" exposure to fluoride. However, none of these promoters or agencies has explained what is meant by the word "high" or attempted to quantify the term in any meaningful way. To do this requires a consideration of the *margin of safety.*

The concept of margin of safety is normally used by toxicologists, pharmacologists, and regulatory officials when establishing so-called safe levels of a known toxic substance to which the public may be exposed. Such a margin of safety (or safety factor) is set to ensure protection for everyone from an identified or anticipated harmful effect. This margin of safety has to take into account the full range of sensitivities to a toxic substance that can be anticipated in any human population (*intraspecies variation*). In the case of fluoride, an extra safety factor will be needed when setting a safe level for fluoride in water (either natural or added) to take into account the full range of exposure for a population drinking uncontrolled amounts of water and getting fluoride from other sources as well.

Typically, to take into account intraspecies variation, the lowest level or dose at which toxicity is observed (i.e., *lowest observable adverse effect level,* or LOAEL) is divided by 10 to set the margin of safety. This factor of 10 assumes that the most sensitive person is ten times more sensitive than the least sensitive.

Sometimes more conservative regulatory agencies insist on working from a *no observable adverse effect level,* or NOAEL. If that is not available, they require that a margin of safety of 100, not 10, be applied to the LOAEL.

Sometimes a margin of safety lower than 10 is used if data have been collected on an adequate range of doses from studies in very large populations. In such a case it is assumed that enough people have been observed to cover the full range of human sensitivity. However, in the case of fluoride, many of the studies finding adverse effects have involved relatively small study groups. Such studies would not cover either the full range of anticipated sensitivity or the full range of dose when a much larger population is exposed.

The people who need special protection in the case of exposure to fluoride include the very young, the very old, those with poor diet (including borderline iodine deficiency), those with poor kidney function (which reduces the ability to excrete fluoride), those who consume above-average quantities of water (athletes, diabetics, etc.), and infants who are fed formula that has been reconstituted with fluoridated water.

Based on current levels of exposure and the levels at which effects were shown to occur in the 2006 NRC report,[8] it is hard to see how a scientifically defensible safety factor could yield a safe level for fluoride in water of more than 0.1 ppm. Indeed, Dr. Robert Carton, a former risk assessment specialist at the Environmental Protection Agency (EPA), has argued, based on the NRC findings, that the maximum contaminant level goal (MCLG) for fluoride should be set at zero, as has been done for both lead and arsenic.[9] This is what we believe a scientific margin-of-safety analysis would show.

Those who claim that the practice of water fluoridation is safe for *everyone* have a clear obligation to demonstrate that by performing a careful margin-of-safety analysis for the adverse health effects reviewed and summarized in the 2006 NRC report.[10] Such a demonstration would have to include the rationale for choosing the most appropriate (i.e., most sensitive) end point and LOAEL for that end point (the end point being a known or reasonably anticipated health effect) for all those health effects discussed by the NRC report.

It is reckless to continue promoting fluoridation when studies indicate that thyroid function may be lowered at 2.3 ppm,[11] IQ in children may be lowered at levels as low as 1.9 ppm[12, 13] or even at 0.9 ppm if there is borderline iodine deficiency,[14] and hip fractures in the elderly may be increased at levels as low as 1.5 ppm and tripled at levels over 4.3 ppm.[15, 16] Unless all these effects can be dismissed because all the relevant studies have been shown to be fatally flawed, there is clearly no adequate margin of safety to protect the whole population from those end points. Thus, the practice of fluoridating the public water system should be discontinued. Furthermore, if the relevant studies have faults but still raise plausible doubts about safety, the program should be stopped until research yields reliable conclusions (the precautionary principle; see chapter 21).

Not a New Idea

The application of a margin-of-safety analysis to water fluoridation is not a new idea. As long ago as 1956, Benjamin Nesin, a prominent water engineer, indicated that the safety factors discussed at the time offered inadequate protection. Focusing particularly on the range of doses one could anticipate across the whole population, he wrote the following:

> The proponents have tried to demonstrate various factors of safety which are patently naive . . . It has been customary to consider a minimal factor of safety of not less than 10 for substances which are admitted to water supplies. This would mean that ten times the amount of the proposed substance when present in the water supply would be definitely without harm to human or beast. It is obvious from the knowledge of fluoride toxicity that such factor of safety cannot be established when fluoride is added to the public water supply at the level recommended by the proponents of fluoridation. In view of the fact that the range of water consumption may vary over a ratio of 20 to 1 the insistence of a safety factor of 10 is exceedingly moderate.[17]

Inadequate Margin-of-Safety Calculations

To date, the margins of safety used by agencies in the United States (and other fluoridating countries) for fluoride have been woefully inadequate. We examine a few of these.

EPA and the MCLG

The U.S. EPA's Office of Drinking Water's 1986 derivation of the 4 ppm maximum contaminant level goal (MCLG) for fluoride in drinking water[18] is scientifically flawed. The EPA's Office of Prevention, Pesticides and Toxic Substances explained the derivation of the current MCLG by the EPA's Office of Drinking Water as it was preparing to permit sulfuryl fluoride as a new food fumigant:

> For fluoride, both the MCL and the MCLG have been set at 4.0 ppm in order to protect against crippling skeletal fluorosis. The MCLG was established in 1986 [*Federal Register* 51, no. 63] and is based on a LOAEL of 20 mg/day, a safety factor of 2.5, and an adult drinking water intake of 2 L/day. The use of a safety factor of 2.5 ensures public health criteria while still allowing sufficient concentration of fluoride in water to realize its beneficial effects

in protecting against dental caries. The typical 100x factor used by the HED [the EPA's Health Effects Division] to account for inter- and intra-species variability have been removed due to the large amounts of human epidemiological data surrounding fluoride and skeletal fluorosis.[19]

Having explained this derivation of the MCLG of 4 ppm, the Office of Pesticides then used it as a basis to determine tolerances for fluoride residues left on foodstuffs treated with sulfuryl fluoride. We discuss the way they did this in three different health risk assessments in the section "EPA Pesticide Division" below. But first let us break down the 1986 derivation of the MCLG by the EPA's Office of Drinking Water into its component parts:

1. The end point chosen was crippling skeletal fluorosis.
2. The LOAEL offered for this was 20 milligrams per day.
3. The safety factor offered to protect the most vulnerable was 2.5.
4. The amount of water drunk per day was 2 liters.
5. The only source of fluoride considered was water.

The EPA's (Office of Drinking Water) calculation was as follows: 20 milligrams per day divided by 2.5 (safety factor) equals 8 milligrams per day. If one assumes that a person drinks 2 liters of water a day, the supposed safe level is 4 milligrams per liter, because if someone drank 2 liters of water at that level, they would receive the supposed safe level of 8 milligrams of fluoride. Thus the EPA arrived at an MCLG of 4 ppm.

There are six things wrong with the EPA's derivation. It is hopelessly wrong at all five steps, and two mistakes are made on one of those steps. Even at the time, the inadequacies of the derivation were pointed out by some EPA scientists, including Dr. Robert Carton, who claimed that it was manipulated for political reasons.[20] Today, with the benefit of more research findings, the inadequacies are even more glaring. We now examine each step of the calculation and the six places where the EPA went wrong.

Mistake one: Selecting crippling skeletal fluorosis as the end point of concern. There are two problems with the EPA's selection of *crippling* skeletal fluorosis as the only end point of concern. First, even if the EPA wished to focus on fluoride's impact on the bone it was both unscientific and contrary to common sense to focus solely on the *crippling* phase of skeletal fluorosis. More sensitive end points were known in 1986 and these include the earlier stages of skel-etal fluorosis as well as bone defects (see chapter 17). Second, in 1986, there was evidence available that fluoride could have impacts on thyroid function at levels far lower than those that caused crippling skeletal fluorosis[21, 22] (see chapter 16).

As far as skeletal fluorosis was concerned, a lot of observable damage occurs to the bone and connective tissue before the *crippling* phase is reached. The existence of arthritic symptoms in the pre-crippling stages of the disease has been widely reported in the literature prior to the EPA's 1986 determination of the MCLG[23-28] (see chapter 17). While not everyone with pre-crippling clinical fluorosis will experience arthritic pain, the evidence is clear that *some* people will. Thus the EPA should have selected *pre-crippling* clinical effects as a more sensitive end point of concern. Indeed, the 2006 NRC panel recom-mended to the EPA that stage II of skeletal fluorosis be considered an adverse health effect (see chapter 14).

According to the NRC, "The committee judges that stage II is also an adverse health effect, as it is associated with chronic joint pain, arthritic symptoms, slight calcification of ligaments, and osteosclerosis of cancellous bones."[29]

In addition, as far back as 1956, researchers had found that cortical bone defects were significantly higher in children in fluoridated Newburgh, New York, compared to unfluoridated Kingston[30] (see chapter 17).

Mistake two: Using a LOAEL of 20 mg/day

If the EPA had used cortical bone defects as the most sensitive end point then the LOAEL should have been selected between 1 and 2 mg/day. This assumes that children in fluoridated Newburgh were drinking one to two liters of water per day and that water was their main source of fluoride.[31]

If the EPA had selected lowered thyroid function as the most sensitive end point, then the study by Bachinskii et al. would indicate a LOAEL in the range of 2.3 to 4.6 mg/day.[32] This again assumes that those who had expe-rienced lowered thyroid function drinking water at 2.3 ppm fluoride were drinking between one to two liters of water per day.

If the EPA had selected a pre-crippling stage of skeletal fluorosis it is hard to see how they could have selected a LOAEL larger than 10 mg per day and probably considerably less. So whichever adverse health effect the EPA had selected, of the several options available, it is clear that 20 mg per day was far too high to be protective.

Mistake three: Failure to use an adequate safety factor.

Even if we ignore the inadequate LOAEL used by the EPA, the fact remains that the agency failed to apply an adequate safety factor to even that LOAEL to allow for the range of vulnerability to any toxic substance in a human population.

To claim that the normal safety factor of 100 was dropped because of "the large amounts of human epidemiological data surrounding fluoride and skeletal fluorosis" is wrong on two fronts. First, the EPA ignored the large amount of data on this issue from India and China, which have areas where both dental and skeletal fluorosis are endemic. Bone effects have been observed in India at levels of fluoride in water ranging from 1 ppm to 3 ppm where there is poor nutrition.[33] Second, the agency derived the LOAEL of 20 mg/day largely from Kaj Roholm's work, which was based on a small sample of otherwise healthy male industrial workers.[34] One needs a much larger safety factor to cover the whole range of sensitivity anticipated in a large human population.

Mistake four: Dropping the normal safety margin to protect the fluoridation program.

The EPA pesticide division, in the quote above, made it very clear why the standard protective safety factor of 10 or 100 was sacrificed in the EPA water division's calculation, stating that it was to allow "sufficient concentration of fluoride in water to realize its beneficial effects in protecting against dental caries."[35] In other words, the EPA admitted that its derivation involved protecting the water fluoridation program. This kind of thinking may have been appropriate when the agency moved from an MCLG (a goal) to an MCL (a standard), but it was inappropriate to use such reasoning in determining the MCLG. For an MCLG, the task is to determine an *ideal* safe level based on scientific studies of toxic end points and to apply an appropriate safety factor *to protect the most vulnerable*. The EPA should not have allowed the *purported* benefit of the fluoridation program to interfere with what should have been a scientific determination of the ideal goal to protect everyone from "known or reasonably anticipated health effects," as mandated in the Safe Drinking Water Act.

It should be noted that, as requested by the EPA,[36] the 2006 NRC report[37] ignored any discussion of the benefits of the water fluoridation program when the NRC panel members set out to provide the toxicological data that could be used by the EPA to determine a new MCLG.

There are two more problems when we move from the supposedly safe level of 8 milligrams per day (20 mg/day divided by 2.5) to an MCLG of 4 ppm.

Mistake five: Assuming that people drink only 2 liters of water a day.
The assumption that people drink only 2 liters of water per day is clearly wrong. Although that may be the average consumption, the MCLG has to protect *everyone*, including above-average water drinkers. In fact, millions of people drink far more than 2 liters per day. Indeed, some agencies, such as the Food and Nutrition Board (FNB) of the Institute of Medicine, now recommend that males over the age of eighteen drink 3 liters of water per day.[38] Also according to the FNB, over 5 percent of males between the ages of nineteen and fifty consume at least 5 liters of water a day, while 1 percent consume at least 9 liters a day. Over 5 percent of adult females consume over 4 liters a day, while 1 percent of females consume over 5.5 liters a day.[39]

At most, the EPA's use of the 2-liter consumption figure is designed to protect the average person, not everyone—and certainly not the above-average water drinker.

Mistake six: Not making allowance for fluoride exposure from other sources.
Other sources of fluoride include food and beverages processed with fluoridated water,[40–43] fluoridated dental products,[44, 45] mechanically deboned meat,[46] teas,[47–50] pesticide residues on food,[51] and wine.[52, 53] An estimate of the total ingested fluoride should have been subtracted from the 8 mg/day before proceeding to the calculation of the safe water concentration (MCLG).

People attempting to perform a risk assessment run into another daunting problem at this stage. If they estimate a more appropriate safe daily dose (e.g., 1 or 2 mg/day), they then find that a conservative estimate for the total fluoride obtained from other sources may already exceed this safe level. How can they then proceed to a non-zero safe level in water? The simple answer is, they cannot. If it is concluded that some people are already getting above the determined safe level from other sources, we cannot allow any fluoride *to be added* to our water. In other words, one is forced to set the MCLG at zero (as has been done for arsenic and lead). This would rule out the deliberate addition of fluoride to the water and instead shift the whole focus onto the federally enforceable maximum contaminant level (MCL) and the converse issue of how much it would cost some communities with high natural levels of fluoride to reduce those to some compromise level.

Reaction to the MCLG.

Every assumption used by the EPA water division to determine the 1986 MCLG of 4 ppm was inadequate, unscientific, and clearly designed to produce an MCLG that would protect the fluoridation program rather than human health. The manipulations outraged professional employees at the EPA, leading their union to file a "friend of the court" brief in support of the National Resources Defense Fund's application for an injunction against the 1986 MCLG for fluoride.[54]

Focusing on only one of the mistakes discussed above (the choice of end point), the 2006 NRC panel found that the 4 ppm MCLG was not protective of health and recommended that the EPA determine a new MCLG.[55] After four years, as of the time of this writing, the EPA had yet to do that.

Food and Nutrition Board

It came as a considerable shock in 1997 when the Food and Nutrition Board (FNB) of the Institute of Medicine (IOM) announced that it was setting "adequate intakes" (AIs) and "upper tolerance limits" (ULs) for fluoride along with magnesium, calcium, phosphate, and vitamin D.[56] It was a shock because there is no evidence that fluoride is an essential nutrient, as are the other substances appearing on this list, and because its predominant action in fighting tooth decay is topical, not systemic.[57, 58]

In response to a letter sent by about a dozen scientists complaining about this treatment of fluoride as a nutrient, the directors of both the IOM and the National Academy of Sciences made it very clear that they did not consider fluoride a nutrient and instead described it as a "beneficial element" (see chapter 1).[59] However, the FNB proceeded as if it were, indeed, a nutrient.

In determining the UL for fluoride, the FNB, like the EPA ten years before, considered skeletal fluorosis as the only adverse health effect of concern. However, the board dropped the LOAEL to "10 mg/day for 10 or more years." While that was clearly an improvement over what the EPA did in 1986, the board then did something quite inexplicable (at least on scientific grounds). In deriving a UL from this LOAEL, it applied a safety margin of *1.0*—meaning there was *no* uncertainty in applying this so-called safe level to a large segment of the whole population. The terminology the board used was "uncertainty factor" (UF) of 1.0.[60] Thus it was that the FNB resolved that, for anyone eight years of age or older, it would be safe to consume 10 mg/day for a lifetime. That is a preposterous notion, best explained by the need felt by yet another agency to protect the U.S. water fluoridation program at whatever cost to scientific credibility or the public's health.

The Fluoridation Forum

We discuss Ireland's 2002 Fluoridation Forum report in some detail in chapter 24. Suffice it to say here that this panel simply copied the Food and Nutrition Board's approach of applying a safety factor of 1.0 to an LOAEL in deriving an upper tolerance level (UL) of 10 mg per day.[61]

EPA Pesticide Division

However bad the science used by the EPA's Office of Water in its derivation of the MCLG of 4 ppm, it pales compared to the outrageous manipulations the EPA's Office of Pesticides applied to the same MCLG in deriving a so-called *safe* reference dose (RfD) for infants. In three successive risk assessments,[62–64] the EPA Office of Pesticides derived three different RfDs for infants: 0.114 mg/kg/day, 0.57 mg/kg/day, and 1.14 mg/kg/day. The final one, 1.14 mg/kg/day, is *ten times higher* than the RfD for adults.[65] That is indeed a remarkable conclusion.

Here we examine the three different methods used by the EPA Office of Pesticides to derive these three different RfDs for infants. It is important to note that the second and third derivations came as a consequence of interventions by the Fluoride Action Network (FAN), the Environmental Working Group (EWG), and Beyond Pesticides (BP). Ironically, even though the EPA arrived at three different RfDs for infants the starting point for their calculations was the same in each case: the EPA Office of Drinking Water's 1986 derivation of the MCLG (4 ppm). If readers are puzzled as to how the EPA in good conscience could derive three different end points beginning with the same starting point, so are we!

This is how the EPA Pesticide division says it did this.

In the *first* health risk assessment, it assumed that the RfD for children was the same as adults: 0.114 mg/kg/day. The latter is obtained by dividing the so-called "safe dose" for adults used in the 1986 derivation of the MCLG (8 mg/day) by an adult's bodyweight of 70 kg. 8 mg/day divided by 70 kg = 0.114 mg/kg/day.

In the *second* health risk assessment (after FAN intervened and had shown that some children are already exceeding this dosage of 0.114 mg/kg/day) the EPA used a different approach in order to derive a different RfD for infants.

For this the EPA used a back-calculation from the notion that if 4 ppm fluoride in water would be safe for everyone, then it would also be safe for a 7-kg infant. Assuming such an infant consumed one liter of water per day, the EPA estimated that it was safe for a 7-kg child to ingest dose of 4 mg/day (i.e. one liter of water at 4 ppm contains 4 mg of fluoride). Dividing 4 mg/day by an infant's bodyweight of 7 kg would yield a RfD of 0.57 mg/kg/day. This is now *five* times the RfD for an adult.

In the *third* health risk assessment, after FAN, EWG, and BP had intervened again, the EPA assumed that if 8 mg/day was safe for a 70-kg adult it was *also* safe for a 7-kg infant. Such an assumption flies in the face of basic toxicology and common sense. It is akin to saying that if 1000 mg/day of aspirin is safe for an adult it is *also* safe for an infant. This is patently absurd. However, it allowed the EPA to derive a third RfD for infants even higher than the previous ones. If one divides 8 mg/day of fluoride by the bodyweight of an infant (7 kg) one arrives at an RfD for infants of 1.14 mg/kg/day, which is now *ten* times the RfD for an adult!

All this was done, we believe, in an effort to set very high tolerance levels for fluoride residues left by the use of Dow AgroSciences' sulfuryl fluoride fumigant on food in warehouses and processing plants. Protecting Dow's interests was apparently more important than protecting the health of babies or infants. FAN, EWG, and BP continue to appeal the EPA's approval of the new fluoride tolerance limits for sulfuryl fluoride use based on these highly dubious calcuations. Because of the long time that the EPA has taken in responding to several appeals on this matter, it is expected that the issue will end up in court.

As a consequence of these scientifically unjustifiable manipulations of the reference dose for infants, the EPA's permitted tolerances (i.e., of fluoride residues left after sulfuryl fluoride treatment) have risen from the previous level of 7 ppm (used for cryolite applications on fruit and vegetables) to levels on over six hundred foods (and many more if we include processed foods) that range from a low of 5 ppm for dried raisins to a high of 125 ppm for wheat flour.[66] Since wheat flour is used in everything from cakes to pizza dough, these tolerances will greatly increase the total dose of fluoride that the average American gets from all sources combined. In this last application for increased tolerances the EPA permitted Dow to have a tolerance (i.e., residue) of 900 ppm fluoride on powdered eggs. Not surprisingly this tolerance appears to have been withdrawn because as FAN pointed out even a modest consumption of eggs at this level could make someone acutely ill.

Summary

Proponents tend to use phrases like "high doses" and "not relevant to water fluoridation at 1 ppm" to dismiss concerns about harm caused by fluoride in areas endemic for fluorosis, arguing that the relatively high doses in these studies make the results irrelevant for exposures at 1 ppm concentration. They seldom discuss the concept of *margin of safety*, which is absolutely essential to determine a safe dose sufficient to protect everyone in society from a substance known to cause harm. When government agencies have been forced to address the margin-of-safety issue for fluoride's adverse health effects, they have invariably used safety factors that cannot be defended scientifically. In addition, they have often violated the very procedures they used in permitting or regulating other chemicals or pollutants. The worst example of an unacceptable manipulation of science in this respect has come from the EPA's Office of Pesticides in the help it has given Dow AgroScience in its efforts to use sulfuryl fluoride as a fumigant on food in warehouses and processing plants. Just as fluoride has been dubbed the "protected pollutant," we can now add that water fluoridation is the "protected practice" and sulfuryl fluoride is the "protected fumigant."

All of this represents very poor science. We return in chapter 22 to other examples of the dubious calculations that have characterized the promotion of fluoridation for over sixty years.

• 21 •

The Precautionary Principle

The precautionary principle (PP) has come into play, particularly in Europe, because it has been found that in the time it takes to get definitive, scientific proof that a chemical or practice has caused harm, the health of some people has been damaged irreversibly. This was the case with lead, benzene, asbestos, and smoking. The PP acknowledges this problem and posits the notion that when there is reasonable doubt about safety, we should err on the side of caution and *not* insist on absolute evidence of harm before eliminating or rejecting a substance or practice.

Joel Tickner and Melissa Coffin state the PP clearly: "If there is uncertainty, yet credible scientific evidence or concern of threats to health, precautionary measures should be taken. In other words, preventive action should be taken on early warnings even though the nature and magnitude of the risk are not fully understood."[1]

For more on the PP, readers may wish to consult the book *Protecting Public Health and the Environment: Implementing the Precautionary Principle.*[2]

Applying the Precautionary Principle

Use of the PP is not without its critics, especially from those who fear that blanket use of the principle could block any form of industrial or economic development.[3-5] Clearly, unless the PP is to stymie progress, it should not be applied in a cavalier fashion; certain criteria should be met before it is invoked. We offer the following criteria to be considered in the case of water fluoridation:

1. *Is the risk of harm plausible?* YES. There is no adequate margin of safety for known detrimental health effects at moderate to high doses sufficient to protect everyone consuming fluoridated water and fluoride from other sources (see chapter 20).

2. *Is the evidence of harm supported by a number of peer-reviewed, published studies?* YES. Many such studies are reviewed in the 2006 NRC report[6] (see chapters 14–19).

3. *Is the potential harm serious?* YES. Arthritis affects about 46 million Americans. Hip fractures are very serious for the elderly and can lead to a permanent loss of independence and even to an early death (see chapter 17). Hypothyroidism brings with it a litany of problems, including lethargy, depression, and obesity (see chapter 16). Lowering IQ in children has serious consequences both for individuals, by robbing them of their full potential, and for society, by reducing the number of highly intelligent people and increasing the number of mentally handicapped (see chapter 15). Even the one adverse effect that is not denied by proponents—dental fluorosis—can lead to a loss of self-esteem, especially in teenagers (see chapter 11).

4. *Are the effects reversible?* MANY ARE NOT. A change in the intellectual development of a child in his early years cannot be erased. Fluoride steadily accumulates in the bone over a lifetime of exposure. If the source of fluoride is removed, the fluoride will gradually leave the bone, but the estimated half-life is very long, up to twenty years (see chapter 12). Treatment is possible for a fractured hip bone, but it can be difficult for the patient to make a full recovery.

5. *Is the public being fully informed of the potential health risks?* NO. The very opposite is occurring. Spokespersons for local, state, and federal health agencies deny any health risks at all.

6. *Does the proposed intervention achieve the desired benefit?* QUESTIONABLE. As we saw in chapters 6–8, the evidence that swallowing fluoride actually reduces decay in the permanent teeth is weak.

7. *How significant are the consequences if the practice is halted?* NOT VERY. At least four modern studies conducted in Finland, East Germany, Cuba, and British Columbia found that in communities that stopped fluoridation, tooth decay rates did not go up (see chapter 2).

8. *Are there alternatives?* YES. The vast majority of European countries do not fluoridate their water, and yet, according to World Health Organization figures, their children's teeth are as good if not better than children's teeth in fluoridating countries.

In summary, all these sensible criteria for applying the PP to the implementation of fluoridation are easily met.

The Precautionary Principle and Fluoridation

In the March 2006 issue of the *Journal of Evidence-Based Dental Practice,* Tickner and Coffin examined the water fluoridation controversy in the context of the PP. According to those authors, the PP has become a core guiding principle of environmental health regulations in Europe. They noted, "The need for precaution arises because the costs of inaction in the face of uncertainty can be high, and paid at the expense of sound public health."[7]

They wrote that when determining whether the PP should be applied to fluoridation, one should consider the following questions:

- Whether there are other ways of delivering fluoride besides the water supply
- Whether fluoride needs to be swallowed to prevent tooth decay
- Whether tooth decay has dropped at the same rate in countries with and without water fluoridation
- Whether people are now receiving fluoride from many other sources besides the water supply
- Whether studies indicate fluoride's potential to cause a range of adverse systemic health effects
- Whether, since fluoridation affects so many people, "one might accept a lower level of proof before taking preventive actions"[8]

While the authors never state their personal opinion on water fluoridation, their analysis confirms our view that the practice is incompatible with the PP.

Summary

In advance of any application of the precautionary principle, it is important to lay out and make transparent the important criteria that first need to be satisfied. We, as well as specialists in the field, have done this, and it is clear that the practice of water fluoridation is a violation of the precautionary principle on all the criteria presented.

PART SIX

The Promoters and the Techniques of Promotion

In chapter 22, we summarize the evidence, much of it covered in earlier chapters, that fluoridation has been propagated for over sixty years using poor science. In chapter 23, we examine some of the promoters' strategies and tactics that have kept this outdated policy alive for so many years. In chapter 24, we critique some of the self-serving reviews commissioned or conducted by pro-fluoridation government agencies. In chapter 25, we identify and respond to the "chestnuts" used to promote fluoridation, along with less frivolous arguments. In chapter 26, we venture into the very tricky area of trying to understand what motivates the proponents of fluoridation.

• 22 •

Weak and Inadequate Science

We saw in chapters 6–8 that evidence for the notion that swallowing fluoride (as opposed to applying it topically) reduces tooth decay is very weak. The exaggerated claims of fluoridation's benefits have been supported by very dubious science, but the matter does not stop there; poor science has characterized the whole promotion and defense of the fluoridation program over its long history. Some of this we discussed in chapters 9 and 10, where we saw how little science existed on the safety of fluoridation before the U.S. Public Health Service (PHS) endorsed it in 1950, a decision that was a key step in the Great Fluoridation Gamble. That gamble was based on the *belief* that somehow ingested fluoride could damage the growing tooth (causing dental fluorosis) without damaging any other tissue in the body, even the delicate tissues of a newborn baby.

After the PHS endorsed fluoridation in 1950, other professional bodies swiftly followed with their own endorsements. Promoters have used those endorsements as a substitute for well-conducted science ever since. In the following paragraphs we discuss several other examples of the poor science, evasions of science, and poor administration used to promote and defend fluoridation.

The Food and Drug Administration has not been involved.

Today, before a new drug can be approved by the Food and Drug Administration (FDA) for clinical use, it must be rigorously tested for efficacy in randomized clinical trials (RCT). Such trials have been recognized for many years as being the only scientifically reliable way to determine whether a drug actually works. No such requirement existed when fluoridation was introduced in the 1940s and the methodology of testing was haphazard and superficial by modern standards (see chapter 7). Even the conditions and criteria that were put in place for the early fluoridation trials were not always adhered to. Even if those trials had been meticulously conducted, it would have been impossible to exclude a range of possible confounding variables.

In the light of such shortcomings, it is astonishing that, sixty years later, the efficacy of ingested fluoride in preventing dental caries has *never* been tested in an RCT. Nor, as we saw in chapter 2, has the FDA taken any active interest in fluoride, possibly the most extensively taken drug in history.

Another thing the FDA requires when drugs are approved is tracking reports of their possible side effects. Had the FDA been involved at any stage, it would have had to tabulate the many accounts of individuals complaining of fairly common symptoms (e.g., tiredness not relieved by sleep, headaches, rashes, and gastrointestinal problems) that were easily reversed when the source of fluoride was removed (see chapter 13). Had the FDA tracked these complaints, at some point it might have felt obliged to review the issue scientifically. Remarkably, no health agency in the United States or any of the other fluoridated countries has pursued this.

Fluoride exposure is poorly monitored.

There has never been a comprehensive analysis of the fluoride levels in the bones, blood, or urine of citizens in the United States or other fluoridated countries. Based on the sparse data that have become available, however, it is increasingly evident that some people, particularly people with kidney disease, are accumulating fluoride levels in their bones that have been associated with harm to both animals and humans (chapter 18).

In 1991, a panel of the Australian National Health and Medical Research Council (NHMRC) recommended that measurements of fluoride levels in bone be collected. In its recommendation, the panel wrote, "If skeletal fluorosis is occurring at all in Australians, it is likely to be slight, and it will most likely occur in those who drink large amounts of water, or whose renal function is impaired. Studies of bone fluoride collected at autopsy in selected individuals could provide needed reassurance that the current policy is not resulting in hazardous levels of accumulation in bone."[1] In the nineteen years since that recommendation was made, no Australian health authority has sought such reassurance.

Measuring fluoride in urine is a much easier task than measuring fluoride in bone, and yet even that simple procedure to gauge exposure, and overexposure, is not performed on a routine basis in fluoridated countries. When measurements have been made by independent researchers, such as Dr. Peter Mansfield in the UK, the results have been disturbing.[2] Mansfield has found that some urine levels are very high in the UK, perhaps because the British drink a lot of tea, but no one is checking urine fluoride levels in other fluoridating countries, and some of those (e.g., Australia, Ireland, and New Zealand) also have heavy tea drinkers. Someone needs to find out what the total exposure of fluoride is in those countries from all sources (including tea), and the simplest and quickest way to do that would be to measure the fluoride levels in urine.

Few basic health studies have been done in fluoridated communities.

One of the most shocking aspects of the promotion of fluoridation is the failure of the DHHS and health authorities promoting fluoridation in other countries to study, in a comprehensive fashion, the health of individuals and communities that have been exposed to fluoridated water, whether for relatively short periods or over a lifetime.

In chapter 5, we quote Trevor Sheldon's comment from a letter to the House of Lords about there being "a dearth of reliable evidence with which to inform policy"[3] and the surprise of Dr. John Doull (2006 NRC panel chair) at how "we have much less information [on health issues] than we should, considering how long this [fluoridation] has been going on."[4] Note that these comments from independent observers were made fifty-one and fifty-eight years, respectively, after the DHHS endorsed fluoridation.

To be more specific, no studies have been carried out in the United States or most other fluoridating countries to investigate possible relationships between fluoridation and the following:

- *Lowered IQ in children*, even though twenty-three studies published in four different countries have now found an association between moderate and high fluoride exposure and lowered IQ in children (see chapter 15)
- *Alzheimer's disease in adults*, even though one study showed that rats given water containing 1 ppm of fluoride for one year had a greater uptake of aluminum into their brains and the formation of beta-amyloid deposits, which are associated with Alzheimer's disease[5]
- *Lowered thyroid function*, even though doctors used to give fluoride to patients to lower thyroid activity, and millions of Americans today suffer from hypothyroidism or subclinical hypothyroidism, in which there occurs an abnormally low level of thyroid hormone without clinical symptoms or signs (see chapter 16)
- *Increased arthritis rates in adults*, even though an estimated 46 million Americans have arthritis, and the first symptoms of poisoning of the bones by fluoride are identical to the first symptoms of arthritis (see chapter 17)
- *Bone fractures in children*, even though the first health study of children exposed to fluoridation[6] showed an increase in cortical bone defects and a study from Mexico[7] showed a positive linear correlation between the severity of dental fluorosis (a biomarker of fluoride exposure before the permanent teeth have erupted) and the frequency of bone fractures

in children (see chapter 17; although the Mexican study had method-ological weaknesses, its approach of using dental fluorosis as a simple and noninvasive biomarker was sound [see the following section], and authorities in fluoridating countries should have attempted to repeat at least that aspect of the study)

- *Lowered melatonin levels and earlier onset of puberty*, even though it has been shown that fluoride accumulates in the human pineal gland,[8] and lowered melatonin levels commensurate with earlier onset of puberty have been observed in animals exposed to fluoride from birth,[9] and the earlier onset of menstruation was observed in the fluoridated population in the Newburgh-Kingston trial (see chapters 10 and 16)
- *Irritable bowel syndrome*, and the many other common complaints that, in some individuals, apparently are triggered by fluoride exposure (see chapter 13)

Dental fluorosis is not used as a biomarker in epidemiological studies to investigate the effect of fluoride on children.

It is well known that the severity of dental fluorosis indicates the level of overexposure to fluoride in children prior to the eruption of their secondary teeth. This presents an ideal—and *obvious*—biometric measure of exposure for epidemiological studies on children, as illustrated by the Mexican study on bone fractures discussed in chapter 17.[10] We are not aware of any studies in fluoridated countries, with the single exception of Morgan et al.,[11] that have used that biometric measure.

Animal and biochemical studies are largely discounted.

Many reviews of the fluoridation issue exclude any consideration of animal or biochemical studies. Yet these are routinely used by toxicologists to tease out the potential harmful effects of a suspected toxic substance. The only recent review by an agency in a fluoridated country that has considered animal and biochemical studies was done by the U.S. National Research Council[12] (see chapter 14).

What animal and biochemical studies do is help establish the biological plausibility of epidemiological findings. Thus, they provide a valuable contri-bution to a weight-of-evidence analysis. Clearly, such an analysis is more likely to be meaningful to authorities who have some sympathy for the precaution-ary principle (chapter 21), as opposed to those who insist on absolute proof of harm before acting.

More effort has gone into studying fluoride's impact on the teeth than on any other tissue.

A vast proportion of the budgets assigned to studying the effects of fluoride in fluoridated countries has gone into studying its effects on the teeth. For example, in the UK in 2002, a committee appointed by the Medical Research Council (MRC) to follow up on the York Review[13] recommended a higher priority for further research on dental fluorosis than for research on the possible effects of fluoride on the brain, the endocrine system, or the kidneys.[14] It made no recommendation to attempt to replicate the IQ studies carried out in China, even though several of those studies had already appeared in English[15–18] and other studies referenced in them had been published in Chinese journals. Nor did it recommend studies on the pineal gland, even though it was well aware of Luke's work in that field.[19, 20]

Less effort has gone into replicating studies that found harm than into discrediting them.

Fluoridated countries have spent more time and money in attempts to discredit the methodologies of studies that have found harm than on any effort to replicate the findings. A classic example of this occurred in February 2009, when the Strategic Health Authority (SHA), pushing for fluoridation in Southampton in the UK, hired a firm of consultants with extensive experience in government work, Bazian Ltd., to handle eighteen studies that demonstrate a lowering of IQ associated with moderate to high exposure to fluoride, provided to the SHA by Paul Connett, and to dismiss the relevance of the 2006 NRC review[21, 22, 23] (see chapters 14 and 15).

No effort has been made to follow up claims by many individuals that they are sensitive to fluoride.

Proponents of fluoridation have tended to treat the issue of fluoride sensitivity as only a possible allergic reaction and not as a response to a toxic substance. Health agencies in fluoridating countries have made no effort to pursue this matter scientifically even when urged to do so by independent observers and bodies like the Australian National Health and Medical Research Council in 1991[24] (see chapter 13). Most doctors are apparently unaware that a problem of sensitivity to fluoride exists.

Key health studies have been entrusted to researchers in dental schools, who have a bias in the matter.

When fluoridating countries finance studies on health concerns—for example, the possible relationship between fluoridation and hip fractures or bone cancer in young men—such studies are frequently given to dental schools, which clearly have a conflict of interest in this matter. To their credit, some dental researchers (e.g., Luke, Li, and Bassin) have risen above their "loyalty" to the fluoridation program and have objectively reported adverse effects.[25-28] But that has not always been the case, and when a huge amount of government funding is at stake, more care should be taken to make sure that those who are funded do not have an obvious vested interest in the outcome. The dangers are clearly illustrated in chapter 18, where it is pointed out that the U.S. National Institute of Environmental Heath Sciences (NIEHS) funded a known fluoridation advocate, Professor Chester Douglass, to investigate the very sensitive issue of a possible relationship between osteosarcoma and exposure to fluoridated water.

When studies find harm, promoters try to discredit either the author or the methodology used.

When studies finding evidence of harm do emerge in fluoridated countries, often efforts have been made to prevent their publication or, if that does not work, to attack the methodology (often privately) or undermine the credibility of the primary author. Such was the experience of George Waldbott, Alfred Taylor, Ionel Rapoport, and others in the United States.[29] The response sometimes goes as far as termination of employment, as in the case of Dr. Phyllis Mullenix (see chapter 15). Such tactics, incidentally, are by no means limited to fluoridation; they are quite characteristic of areas where science impinges on powerful political and financial interests.[30]

The American Dental Association dismisses all *evidence of harm.*

In the fluoridation promotion piece of the American Dental Association (ADA) titled *Fluoride Facts,* nearly every piece of evidence indicating harm is described as not meeting "generally accepted scientific knowledge."[31] However, the ADA has violated normal scientific procedures again and again. One violation is the manner in which the ADA dismissed the work of Dr. Stan Freni.

After reviewing the many animal studies indicating that fluoride affected the reproductive system, a subject he reviewed for the important Department of Health and Human Services report of 1991,[32] Freni decided to compare fertility rates in counties in the United States as a function of fluoride levels in the drinking water. He found that fertility rates were lower in counties with

3 ppm or more fluoride in their water. His conclusion was that this might be relevant to water fluoridation of 1 ppm when that is factored into the total dose of fluoride a person might ingest from all sources.[33]

This is how the ADA handled Freni's finding: "One human study compared county birth data with county fluoride levels greater than 3 ppm and attempted to show an association between high fluoride levels in drinking water and lower birth rates.(271) However, because of serious limitations in design and analysis, the investigation failed to demonstrate a positive correlation.(272)"[34] Reference 272 is a "personal communication" from Thomas Sinks dated two years before Freni's paper was published. Sink's critique was never sent to Freni for his response.[35]

Another example of the ADA's unscientific behavior was its eagerness to dismiss the relevance to water fluoridation of the 2006 507-page National Research Council review[36] on the very day it was published[37] (see chapter 14). The CDC followed suit six days later.[38] Neither body had had the time to review the scientific analysis within the report thoroughly.

On safety, fluoridation promoters work backward.

Time and again fluoridation promoters like the ADA and the CDC give the impression that they are working backward from the firm belief that fluoride at 1 ppm *cannot possibly (and must not)* do any harm to health.

The normal application of the scientific method requires the scientist to collect data, propose an explanation for any apparent relationship (this is called developing a hypothesis), and then test the hypothesis by making predictions, which are tested by further data collection (experiments). If the further data continue to be consistent with the hypothesis, then it is elevated to the status of theory. Even at that point, to paraphrase Thomas Huxley, an ugly fact can destroy a beautiful theory.

In the case of water fluoridation, the hypothesis that drinking water at 1 ppm was both safe and effective was quickly elevated to an accepted theory and, within the pro-fluoridation establishment, became virtually inscribed in stone as an irrefutable "law" when the U.S. Public Health Service endorsed the practice in 1950 (see chapters 9 and 10). Since then proponents have appeared to work in the opposite direction from true scientists. They start with the conclusion that fluoridation is safe and effective and simply leave out the hypotheses and the experiments. In other words, fluoridation is not a public health policy based on science so much as a practice propagated as a "belief system."

Absence of study *is used to imply* absence of harm.

It has been clear from the very beginning of fluoridation of public water systems that not *sound science* but a *dearth of science* has been used to demonstrate safety. For example, in 1952, Dr. John Knutson stated that the best evidence that fluoridation was safe was the fact that millions of people had been drinking naturally occurring fluoride in their water without visible signs of harm[39] (see chapter 10). The same notion was repeated by Harold Hodge in 1963.[40] Such assertions, however, are based on anecdotal, not scientific, evidence. Even today, promoters trivialize the issue by implying that the *absence of study* is the same as *absence of harm.* For example, in April 2007, Dr. Peter Cooney, the chief dental officer for Canada, told an audience in Dryden, Ontario, that, although Dryden had been fluoridated for forty years, he had walked down the town's main street that afternoon and did not see anyone "growing horns."[41]

Summary

We have summarized a long list of examples of the poor science involved in promoting and protecting the fluoridation program. These include the use of endorsements in place of scientific evidence; the failure to involve a proper regulator such as the FDA; the poor monitoring of the accumulation of fluoride in the bones of individuals exposed to fluoride; the paucity of basic health studies in fluoridated communities; the failure to use dental fluorosis as a biomarker in epidemiological studies, especially on health effects in children; the frequent discounting of animal and biochemical studies; the excessive attention to studies on teeth while other tissues are largely ignored; the efforts to discredit any study that finds harm; the lack of concern for those who appear to be particularly sensitive to fluoride; the granting of highly sensitive studies such as those of osteosarcoma and hip fractures to dental schools rather than independent researchers; and the assumption that an absence of study means absence of harm.

The many activities of the ADA and other promoters appear to flow backward from the notion that fluoridation has been *ordained* safe and effective and that any evidence to the contrary must be flawed in some way. These examples of poor science are best explained by the need to protect the program at all costs. We discuss some of the possible motivations behind this unscientific stance in chapter 26. In the next chapter, we review the tactics used by fluoridation promoters, tactics that merely underline their inability to prove their case scientifically. If the science were in their favor, many of their tactics would be unnecessary.

Promoters' Strategies and Tactics

We have seen in the course of this book how poor the science is that promoters claim supports the notion that fluoridation is an acceptable medical practice and is both *safe* and *effective*. At this point, we expect that many of our readers are left wondering how on earth the promoters of this program have been able to get away with that claim for over sixty years. There are two simple one-word answers to that question: power and prestige. The promoters have the political power of the U.S. government (and the governments of other countries where fluoridation is practiced), and they have the prestige that goes with professional bodies and professional status. They exercise this power and prestige through two chains of command, as we outline below. The overarching strategy that proponents use to protect the fluoridation program is to exploit these two chains of command to keep the media, decision makers, and dental, medical, and other professionals away from the primary scientific literature.

The Chains of Command

The two chains of command that relentlessly promote fluoridation are the government's public health service network and the national dental association's professional network. One reaches down to every state health department and eventually every local governmental health official. The other reaches down to every state and local dental association and thence to nearly every dentist.

Once these chains of command were captured at the top (which occurred in the United States in 1950; see chapters 9 and 10), fluoridation-promotion policy could move down from their headquarters to every town in every fluoridating country. Moreover, each chain of command is self-perpetuating. Since 1950, the belief system that supports water fluoridation (it has never been based on science; see chapters 9, 10, and 22) has been passed on to each new generation of dentists and public health bureaucrats. Most courses at dental schools and public health programs do not challenge the dogma of the "safety and effectiveness" of fluoridation. Fluoridation is promoted as a crusade. Within the links of the governmental and dental chains of command, it seems to be the norm to accept recommendations from above, almost without question. In fact, to question policy, especially that of fluoridation, is not a healthy move for career advancement.

We see here the potential of a handful of people to influence the actions and opinions of a vast number of public health, dental, and medical professionals in their own countries and around the world. What makes this disturbing is that the vast majority of rank-and-file professionals have little time to examine the issue for themselves, at least not in detail. Moreover, those who do and speak out against fluoridation are treated so badly it discourages others from following suit. By and large, the dentists and doctors at the bottom end of these chains of command believe, or behave as though they believe, what they are told either by their parent government health body or by their professional organization. There is very little independent or rational discussion or intervention. Self-serving reviews by government agencies also go a long way to convince even intelligent, but busy, professionals that fluoridation is safe and effective and keep them in line (see chapter 24). Sadly, despite lacking firsthand knowledge of the issue, many seem to have little problem repeating the "safe and effective" mantra in public.

Together or separately, the two chains of command can generate letters to the editor, fund a PR campaign, provide a small group to lobby newspaper editors behind closed doors, or turn out a posse of dentists and health officials in any community where fluoridation is newly proposed or threatened.

Two Personal Stories
Two stories from Paul Connett's experience illustrate prestige and power in action at each end of the chain of command.

Prestige at the Bottom of the Chain of Command
The first story emerged on the very first day of Paul Connett's involvement with this issue nearly fourteen years ago. In July 1996, at a meeting of the Canton, New York, village board, Dr. Connett heard local citizens say that although they weren't scientists, they "trusted" their doctor on the safety of fluoridation. After the meeting, Dr. Connett offered copies of three scientific articles to one such doctor who happened to be present. He refused to take the copies, saying that he did not have time to read the literature. What was troubling to Dr. Connett was not just that the doctor was unwilling to read the articles, but that he was quite content to have the public trust his judgment on a matter for which he was not prepared to do the research.

Power at the Top of the Chain of Command

The second experience came when Dr. Connett met Dr. Robert Hall, chief health officer for Victoria, Australia. When Connett asked if Hall had read the "50 Reasons to Oppose Fluoridation" statement[1] he had sent ahead of the meeting, Hall responded that he had but it had not changed his opinion on fluoridation. When Connett asked him if he would provide a written response to the "50 Reasons," Hall replied, "Neither I, nor my staff, have any intention of doing that." Adding irony to Dr. Hall's refusal was the fact that the Victoria government had hired a public relations company to produce a booklet providing answers to "frequently asked questions on fluoridation." Clearly, the health department was better at answering its own "selected" questions than real questions from opponents.

The Tactics Examined

Various tactics have been used regularly by the two chains of command to keep doctors, dentists, scientists, the media, and decision makers away from the science that shows that fluoridation is neither safe nor effective. Moreover, even when local officials are skeptical about fluoridation, they are easily intimidated when professionals from the community turn out in force. We discuss some of these tactics in the sections that follow.

Promoters use the authority of endorsements.

Fluoridation is promoted today just as it was nearly sixty years ago: with endorsements. These endorsements, however, are highly suspect. As shown in chapter 9, when the U.S. Public Health Service (PHS) endorsed fluoridation in 1950, it was mainly reacting to political pressure. Even though the supporting science was weak, many professional associations, including the American Dental Association (ADA), the American Public Health Association (APHA), and the American Medical Association (AMA), quickly followed suit, still without solid scientific evidence that the practice was safe or effective (see chapter 10). Between 1950 and 1960 the endorsements kept rolling in, and today the ADA boasts a list of nearly one hundred organizations that endorse fluoridation.[2]

While it is clear that these organizations have mobilized very little science of any substance to support their endorsements, for many people, who do not have the time to study the details of this issue for themselves, the strategy of using endorsements is very effective.

Emblematic of the subservience to authority is the use made of the statement by the Centers for Disease Control and Prevention (CDC), mentioned previously, that fluoridation is one of the "ten great public health achievements" of the twentieth century.[3] Hardly a day goes by without this being cited somewhere in the world by a journalist, editor, or government official. The statement provides a very convenient shield behind which proponents, including those who have not read a word of the primary literature, can conveniently hide.

However, if those who so casually bandy this statement around spent a little time reading the supporting document,[4] they would be surprised to find how little substance there is behind that lofty declaration.[5] For example, the CDC document ignored all published studies from 1993–1999 that reported adverse effects, citing a single review that was already six years old when the CDC statement was issued in 1999.[6] Moreover, the evidence offered for effectiveness would have made an undergraduate blush (compare figures 6.1 and 6.2). But the CDC gets away with it because the agency has authority. Whether it deserves to be considered an authority on fluoridation is a different matter. Most people are unaware of how biased the CDC is on this matter.

The media are easily taken in by proponents' authority.

What makes this situation dangerous is that, while they may not be well informed on the matter, dentists and doctors are highly influential in their local communities. Their opinions are usually taken as gospel by the local media, decision makers, and members of the public. In a 1979 white paper produced by its Council on Dental Health and Health Planning,[7] the ADA illustrated the powerful influence that the authority of local dentists and other health professionals has on the media when it quoted the editor-in-chief of the *Winona [Minnesota] Daily News*, which published features and editorials favorable to fluoridation:

> Historically on the area scene, the dental society has been the pioneer and leader among the professional groups in communicating to the public helpful information in its professional area of responsibility. We have always tried to cooperate . . . The decade-ago campaign for fluoridation had our support not so much because we favored it, but because the dental society had established credibility with us and with the community.[8]

Even when local officials are skeptical about fluoridation, they are easily intimidated when local media support it and disparage those who oppose it.

The vast majority of people innocently believe that their doctor, their dentist, and the CDC, ADA, and AMA would not promote this practice unless they had studied the issue long and hard and were *certain* it was safe and effective. However, "certainty" in the absence of knowledge should carry no weight.

The unsatisfactory situation in which authority trumps rational argument is made even worse when local journalists are prepared to do little more than quote one sentence from each side, especially if one of those sentences is the infamous CDC quote above.

The promoters' interests are served in two ways by the media. First, few journalists go deeper than a superficial treatment, frequently giving deference to the proponents' presumed authority. Second, proponents make a special effort to get one-on-one sessions with editors. The resulting editorials can be so one-sided and derogatory of opponents of fluoridation that they can be truly disheartening to those who have worked hard to make a more balanced and objective assessment of the science available to the public. Of course, the opponents' case is not helped by a handful of people who talk about fluoridation as a "plot to limit world population." Their unsubstantiated passion serves to make the white-coated supporters of fluoridation look very reasonable indeed. It also makes it more difficult for the scientific case *against* fluoridation to get a hearing.

Promoters denigrate and intimidate opponents.

Hand in hand with elevation of the authority of the promoters goes the denigration of opponents. Denigrating fluoridation opponents is not hard to do if the unscrupulous proponents focus on the hysterical fringe of the antifluoridation movement and ignore the rational majority. In 1976 Dr. Stephen Barrett, the director of DentalWatch and Quackwatch, described opponents of fluoridation as "poison-mongers."[9] The label is ironic when one considers that opponents are largely unpaid—indeed, many have to dig deep into their own pockets to oppose this practice—have nothing to "monger" (sell), and are trying to take a poison out of the water, not put it in!

DentalWatch Online posts a paper dated 1999 by Michael Easley, DDS, MPH, a member of the advisory board of the American Council of Science and Health (see chapter 26), in which he variously describes opponents as "health terrorists," "fluorophobics," and "antiscience messengers" and accuses them of using "innuendo," "half-truths," "scare words," and "The Big Lie." He declares, "Like parasites, opponents steal undeserved credibility just by sharing the stage with respected scientists who are there to defend fluoridation."[10]

Easley takes the argument one step further and aims an intimidating warning to dentists and doctors not to step out of line on this matter when he adds: "Unfortunately, a most flagrant abuse of the public trust occasionally occurs when a physician or a dentist, for whatever personal reason, uses their professional standing in the community to argue against fluoridation, a clear violation of professional ethics, the principles of science and community standards of practice."[11]

Abusive and intimidating language is the last refuge of those who are unable to argue credibly, and it was such language that made Paul Connett realize, quite early in his efforts to examine both sides of the issue, that there must be something wrong with the proponents' case.[12]

Promoters claim there is no debate.

In October 2009, Colleen Wulf of the Ohio Department of Health explained to a councilor in Athens, Ohio, why she would not debate Dr. Paul Connett:

> Our reasoning for not participating in debates on fluoridation is simple. Debates give the illusion that a scientific controversy exists. All major dental and public health associations . . . support the practice of fluoridation. Community water fluoridation has been recognized as one of the ten great public health achievements of the 20th century. Debates and public hearings give the vocal minority a forum to spread misinformation and fear.[13]

But no scientific subject is ever beyond debate. There is always the possibility that an ugly fact will destroy a beautiful theory. As the French writer Joseph Joubert (1754–1824) wrote, "It is better to debate an issue without resolving it, than to resolve an issue without debating it."

In Australia, the Victoria government has posted on its Web site the following explanation as to why it will not debate the issue:

> The Department of Human Services, along with key partners, including the Australian Dental Association and Dental Health Services Victoria, are unanimously of the view that public debates about water fluoridation, including debates about the relative scientific merits of particular pieces of research, provide little or no value to members of the public with a genuine interest in learning more about water fluoridation.[14]

The alternative it offers consists of professionally produced leaflets that give only one side of the issue. When asked to respond to specific questions from opponents, the department refuses to do so. For example, after over nine months, Dr. John Carnie, chief health officer of the Victoria Department of Human Services, has failed to respond to eight specific questions posed to him by nineteen professionals, that were published in an open letter in the newspaper of a community threatened with forced fluoridation.[15]

Promoters discourage professionals from investigating this matter for themselves, even while actively encouraging them to promote the practice.

The American Dental Association gave some extraordinary advice to its members in the same 1979 white paper cited above. The ADA Council on Dental Health and Health Planning wrote, "Individual dentists must be convinced that they need not be familiar with scientific reports and field investigations on fluoridation to be effective participants and that non-participation is overt neglect of professional responsibility."[16]

We are sure that many readers are shocked to learn that the ADA believes that professionals need not be on top of their subject to promote a practice that has the potential to affect the health of millions. Such an upside-down definition of *professionalism* would be more appropriate in *Alice in Wonderland* than in a communication to members of a professional organization.

Promoters make declarative statements about the "safety" and "effectiveness" of fluoridation without citing the primary literature.

One of the key features of propaganda is repetition. It is very noticeable in their public statements on fluoridation how frequently promoters use the phrase "safe and effective," as if saying this enough times would make it so. Normally, a listener might anticipate that such declarations would be accompanied by scientific evidence, but it is one of the beauties of "authority" that as long as a proponent is wearing a white coat or holds a high office, and he makes his assertions with confidence, many people will believe him.

An interesting example of an "official" declarative statement is in a short video clip by Dr. Poul Erik Petersen, the oral health director for the World Health Organization's Department of Chronic Diseases and Health Promotion. The video was released at the time of the Chicago celebration by the ADA and the CDC of the sixtieth anniversary of fluoridation in July 2005. In a nutshell, this four-minute video exemplifies the problem faced by those trying to stop fluoridation. Apparently decent, intelligent, and caring professionals who hold important positions, like Dr. Petersen, can look the camera straight in the lens and make categorical claims about the safety and effectiveness of fluoridation without blinking an eye. This video can be viewed online.[17]

Maybe Petersen and others promoting fluoridation actually believe what they are saying. Whether they do or not, however, they seldom feel the need to back up their comments with references to the primary literature or express the slightest reservation about what they are recommending. They issue no caveats; they suggest no doubts. The program is promoted with absolute confidence and certainty. Such certainty simply does not exist on any scientific question. But certainty is important when a policy is being aggressively promoted. Promotion does not sit well with uncertainty (see chapter 26).

Dental journals show little interest in publishing articles that indicate any dangers from fluoridation or editorials critical of the practice.

It is rare to see an article in a mainstream dental, medical, or even scientific journal challenging or criticizing fluoridation. Articles by Mark Diesendorf, Bette Hileman, and Dan Fagin provide some notable exceptions.[18-20]

Articles published in the journal Fluoride *are not listed in the search engine Medline/PubMed.*

Ironically, the one specialist journal, *Fluoride,* that deals with all aspects of fluoride research has not been readily available to mainstream readers of the medical or scientific literature. The International Society for Fluoride Research (ISFR), which publishes *Fluoride,* was set up in 1968 by Dr. George Waldbott (see chapter 13) as a forum for research on fluoride, particularly its biological effects. It is fair to say that both Waldbott and subsequent editors of the journal have been of an anti-fluoridation persuasion and have expressed that point of view in editorials. However, the editorial board covers a wide range of interests and includes a large representation from countries that have no interest in fluoridation but on the contrary suffer from an excess of fluoride in their groundwater.

The journal provides a platform for the publication in English of work from such countries, some of which, by documenting the harmful effects of naturally occurring fluoride, argue by implication against artificial fluoridation. (All articles published in *Fluoride* after 1998, and for several previous years, are available online to read or download at no cost.)[21] But many articles have little or no relevance to fluoridation. This has not stopped promoters of fluoridation from labeling the journal as an "anti-fluoridation magazine" and dismissing its entire contents. Many journals take editorial positions, but the editors of *Fluoride* have been careful of their own opposition to fluoridation and willing to publish well-written articles and guest editorials that take a pro-fluoridation position.

The real issue is that *Fluoride* carries a lot of information on fluoride's health effects that promoters prefer to keep hidden. For example, it was the first journal published in English to make available the IQ studies from China, and in two special issues it has recently published nineteen other articles on the brain, recently translated from the original Chinese versions (see chapter 15).

Several U.S. reports on fluoride published by the Agency for Toxic Substances and Disease Prevention;[22] the National Research Council of the National Academies;[23] and TOXNET,[24] hosted online by the U.S. Library of Medicine and the National Institutes of Health, cite papers published in *Fluoride*. The 2006 NRC review, the most important report on the toxicology of fluoride published in the United States, cited *Fluoride* more than any other journal.[25] But for whatever reason, *Fluoride* has been kept off the list covered by PubMed, the most popular online search engine of the medical literature (it is, however, covered by the Science Citation Index).

It is difficult to avoid the suspicion that the PubMed exclusion is an act of censorship, considering the hostility of powerful dental interests within the U.S. Department of Health and Human Services. Moreover, the exclusion smacks of a double standard when the same search engine covers dental journals such as *Dentistry Today*, which is considered by dentists as a trade magazine with little evidence of being a scientific journal.[26]

In general, promoters oppose local referenda on fluoridation and push for mandatory fluoridation on a statewide basis.

Proponents have learned that even with their huge budgets and some of the tactics identified above, it is difficult for them to win if the matter goes to referendum, especially if the press does a good job of covering both sides of the issue. Notable examples of where citizens have won victories against fluoridation, even though being vastly outspent by proponents, are Worcester, Massachusetts;[27] Bellingham, Washington;[28] and Juneau, Alaska.[29] Thus, over recent years, proponents in the United States have preferred to use their political and financial power to introduce mandatory fluoridation by legislation at the state level.

As indicated in chapter 1, we are conscious that local decisions by referendum are not ideal since they transfer to our neighbors a decision (consent to medication) that we should make as individuals. However, they are a large step better than mandatory statewide fluoridation, an oppressive measure that effectively bypasses any local discussion or control.

Recently, the Louisiana Dental Association (LDA) used both a high-powered PR firm and a lobbying firm to help pass a statewide mandatory fluoridation bill with very few citizens in Louisiana knowing what was happening. Only now are a small number of citizens finding out about it, a possibly ominous portent of what may occur in other states. According to the director of the LDA:

> "Tap Into a Healthier Smile" is the theme for the LDA's new public affairs campaign to broaden public, media and governmental awareness of the benefits of community water fluoridation and lay the groundwork for passing legislation in 2008 that could bring fluoridated water to virtually everyone in Louisiana.
>
> The campaign is a partnership with the ADA and part of the State-Based Public Affairs Program initiated by the ADA earlier this year. With ADA funding, the LDA has hired a leading Louisiana communications firm, Creative Communications, Inc. (CCI) from Baton Rouge, to direct the public relations aspects of the project. We've also engaged our lobbying firm, Roedel Parsons, et al., in a new, separate contract to handle the campaign's governmental relations aspect.[30]

While citizen groups have held off these attempts in the past, one wonders how long they can keep such efforts at bay. The two chains of command relentlessly renew themselves; dental schools keep producing wave after wave of new dentists who have heard only one side of the story; and in the United States each state health department has a dental director who spends a considerable amount of his or her time and budget promoting and defending fluoridation.

Currently, citizens in New Jersey, Oregon, and Pennsylvania are facing renewed attempts to introduce mandatory fluoridation in their states. Promoters are also preparing to push for mandatory fluoridation in several New England states, including Massachusetts.

The approach of going after a large jurisdiction rather than winning one community at a time also occurred recently in the state of Queensland, Australia. Since the 1960s, the majority of communities in the state (including the capital, Brisbane) have resisted fluoridation. Then, almost out of the blue, the newly appointed (not elected) premier of Queensland, Anna Bligh, announced that she was going to introduce mandatory fluoridation to the state. Her party has a large majority in parliament, so once the bill was introduced, it sailed through, even though the same party had voted against a similar bill introduced by the opposing party a few years before.[31]

Opponents of fluoridation in Queensland have been stunned at how fast they lost the whole state, when in the relatively recent past they were able to keep proposals out of their individual communities. Many believe that in this process they lost their democratic rights. Some are preparing to do battle on constitutional grounds.

Meanwhile, in other Australian states, particularly New South Wales and Victoria, equally authoritarian efforts are being made to force fluoridation on communities, even when those communities have made it clear that they do not want the measure. Wendy Varney has written an excellent book on fluoridation in Australia[32] and has recently updated her thoughts in an essay posted on the Web site of the Fluoride Action Network.[33]

In the UK the percentage of the population drinking fluoridated water held steady at about 10 percent for many years. Little expansion occurred because (1) most communities made it clear that they did not want the measure and (2) private water companies were fearful of liability.

Then in 2003, the Labor government passed a new Water Act that indemnified the private water companies against any lawsuits. According to a report in *The Guardian*, the government changed the law "to enable health chiefs to order, rather than request, water companies to add fluoride."[34] Moreover, the bill took the decision out of the hands of local councils and gave the sole authority to initiate fluoridation to unelected "strategic health authorities" (SHA). The only requirement was that these authorities organize public consultations before going ahead with a measure.

In the fall of 2008, the South Central SHA demonstrated what a mockery such so-called public consultations could be, when, having heard from the people that 72 percent did not want to be fluoridated, they nevertheless voted unanimously to go ahead to fluoridate much of Southampton and several surrounding communities.[35] They dealt with the many scientific questions posed to them during their so-called consultation by hiring a firm of consultants,[36, 37] which dismissed the "direct" relevance of both the 2006 NRC report (see chapter 14) and eighteen IQ studies (see chapter 15) to fluoridating Southampton. Although citizens in Southampton are doing everything they can to overturn this decision, we may have seen the blueprint of what could happen elsewhere in Britain. The latest news from the UK is that the Southampton council, which had previously supported fluoridation, has voted to ask the SHA "to hold a referendum before fluoride is introduced to the water supply, and for the authority to honour the result of that vote."[38, 39]

Promoters intimidate decision makers when communities try to stop fluoridation.

Whenever there is a suggestion that a community is considering halting fluoridation, a series of orchestrated actions ensue. Letters are sent to the editors of local newspapers warning of the enormous catastrophe that will befall the community if that happens. At the first public meeting held on the issue, a posse of dentists, doctors, and representatives of state or county health departments descend upon the chambers of the city council or other local government body. Most local decision makers cave in under such pressures.

A blogger, Rae Nadler-Olenick, gives a fascinating blow-by-blow account of what happened in Del Rio, Texas, after the town councilors there tried to halt the fluoridation program.[40] What she describes is fairly typical of what has been observed in other communities when decision makers, at the urging of citizens, try to reverse years of fluoridation.

Summary

The two chains of command of the pro-fluoridation lobby, headed by the CDC and the ADA, respectively, and similar bodies in other fluoridating countries, have used a number of different tactics to achieve their overall strategy of keeping the public, the media, and dental and medical professionals away from the primary scientific literature that indicates that fluoridation is neither effective nor safe. Instead of encouraging impartial review of the literature and open debate, fluoridation proponents have tried to win the argument with a combination of extolling their own authority (particularly via endorsements) and dismissing the credibility of their opponents.

While there is no doubt that the various tactics discussed in this chapter have been very effective at protecting the fluoridation program, that protection may have come at a heavy price. These tactics constitute a series of betrayals. The refusal to publish articles that present negative information on fluoridation, the refusal to debate the issue in public, and the refusal to present both sides of the argument to dental and medical students all represent a betrayal of what we have the right to expect of science: a free flow of information.

The expectation that dentists should promote fluoridation whether they have studied the issue or not and the disparagement and harassment of those who speak out against the practice constitute a serious betrayal of the standards we have the right to expect from any profession.

Using the authority of governmental office or the prestige of one's profession to confidently assure the public that fluoridation is safe and effective, when such assurance is not based on one's own review of the literature, is the worst betrayal of all: it is the betrayal of the public's trust.

Self-Serving Governmental Reviews

Every so often, particularly when their fluoridation programs are under threat because of renewed public concern, fluoridation-promoting governments organize panels to review the issue. More often than not those panels are selected to deliver the necessary re-endorsements.

In their recent book *Fluoride Wars* (2009), which is otherwise slanted toward fluoridation, Alan Freeze and Jay Lehr concede this point when they write:

> There is one anti-fluoridationist charge that does have some truth to it. Anti-fluoride forces have always claimed that the many government-sponsored review panels set up over the years to assess the costs and benefits of fluoridation were stacked in favor of fluoridation. A review of the membership of the various panels confirms this charge. The expert committees that put together reports by the American Association for the Advancement of Science in 1941, 1944 and 1954; the National Academy of Sciences in 1951, 1971, 1977 and 1993; the World Health Organization in 1958 and 1970; and the U.S. Public Health Service in 1991 are rife with the names of well-known medical and dental researchers who actively campaigned on behalf of fluoridation or whose research was held in high regard in the pro-fluoridation movement. Membership was interlocking and incestuous.[1]

We have already questioned the objectivity of the report by the Department of Health and Human Services[2] in chapter 18. Here we will examine three more recent government-sponsored reviews for which we believe the panels were selected to reach a pre-ordained pro-fluoridation position: the review by the Fluoridation Forum in Ireland (2002),[3] the review by the National Health and Medical Research Council in Australia (NHMRC, 2007),[4] and the review by Health Canada (2008, 2009).[5,6]

Fluoridation Forum
A fairly recent example of a panel stacked with pro-fluoridation experts and government employees is the Fluoridation Forum in Ireland, which

published its "review" in 2002.[7] Paul Connett was able to watch that process closely.

The Republic of Ireland is the only country in Europe that has mandatory fluoridation. By 2000, over 70 percent of the Irish population was drinking fluoridated water. In Northern Ireland (part of the UK and separate from the Republic of Ireland), by contrast, no fewer than twenty-six of twenty-seven councils had rejected a renewed bid to fluoridate in the late 1990s. So intense was the opposition that the whole political spectrum from Sinn Féin to Ian Paisley had gone on record in opposition to fluoridation. Meanwhile, news of the furor spread to the Republic of Ireland, and several anti-fluoridation groups sprang up there, including the 150-member Irish Dentists Opposed to Fluoridation. Also involved was the environmental group VOICE for the Irish Environment.

As a result of the political waves generated by this movement against fluoridation, the Irish Department of Health and Children organized a forum to review the matter. This was called the Fluoridation Forum. In October 2000, Hardy Limeback, PhD, DDS, and Paul Connett, PhD, were invited to present their concerns about water fluoridation to the Irish panel. They accepted.

Fluoridation opponents in Ireland were upset to hear that Connett and Limeback had agreed to testify. They believed that most of the forum members had been hand-picked to "whitewash" fluoridation, and that, by testifying, Limeback and Connett would give an illusion of legitimacy to any report the forum produced.

Connett and Limeback were in a dilemma. Although they also suspected that the forum was merely a rubber stamp for government policy, they both had a strong desire to bring the best science available before its members. Had they chosen not to appear, proponents could have argued that there was no valid scientific case to be made against fluoridation, and the issue would have been lost by default.

In the face of fierce opposition, they proceeded to testify. In giving his testimony, Connett explained to the panel members that many citizens felt the forum was fixed. Then he offered the panelists a challenge whereby they might demonstrate that they really did intend to perform an objective review of the issue. He presented a document titled "50 Reasons to Oppose Fluoridation"[8] and asked the panel to prepare a written, scientifically documented response to the document and make it publicly available.

Initially, the panel agreed to respond to the document and set up a subcommittee for the purpose. Forum minutes over the next year indicate several exchanges about the progress being made. However, shortly before the forum's report was completed, it was announced that the panel had not had time to provide a written response to Connett's "50 Reasons" but would address the issues in the body of the report. However, that did not happen.

The final report was one of the worst reviews ever conducted concerning the potential health effects of fluoridation. This was all the more shocking as not a single health study has been conducted in Ireland since mandatory fluoridation was introduced in 1963.

In its 296-page review, the panel devoted only seventeen pages to health issues, with most of their comments coming from other reviews. Fewer than two pages were devoted to *primary* health studies, and there the panel focused on just one issue: bone fractures. The three primary studies on bone fractures mentioned briefly by the forum panel did not even include the study by Li et al.[9] on which Connett placed special emphasis in his presentation. The Li study was published *after* Connett testified (he had received a pre-publication copy in his role as an invited peer reviewer of the York Review) but *before* the Fluoridation Forum published its report in 2002. Besides that important study, the panel ignored all of the other primary health studies referenced by Limeback and Connett. Incredibly, the forum spent less space examining the primary literature on health than on illustrating what a pea-sized amount of toothpaste looks like on a toothbrush.

Subsequently, a group of eleven scientists, including Limeback and Connett, issued a detailed critique of the forum's report.[10] After a delay of over three years, in 2005, an anonymous critique of "50 Reasons to Oppose Fluoridation" appeared on Ireland's Department of Health's Web site,[11] to which Connett responded.[12]

Australian National Health and Medical Research Council

Another entity that delivers reports on fluoridation to fit in with government policy is the Australian National Health and Medical Research Council (NHMRC). This agency is part of the Australian federal government and has endorsed fluoridation since 1958.

In 2007 the NHMRC produced a systematic review that purported to demonstrate the safety and effectiveness of fluoridation.[13] This report has been used extensively in Australia in efforts to get more communities fluoridated there, especially in Queensland. However, the NHMRC report is little more than a duplication of large chunks of the York Review,[14] but without the caveats the York Review provided.[15]

To circumvent the science, the NHMRC had to find a way around the extensive evidence of harm given in the report from the U.S. National Research Council of the National Academies (NRC) published the previous year.[16] The only reference the NHMRC made to the NRC report was the following brief comment that appeared in the introduction to the report:

> The reader is also referred to recent comprehensive reports regarding water fluoridation by the World Health Organization (WHO, 2006) and the National Research Council of the National Academies (NAS, 2006). The NAS report refers to the adverse health effects from fluoride at 2–4 mg/L, the reader is alerted to the fact that fluoridation of Australia's drinking water occurs in the range of 0.6 to 1.1 mg/L.[17]

This was political sleight of hand. Although the authors did not actually state that the NRC report was irrelevant to Australia, they encouraged the reader to draw that conclusion. As we explain in chapter 14, the NRC report is very relevant to fluoridation. However, with one sentence, the NHMRC served up a convenient excuse for dodging any need to review the NRC report, acknowledge its findings, or bother about any of its 1,100 references. While this certainly made the NHMRC's task easier, the result was hardly the kind of analysis the Australian public had a right to expect from this government-financed agency.

Moreover, while claiming that there was no evidence to support any health effects from fluoridation at 1 ppm, nowhere did the NHMRC acknowledge that practically no health studies had been conducted on this matter in Australia or, indeed, in any other fluoridating country. By ignoring the NRC report,[18] the council members largely ignored the voluminous material on the health effects observed in areas endemic for fluorosis published in nonfluoridated countries. They reviewed no animal or biochemical studies and no clinical trials. They examined only studies in English (thus ignoring the important Chinese literature). They devoted more pages to the study of teeth than to the study of other tissues and organs combined. In fact, they devoted ten times more space to studies on teeth than to those on bone or brain (see table 24.1). Overall, they included over three times more citations from dental journals than nondental journals. They give the levels of fluoride in water, soil, air, food, tea, and baby formula but somehow overlook the all-important level in mother's milk. See chapter 18 for the way they downplayed Elise Bassin's findings on osteosarcoma.[19, 20]

Despite its huge limitations and bias, this 2007 NHMRC review has been very influential in efforts to fluoridate more towns in Australia. Here is an excerpt from a letter by the premier of Queensland, Anna Bligh, explaining why her government has imposed mandatory fluoridation on the state:

> I would like to reassure you that my Government did not take this decision lightly. At all times the health and safety of Queenslanders has been our paramount concern, and we have based our decision on the overwhelming amount of credible, peer-reviewed medical and scientific evidence, from long-term use around the world, that shows that fluoridation is a safe, proven and effective preventive health measure to combat tooth decay and improve oral health.
>
> The most recent review by Australia's National Health and Medical Research Council found that fluoridation does not cause bone fractures, allergies or cancer or other adverse health effects.[21]

Health Canada: Expert Panel, 2008; Health Canada Report, 2009

Our third example of a self-serving review comes from a two-part review by Health Canada in 2008 and 2009 that was undertaken at a time of growing opposition to fluoridation in Canada.[22, 23] Quebec City, as well as three towns in the Niagara region of Ontario, had recently stopped fluoridation after many years. Several other major cities in Canada were also actively engaged in reviewing their programs, including Hamilton, London, Oakville, Sarnia, and Waterloo in Ontario and Calgary in Alberta.

The panelists for this Health Canada review were perhaps the most biased that could have been selected. Four of the six (Steven Levy, Christopher Clark, Michel Levy, and Jayanth Kumar) are dentists and well-known promoters of fluoridation, and the remaining two (Robert Tardif and Albert Nantel), along with dentist Michel Levy, were engaged in writing a pro-fluoridation report for the Institut National de Santé Publique du Québec at the time of their selection.[24] It must have been clear to those at Health Canada who selected this panel where their sympathies lay.

A shocking omission from the panel was that of Hardy Limeback. Both Limeback and Jayanth Kumar served on the 2006 NRC panel,[25] but Health Canada selected Kumar from New York over Limeback from Toronto. Limeback was eminently qualified for such a review. He holds both a DDS and a PhD in

Table 24.1 Number of pages in agency reviews devoted to different tissues and systems of the body

Agency (date)	Teeth	Bones	Brain	Endocrine System	Kidneys	Osteosarcoma or Other Cancer
Fluoridation Forum (2002)	50	5	0*	0*	0*	0*
NRC (2006)	28	50	19	105	12	36
NHMRC (2007)	106	12	<1	<1	<1	13
Health Canada (2009)	6	5	3	<1	<1	6

*These figures do not include primary references included in other reviews cited.

biochemistry; he is the former president of the Canadian Association for Dental Research and a professor and head of preventive dentistry at the University of Toronto and has his own dental practice. However, he does not support fluoridation. Kumar does and strongly. If both had been selected, it would have been a demonstration that Health Canada wanted a balanced review. However, Health Canada selected no dissenting voice. The result was entirely predictable.

The six members met in Ottawa in January 2007, and their five-page report was published on Health Canada's Web site in April 2008, at the very time there was an intense debate going on about whether Hamilton, Ontario, would stop fluoridating its water. Here are some excerpts from the report:

> *Cancer:* Weight of evidence does not support a link between exposure to fluoride and increased risks of cancer. It is important to avoid any generalization and overinterpretation of the results of the Bassin *et al.* paper and to await the publication of the full study before drawing conclusions and particularly before influencing any related policy . . .
>
> *Intelligence Quotient:* Weight of evidence does not support a link between fluoride and intelligence quotient deficit. There are significant concerns regarding the available studies, including quality, credibility, and methodological weaknesses such as the lack of control for confounding factors, the small number of subjects, and the dose of exposure . . .

> The current Maximum Acceptable Concentration (MAC) of 1.5 mg/L of fluoride in drinking water is unlikely to cause adverse health effects, including cancer, bone fracture, immuno-toxicity, reproductive/developmental toxicity, genotoxicity, and/or neurotoxicity.[26]

We have already commented on the use of Chester Douglass's letter promising a "full study" that would refute Elise Bassin's findings on osteosarcoma (see chapter 18)—a promise still unfulfilled after four years.[27] It was nearly two years overdue when the expert panel met. However, the promise of a study was used by that panel to nullify any concerns about the possibility that drinking fluoridated water might be increasing the number of young men who contract that frequently fatal bone cancer.

In September 2009, Health Canada published a draft report that relied heavily on the findings of the 2008 expert panel.[28] The report concludes that the MAC level of 1.5 ppm for fluoride should remain unchanged, thereby protecting Canada's fluoridation program. The authors of this report called the findings on neurotoxicity "controversial," but their analysis suggested that they were unaware of most of the studies that have been published in this area. They cited only five out of the twenty-three studies on lowered IQ and cited no studies that did not find that association. In support of their conclusion that "the significance of these studies is uncertain," they referenced reviews[29–31] that had appeared several years *before* the bulk of the IQ studies were published. Such a cavalier neglect of the primary literature is even more inexcusable since a joint conference was held by the International Society for Fluoride Research and the Fluoride Action Network on this very subject at the Mississauga campus of the University of Toronto over a year before the 2009 Health Canada report was released. Moreover, a press conference at which the significance of the eighteen of the twenty-three studies on fluoride and IQ that have been translated into English were discussed by scientists attending the conference received major national media coverage.[32, 33]

Summary

An examination of several reviews of fluoridation conducted by panels selected by pro-fluoridation governments (e.g., Fluoridation Forum in Ireland, 2002; NHMRC in Australia, 2007; and Health Canada, 2008 and 2009) indicate a clear bias toward supporting government policy. In any review of this type the outcome is largely dependent on the nature of the panel selected, and in many cases it is fairly obvious from the panel's makeup what the outcome of its review will be. These reviews amount to little more than self-fulfilling prophecies, once again illustrating the hold that politics has over genuine science in this matter.

A Response to Pro-Fluoridation Claims

Proponents of fluoridation have made a number of claims that have been effective with an ill-informed public. However, when those claims are examined carefully, they are found to have little merit. Although opponents have pointed out the weaknesses and fallacies in some of these "chestnuts" over the many years of this debate, they continue to crop up. Let's take a look at them.

Claim 1: There is no difference in principle between chlorination and fluoridation.

This is wrong. Chlorination treats water; fluoridation treats people. Water is treated with chlorine to make the water safe to drink. It kills the bacteria and other vectors that carry disease. Chlorination is not without its critics, but millions of lives have been saved by this process.

Fluoridation, on the other hand, is not used to make the water safe. It simply uses the public water supply to deliver medicine. Such a practice is rare, indeed, for obvious reasons. Once medicine is added to tap water, key controls are lost. You cannot control the dose, and you cannot control who gets the medicine. Moreover, you are forcing medication on people without their informed consent and, especially in the case of low-income families, without their ability to avoid the medicine if they wish.

Claim 2: Fluoride is "natural." We are just topping up what is there anyway.

Natural does not necessarily mean good. Arsenic, like fluoride, leaches naturally from rocks into groundwater, but no one suggests topping that up. Besides, there is nothing "natural" about the fluoridating chemicals, as they are obtained largely from the wet scrubbers of the phosphate fertilizer industry (see chapter 3). The chemicals used in most fluoridation programs are either hexafluorosilicic acid or its sodium salt, and those silicon fluorides do not occur in nature. What is more, under international law they cannot be dumped into the sea, yet a dilution of about 180,000 to 1 is supposed to protect against all harm when the same chemicals are added to the domestic water supply. In chapter 3, we discussed the language used in a recent Q&A pamphlet from the Victoria (Australia) Department of Human Services in an effort to persuade citizens that the chemicals used in fluoridation are not hazardous waste products of the fertilizer industry.

Claim 3: Fluoride is a nutrient.

As we explained in chapter 1, in order to establish that a substance is an essential nutrient, a researcher has to remove the substance from the diet and demonstrate that disease results. This has not been shown to occur with a lack of fluoride, nor is fluoride known to contribute to any normal metabolic process.

Claim 4: Fluoridation is no different than adding iron, folic acid, or vitamin D to bread and other foodstuffs.

There is a world of difference:

1. Iron, folic acid, and vitamin D are known essential nutrients. Fluoride is not.
2. All of those substances have large margins of safety between their toxic levels and their beneficial levels. Fluoride does not.
3. People who do not want those supplements can seek out foods without them. It is much more difficult to avoid tap water.

Claim 5: The amount of fluoride added to the public water system, 1 ppm, is so small it couldn't possibly hurt you.

Promoters use analogies such as 1 ppm is equivalent to one cent in $10,000 or one inch in sixteen miles to make it appear that we are dealing with insignificant quantities of fluoride. Such analogies are nonsensical without reference to the toxicity of the chemical in question. For example, 1 ppm is about a million times higher than the safe concentration to swallow of dioxin, and 100 times higher than the safe drinking water standard for arsenic; it is also up to 250 times higher than the level of fluoride in mother's milk[1] (see chapter 12).

Claim 6: Everything is toxic given a high enough dose, even water.

This is correct, but one has to be careful when using the word *high*. Fluoride is extremely toxic, especially for young children, as the following quote from Dr. Gary Whitford, a leading fluoride researcher at the Medical College of Georgia, illustrates:

> It may be concluded that if a child ingests a fluoride dose in excess of 15 mg F/kg, then death is likely to occur. A dose as low as

5 mg F/kg may be fatal for some children. Therefore, the probable toxic dose (PTD), defined as the threshold dose that could cause serious or life-threatening systemic signs and symptoms and that should trigger immediate emergency treatment and hospitalization, is 5 mg F/kg.[2]

Thus, according to Whitford, a 7 kg infant could be killed by a dose of just 35 milligrams of fluoride. To get such a dose would require swallowing 35 liters of water at 1 ppm (1 mg per liter). No infant could possibly drink 35 liters of water in one sitting, so we are *not* talking about killing babies with fluoridated water. But there is a world of difference between a *chronic* toxic dose and a lethal dose. What we are particularly concerned about is the impact of consuming water at 1 ppm *over an extended period of time*. In the case of infants, a huge concern is the possible impact on their mental development over the first few years of life, since studies have shown that levels as low as 1.9 ppm fluoride in water are associated with a lowering of IQ in China.[3] In the case of adults, we are concerned about lifelong exposure to levels of 6 mg per day or even lower and what damage that might do to bones and ligaments.[4]

Claim 7: You would have to drink a whole bathtub of water to get a toxic dose of fluoride.

Here again, proponents are confusing a *toxic* dose with a *lethal* dose—that is, a dose causing *illness or harmful effect* as opposed to a dose causing *death*. Opponents of fluoridation are not suggesting that people are going to be killed outright from drinking fluoridated water, but we are suggesting that it may cause immediate health problems in those who are very sensitive (chapter 13) and, with long-term exposure, persistent health problems in others (chapters 14–19).

Claim 8: Fluoridated water is only delivered to the tap. No one is forced to drink it.

Unfortunately, that is not a simple option, especially for families of low income who cannot afford bottled water or expensive fluoride filtration systems. Even those who can afford alternatives cannot easily protect themselves from the water they get outside the home. Fluoridated tap water is used in many processed foods and beverages (soda, beer, coffee, etc.).

Claim 9: Fluoridation is needed to protect children in low-income families.

This is a powerful and emotional argument. However, it ignores the fact that poor nutrition is most prevalent in families of low income, and the people most vulnerable to fluoride's toxic effects are those with a poor diet. Thus, while children from low-income families are a special target for this program, they are precisely the ones most likely to be harmed. Moreover, in chapter 8 we referenced some of the many distressing newspaper accounts of children suffering from tooth decay in low-income areas located in cities that have been fluoridated for over thirty years. Also in chapter 8 we reference the numerous state oral health reports indicating the continued disparity in tooth decay between low-income and high-income families, even in states with a high percentage of the population drinking fluoridated water.

Claim 10: Fluoridation has been going on for over sixty years; if it caused any harm, we would know about it by now.

Such statements would start to be meaningful only if fluoridated countries had conducted comprehensive health studies of their fluoridated populations. Most have not. Only a few health studies have been performed in the United States, most many years ago (see chapters 9 and 10); very few health studies have been performed in Australia, Canada, New Zealand, or the UK; and none has been performed in Colombia, Ireland, Israel, or Singapore (all countries with more than 50 percent of the population drinking fluoridated water). We discussed this and other examples of the very inadequate science involved in the promotion of fluoridation in chapter 22.

Claim 11: According to the Centers for Disease Control and Prevention, fluoridation is one of the top ten public health achievements of the twentieth century.

Most journalists, newspaper editors, and officials who quote this claim have little or no idea how poorly it is supported by the report that supposedly justifies the statement.[5, 6] We have discussed this matter in several places, including chapter 23.

Claim 12: For every dollar spent on fluoridation, $38 is saved in dental costs.

This statement is taken from another report written by members of the Oral Health Division of the CDC.[7] Two of its three authors, Susan Griffin and Scott Tomar, also wrote the report mentioned in Claim 11 above.

Griffin et al. inflated the benefits of fluoridation and ignored the costs of any side effects, including the one effect no one can deny, dental fluorosis. Cosmetic veneer treatment for fluorosis costs upward of $1,000 per tooth. The CDC authors also allowed a loss of earnings of $18 an hour for time off work to get a dental filling. Not all people lose pay when they get dental treatment, and certainly children don't.

Claim 13: The majority of the U.S. population drinks fluoridated water.

This statement is misused to put pressure on communities that do not fluoridate their water. They are led to believe that they are the odd ones out, behind the times, blocking progress. They are not. Only about 400 million people worldwide drink fluoridated water, and most of them live in North America. Globally, those who do are a distinct minority. Only eight countries have more than 50 percent of their population drinking fluoridated water; only 2 percent of the population of Europe drinks fluoridated water (see chapter 5).

Claim 14: The majority of U.S. cities are fluoridated.

There is a far longer list of cities in the rest of the world that do not fluoridate than of cities in the United States that do. Moreover, low-income areas in some major fluoridated cities in America and Australia still have major childhood dental problems (see chapter 8).

Claim 15: Every major dental and medical authority supports fluoridation.

Here we return to the dubious nature of endorsements not backed up by independent and current reviews of the literature. Many of the major associations on the list frequently cited by the American Dental Association endorsed fluoridation before a single trial had been completed and before the first health study had been published, in 1954 (see chapters 9 and 10).

Claim 16: When fluoridation is stopped, tooth decay rates go up.

There now have been at least four modern studies showing that when fluoridation was halted in communities in East Germany, Finland, Cuba, and British Columbia (Canada), tooth decay rates did not go up. This issue was discussed in chapters 5 and 8.

Claim 17: Fluoridation is "safe and effective."

This empty phrase is parroted so many times by pro-fluoridation officials and dentists at meetings considering fluoridation that one begins to wonder if they receive some kind of commission every time it is uttered! Be that as it may, mechanically repeating a phrase, no matter how often, without backing it up with solid supporting evidence does not make it true.

Claim 18: Hundreds (or thousands) of studies demonstrate that fluoridation is effective.

On the contrary, the UK's York Review was able to identify very few studies of even moderate quality, and the results were mixed[8] (see chapter 6).

Claim 19: Fluoridation reduces tooth decay by 20–60 percent.

In chapters 6–8, we examined in detail the evidence for fluoridation's benefits and found it to be very weak. Even a 20 percent reduction in tooth decay is a figure rarely found in more recent studies. Moreover, we have to remember that percentages can give a very misleading picture. For example, if an average of two decayed tooth *surfaces* are found in a non-fluoridated group and one decayed *surface* in a fluoridated group, that would amount to an impressive 50 percent reduction. But when we consider the total of 128 surfaces on a complete set of teeth, the picture—which amounts to an absolute saving in tooth decay of a mere 0.8 percent—does not look so impressive.

Claim 20: Hundreds (or thousands) of studies demonstrate that fluoridation is safe.

When proponents are asked to produce just one study (a primary study, not a governmental review) that has convinced them that fluoridation is safe, they are seldom able to do so. Apparently, they have taken such assurances from others at face value, without reading the literature for themselves. The fact is, it is almost impossible to prove conclusively that a substance has no ill effects. A careful and properly controlled study may show that, under the conditions and limitations of the investigation, no harm is apparent. A hundred such studies may permit a considerable degree of confidence—but in the case of fluoridation, very few studies have even been attempted. As fluoride accumulates progressively in the skeleton and probably the pineal gland, studies need to extend over a lifetime. In chapter 22, we listed the many health concerns that simply have not been investigated in fluoridated countries. Meanwhile, fluoride at moderate to high doses can cause serious health problems, leaving little or no margin of safety for people drinking fluoridated water (see chapter 20).

Claim 21: Opponents of fluoridation do not have professional qualifications.

Some opponents of fluoridation do not have professional qualifications (of course); many do. Many highly qualified doctors, dentists, and scientists have opposed fluoridation in the past and do so today. Currently, over 3,000 individuals from medicine, dentistry, science, and other relevant professions are calling for an end to fluoridation worldwide.[9] Furthermore, many opponents without professional qualifications have educated themselves on the science relevant to fluoridation and are qualified to evaluate many aspects of it.

Claim 22: Opponents of fluoridation are a vocal minority.

In a democratic society, opponents should not have to apologize for being vocal. As far as being a minority is concerned, it is frequently true that for any controversial issue only a minority of people get actively involved. However, it is our experience that the more educated people are on this issue, the more likely they are to oppose fluoridation. Usually, it is only when the matter is resolved by an appeal to "authority," with little resort to scientific information, that proponents prevail.

Claim 23: Opponents of fluoridation use "junk science."

The epithet "junk" is rarely defined and almost entirely subjective. It tends to mean scientific data that the speaker considers (1) inconclusive or (2) inconsistent with his or her personal prejudices. "Junk" is not a term that is used in respectable scientific discourse, but it crops up frequently when science impinges on politics, big business, or the law, where conflicts of interest lead to mudslinging.

Claim 24: Opponents of fluoridation get their information from the Internet.

No one denies that plenty of rubbish appears on the Internet. But just because a published study can be found using the Internet does not invalidate it. In fact, scientists now do much of their reading of the scientific literature online. The Fluoride Action Network maintains a Health Effects Database on its Web site, which provides citations, excerpts, abstracts, and in some cases complete pdf files of many published studies. Proponents would do well to read some of these papers, rather than trying to dismiss them because they are available online.

Claim 25: There is no evidence that fluoride at the levels used in fluoridation schemes causes any health problems.

There are three weaknesses to this argument. First, it does not make clear that fluoridating countries have done few basic health studies of populations drinking fluoridated water. Absence of studies does not mean absence of harm. Second, just because a study is conducted at a higher water fluoride level than 1 ppm does not mean that it is not relevant to water fluoridation. Toxicologists are nearly always extrapolating from high-dose animal experiments to estimate safe doses for humans. In the case of fluoride, we have the luxury of a large number of human studies conducted in countries with moderate to high levels of exposure to naturally occurring fluoride. What is required here is a "margin-of-safety" analysis (see chapter 20) to see if there is a sufficient safety margin between the doses that cause harm and the doses likely to be experienced in fluoridated communities. In our view, there is not. And third, it is not true that there is no evidence of ill effects from fluoride at present levels of fluoridation (see chapters 10–19).

Claim 26: There is no evidence that fluoridation harms the thyroid.

Even though many animal experiments show that fluoride can affect thyroid function, and even though some doctors between the 1930s and the 1950s used fluoride to lower thyroid function in hyperactive patients, governments that promote fluoridation have not taken this issue seriously. Very little research has been supported in fluoridating countries, but two studies raise concerns.[10, 11] See chapter 16 for a full discussion of this issue.

Claim 27: There is no evidence that fluoridation is associated with an increase in hip fractures.

Not true: The evidence is mixed. Some studies show an increase in hip fractures among the elderly in fluoridated areas, and others do not. One of the better studies (Li et al.[12]) showed an increase in hip fractures in the elderly (in a series of villages) as the fluoride levels in the water rose from 1 ppm to 4.3 ppm (see chapter 17).

Claim 28: There is no evidence that fluoride causes cancer.

Again, the evidence is mixed. Some studies show an increase in osteosarcoma (a rare but frequently fatal bone cancer) among young men in fluoridated communities, and others do not. Even though the study results are mixed, a study by Elise Bassin from Harvard, with the most robust methodology to date, has shown a positive relationship between exposure to fluoride in the sixth, seventh, and eighth years of age and a fivefold to sevenfold increased risk of contracting osteosarcoma in young men by the age of twenty.[13] Although a large study has been promised that allegedly rebuts this finding,[14] after four years it has not appeared, nor does it appear in principle to be capable of refuting Bassin's conclusion (see chapter 18).

Claim 29: There is no evidence that fluoride lowers IQ.

There have now been twenty-three published studies showing that moderate to high levels of natural fluoride in source waters are associated with a lowered IQ in children. While proponents point to weaknesses in some of the IQ study designs, what is truly impressive is the fact that, apart from one small study in New Zealand,[15] fluoridated countries have chosen not to replicate them. Moreover, these IQ studies are buttressed by over eighty animal studies that show that fluoride damages the brain, as well as three Chinese studies that show fetal brain damage in areas endemic for fluorosis (see chapter 15).

Claim 30: There is no evidence that any individuals are particularly sensitive to fluoride's toxic effects.

It would be far more accurate to state that governments practicing fluoridation have shown no interest in testing scientifically the many anecdotal reports from citizens (along with case studies published by a number of authors) that they are sensitive to fluoride. Patients complain of a number of symptoms that disappear when the source of fluoride is removed and return when the source is reintroduced (see chapter 13).

Claim 31: Dental fluorosis is only a "cosmetic" problem.

Dental fluorosis is the one condition caused by fluoride that proponents do not deny. However, they commonly claim that the condition is not a health effect but merely a cosmetic effect. Fluoridation opponents, on the other hand, maintain that dental fluorosis—the result of fluoride's interference with the growing tooth cells—is the first visible evidence that fluoride has had an adverse *systemic* effect on the body, and they wonder what other developing tissues may have been affected while the tooth cells were being damaged. Of particular concern are the skeletal system, the brain, and the endocrine system, where damage could be happening without visible telltale signs. Proponents offer no evidence that other tissues have not been affected while dental fluorosis is occurring.

Nor are cosmetic effects necessarily trivial. Moderate dental fluorosis, which involves discoloration of 100 percent of a tooth surface and affects over 1 percent of children living in fluoridated communities,[16] is likely to cause psychological damage to teenagers[17] (see chapter 11) and is very expensive to treat.

Of some pertinence are the CDC's stated objectives of the fluoridation program: "Adjusted fluoridation is the conscious maintenance of the optimal fluoride concentration in the water supply for reducing dental caries and *minimizing the risk of dental fluorosis*" [emphasis added].[18] Regardless of whether the CDC's first objective has been met, with 32 percent of American children now affected by dental fluorosis,[19] the second objective has clearly not been.

Claim 32: Most cases of dental fluorosis are so mild that only a trained professional can recognize the problem.

This may be true of some cases of the *very mild* condition of fluorosis, which impacts over 22 percent of children in fluoridated areas, but is certainly not true of the *mild* condition, which involves up to 50 percent of the tooth surface and affects 5.8 percent of children in fluoridated areas, or the *moderate* condition, which involves 100 percent of the tooth surface and affects over 1 percent of children in fluoridated areas[20] (see chapter 11).

Claim 33: Some cases of dental fluorosis actually improve the appearance of the teeth.

This claim dates back to a famously cynical comment made in 1951 by Dr. Frank Bull, the state dental director for Wisconsin. His remarks are quoted in full in chapter 11, under "Promoters' Spin."

Claim 34: Skeletal fluorosis is very rare in fluoridated countries.

It is difficult for promoters of fluoridation to deny that high natural levels of fluoride have caused severe bone damage in millions of people in India, China, and several other countries. However, proponents insist that skeletal fluorosis is a rare occurrence in countries with artificial fluoridation like the United States. What they really mean by this is that the crippling phase (stage III) of this condition is rare in the United States; they fail to recognize that the earlier phases (stage I and stage II) are associated with pains in the joints and bones, symptoms identical to the early symptoms of arthritis, a condition that affects many millions of adults in the United States (see chapter 17). The 2006 NRC review recommends that stage II skeletal fluorosis be considered an adverse effect: "The committee judges that stage II is also an adverse health effect, as it is associated with chronic joint pain, arthritic symptoms, slight calcification of ligaments, and osteosclerosis of cancellous bones."[21] No fluoridating country has undertaken a study to see if there is a relationship between fluoridation and arthritis (see chapter 17).

Claim 35: Opponents use "scare tactics."

In reality, the potential that fluoride might be causing a number of harms (including osteosarcoma in young men; arthritis and hip fractures in the elderly; lowered IQ in children; and lowered thyroid function) in some of the 400 million people who are drinking fluoridated water daily is indeed worrying (see chapters 10–19). The risks for one individual may be small, but if millions of people drink fluoridated water, a small risk multiplies up to a lot of cases. If we suppose a risk of some harm to 1 in 1,000, that would mean 400,000 cases worldwide or 10,000 in a large city.

Claim 36: Opponents are "poison mongers."

This bizarre claim originates from a piece of work authored by Dr. Stephen Barrett, a retired psychiatrist from Allentown, Pennsylvania, who started an organization called Quackbusters.[22] Another article (coauthored by Barrett) that makes the same silly charge is titled "Fluoridation: Don't Let the Poisonmongers Scare You."[23]

The notion that people opposed to putting a known toxic substance into the drinking water supply are "poison mongers" is *Alice in Wonderland* nonsense. Fluoridation opponents are not selling a poison; in fact, they are not selling anything. It is the proponents, or their friends in the phosphate fertilizer industry, who are doing just that. This is a classic ploy of propagandists: Accuse your opponent of doing exactly what you are doing, or simply take your opponents' arguments and turn them upside down.

Claim 37: Opponents are "conspiracy theorists."

This was true of one faction of the anti-fluoridation movement in the 1950s, whose members believed that fluoridation was a "communist plot," as parodied in Stanley Kubrick's famous movie *Dr. Strangelove*. However, even in those early days many reputable scientists were opposed to fluoridation on scientific grounds and many more on the very rational grounds that it is unethical to deliver medicine through the public water supply, because it removes the individual's right to informed consent to medical treatment. Today, there are still conspiracy theorists around, as there are in almost any field, but most opponents are increasingly well informed.

Claim 38: Opponents are members of a fringe element who propagate discredited myths.

It is true that a *few* people who oppose fluoridation do so based on claims that

Nazi Germany and other totalitarian regimes used it as a method of mind control. There is little evidence that would satisfy a historian to support such claims. The vast majority of fluoridation opponents repudiate such views and base their opposition on science and ethics.

Claim 39: Over sixty countries practice water fluoridation.

A large majority of countries in the world do *not* fluoridate their water. They include China, India, Japan, nearly all the European countries, and almost all the industrialized nations. Only about thirty countries have some percentage of their population drinking fluoridated water, and of those only eight have more than 50 percent of their population doing so (see chapter 5).

Claim 40: The consensus of medical and dental professionals and scientists is that there is no valid debate on fluoridation.

Nothing in science is beyond debate. As far as *consensus* is concerned, we are reminded of what the late Michael Crichton said:

> I regard consensus science as an extremely pernicious development that ought to be stopped cold in its tracks. Historically, the claim of consensus has been the first refuge of scoundrels; it is a way to avoid debate by claiming that the matter is already settled . . . The greatest scientists in history are great precisely because they broke with the consensus . . . There is no such thing as consensus science. If it's consensus, it isn't science. If it's science, it isn't consensus. Period.[24]

Even if there are some areas of science where consensus seems legitimate, Crichton's statement is certainly relevant to the fluoridation debate.

Summary
Proponents of fluoridation possess a wide repertoire of incorrect statements about the science and unfounded generalizations about those who disagree with them. We have reproduced and refuted some of the commoner ones in this chapter.

The Promoters' Motivations

We have put off any analysis of the possible motivations of those promoting fluoridation to the very end of this book. Because it is so difficult to get into other people's minds, this chapter probably raises more questions than answers.

We venture into this problematic area because it is so puzzling to witness the efforts of promoters to fluoridate more and more water supplies, even as the evidence for the effectiveness and safety of fluoridation gets less and less convincing. The zeal with which this matter is still pursued calls for some serious questioning. Why, for example, do promoters do the following:

- Deny the possibility of any adverse health effects from fluoridation?
- Deny the relevance of the 2006 NRC review?
- Fail to do, or call for, the most basic human health studies on soft tissues?
- Fail to investigate a possible relationship between fluoridation and arthritis, hypothyroidism, or Alzheimer's disease?
- Fail to monitor the fluoride in citizens' bones, plasma, and urine?
- Fail to use dental fluorosis as a biomarker to examine health problems in children?
- Dismiss all studies done in other countries that pertain to health effects without attempting to replicate them?
- Refuse to debate the issue in public?
- Fail to conduct a genuine risk-benefit analysis?
- Insist that every man, woman, and child ingest fluoride, while conceding that its predominant mechanism of action is topical?

In short, what is driving the need by so many—from individual dentists to the highest levels of government in fluoridated countries—to keep this practice going at all costs?

Numerous people have tried to answer this question. Possible answers range from factors that influence individual beliefs and behavior to the economic interests of large corporations. Again, much of this is speculative. Two speculations we reject outright are that fluoridation is (1) some sinister plot to "dumb down" the population or (2) part of some worldwide plan to reduce the size of the global population.

Different Professional Perspectives

Edward Groth III, in a commentary contained within Brian Martin's excellent book *Scientific Knowledge in Controversy: The Social Dynamics of the Fluoridation Debate*,[1] describes what he sees as a clash in the fluoridation debate between the *dental public health perspective* and the *environmental health perspective*.[2]

One key difference between the public health and the environmental health perspectives is that the former is interested in providing the *greatest good for the greatest number*, while the latter is concerned about *minimizing* environmental and chemical risks. One focuses on what is safe for the *average* person, while the other is concerned about protecting *everyone*, including the most vulnerable.

One place where we can clearly see the dominance of the public health perspective is in the EPA's derivation of the MCLG (maximum contaminant level goal; see chapter 20). Choosing 2 liters as the amount of water one person drinks each day was an assumption clearly designed to protect an average water consumer, since the EPA knows that *some* people consume much more water than that. Moreover, the EPA's choice of a safety factor of 2.5 (instead of the usual factor of 10) did not take into account the expected variation in sensitivity to a toxic substance in any population. The most vulnerable fall by the wayside. More generally, the refusal of proponents to get into any kind of margin-of-safety analysis is rooted in the notion that it is enough to protect the average person. This attitude is betrayed in simplistic statements such as "If fluoridation was causing any harm, we would know about it by now." The failure of any pro-fluoridation government to investigate in any scientific fashion the many anecdotal reports and case studies indicating that some individuals appear to be very sensitive to fluoride's toxic effects again betrays an attitude of "We are doing some good for the many, why bother about the plight of the few?" The same applies to the dental community, which has always accepted the objective of reducing dental caries for the majority despite increasing dental fluorosis for the few. In all these situations, someone with an environmental health perspective would insist that we should not be imposing a practice on a whole population when we know full well that some individuals will be negatively affected, especially when there are alternative ways of tackling the problem.

Groth concludes that "the two clashing perspectives generally have not received balanced attention in the dispute," preference being given to the public dental health perspective for "largely historical and political" reasons.[3]

The Problem of Promotion

The problem arises when a public health authority sets out to promote a practice. Effective promotion does not mesh well with cautious notes or caveats. Any expressed doubts are seen as a setback for the program. Thus, from the U.S. surgeon general down to local health officials, the practice of fluoridation is promoted with the utmost confidence. It has to be that way. To question the program is to invite its demise. Almost by definition then, promotion of the program requires statements that there are absolutely no dangers, that the practice is extremely effective, and that there is no debate on the science of the matter. Dissent must be stifled.

Bill Osmunson, DDS, MPH, provided a snapshot of the formation of those attitudes when he related an experience while taking his master's degree in public health. He said that he got into an argument with his professor about an issue, and the professor admonished him, "Your job is not to question the science. Your job is to promote the policy."[4]

A Belief System

Most of the rank-and-file supporters of fluoridation programs doubtless believe fluoridation to be safe and effective and hold that position in good faith. Many are genuinely proud of what they see as a great contribution to public health. However, the problem is that for many of those people it has become a "belief system," and not one that can be well argued on the basis of the primary scientific literature.

The late Dr. John Colquhoun, who investigated this issue as part of his PhD thesis,[5] wrote in 1997, "Enthusiasts for a theory can fool themselves very often, and persuade themselves and others that their activities are genuinely scientific."[6] To support his thesis on this, Colquhoun used the well-known text by Thomas Kuhn, *The Structure of Scientific Revolutions.*[7]

The Fear of Losing Prestige

Over fifty years ago, a prominent water engineer had this to say on the matter of "losing prestige" if proponents of fluoridation abandoned the promotion of this practice:

> The continued promotion of water supply fluoridation in [the] face of mounting adverse evidence and criticism requires some evaluation. It seems that the proponents hit upon an idea years ago, which appealed to them, and which they felt was sound. As

their claims of safety were progressively discredited, rather than acknowledge this, they persisted in condoning such evidence. At the same time they were lending their prestige to such equivocation. Certainly the proponents of fluoridation are not intent upon poisoning or harming anyone, however, the dilemma of prestige is a very difficult matter to resolve.[8]

If we run the clock forward to the present, it is very clear that over the last fifty years many leading public health dentists and dental researchers have built their careers and reputations on promotion of this program. Huge reputations are at stake. It takes a person of strong character to change his or her position in public.

The Fear of Losing Credibility

To the reluctance of scientists and others to give up a pet theory, we have to add the concern that bureaucracies have over losing credibility. Abandoning or modifying advocacy becomes harder to do the more vociferously officials have proclaimed the benefits. In the case of the United States, every surgeon general in office since 1950 has championed fluoridation and issued statements of glowing support. The declaration by the CDC in 1999 that fluoridation is one of "the top ten great public health achievements" of the twentieth century[9, 10] is repeated nearly every day somewhere in the world. It is very hard to back down from such lofty rhetoric without losing face and credibility. As Dr. William Hirzy said in a videotaped interview with Michael Connett in 2001:

> Putting this stuff in the drinking water is in essence just a hazardous waste management tool. It has nothing to do with dental health whatsoever. It has to do with defending the reputations of people who have been promoting fluoridation for years and years and years and now find themselves way out on a limb and have nothing more to say except safe and effective, safe and effective, safe and effective, when in fact it is neither safe nor effective. But they can't change. They're riding a tiger and they can't get off.[11]

Also, one has to wonder what other public health practices might be threatened if the CDC or other U.S. Department of Health and Human Services agencies admitted the dangers of water fluoridation, with the sudden loss in credibility—or public trust—that might entail.

The Fear of Liability

Another major reason promoters of fluoridation may be reluctant to stop supporting this practice is fear of liability. If it is admitted that fluoridation causes any harm, there are lawyers waiting in the wings to sue somebody. Many players might be subject to legal action, such as the fluoridated dental-product manufacturers, dental organizations that have endorsed those products, the water utilities that add the fluoride to water, the local councils who are practicing medicine without a license, or the government health agencies that assure everyone that it is safe to ingest fluoride. At the moment, all of these entities are "hanging tough" and presenting a common front; when they sense the battle has been lost, then the finger-pointing will begin over who should shoulder the ultimate blame.

There are ways that governments could abandon fluoridation and avoid or minimize liability. Without admitting any harm, they could halt fluoridation in the name of the precautionary principle, discussed in chapter 21. They could also end it on the perfectly reasonable grounds of the program's declining efficacy and increasing public opposition. But it will only get more difficult as time goes on.

Protecting Economic Interests

Chris Bryson, a former producer and correspondent for the British Broadcasting Corporation, spent ten years writing his book *The Fluoride Deception*,[12] which meticulously documents the collusion between the U.S. Public Health Service, the Fluorine Lawyers Committee, and fluoride-polluting industries in the early promotion of this practice. Bryson stated in a 2004 video interview, "Fluoride science is corporate science, fluoride science is DDT science, it's asbestos science, it's tobacco science, it's a racket."[13]

Bryson's thesis is that fluoridation was a way of changing the image of fluoride from one of the worst air pollutants—responsible for many lawsuits from farmers and others claiming damage from fluoride pollution—in the 1940s to something safe enough to give to children in their drinking water.

Readers of Bryson's fascinating book will have a pretty good notion of why the practice started, but we need another book of that caliber to explain why it continues today. One piece of evidence that industrial interests are still involved is the continued aggressive promotion of fluoridation by the American Council on Science and Health (ACSH).

According to SourceWatch (a Web site produced by the Center for Media and Democracy that describes itself as a "collaborative, specialized encyclopedia of the people, organizations and issues shaping the public agenda"), the ACSH describes itself as "a consumer education consortium concerned with issues related to food, nutrition, chemicals, pharmaceuticals, lifestyle, the environment and health. ACSH is an independent, nonprofit, tax-exempt organization."[14] But SourceWatch indicates that ACSH accepts funding from Coca-Cola, Kellogg, General Mills, Pepsico, and the American Beverage Association, among others. One of the companies also named as supporting ACSH is Alcoa.[15] According to veteran journalist Bill Moyers, host of *Bill Moyers Journal*, broadcast on the Public Broadcasting Service (PBS-TV) in the United States:

> ACSH has been supported in large part by contributions from companies such as American Cyanamid, Chevron, Dow Chemical, DuPont, Exxon, Monsanto and Union Carbide. The organization sends out a continual stream of press releases and reports anchored by one primary theme—that environmental risks, especially the risks of toxic chemicals, are not so great as the public is being led to believe.[16]

Many prominent fluoridation promoters of the past and present have served as ACSH advisers or directors (e.g., Frederick Stare, Michael Easley, and Stephen Barrett). In 1990, the ACSH threatened legal action if any federal agency attempted "to reclassify fluoride from a non-carcinogen to a probable carcinogen."[17] We return to this discussion below when we review the role of the sugar lobby in the promotion of fluoridation.

Industry and Agency Gains

There are certainly a number of powerful entities that gain financially from the continued practice of water fluoridation. However, simply because they gain financially does not mean that they are the driving force behind the continued push for fluoridation, either today or in the past. It is a good place to start, though, if we are to understand fully why, despite the poor evidence of benefit and growing evidence of harm, proponents continue to promote this practice so zealously.

The Sugar Industry

The one economic interest that Bryson did not investigate is the sugar industry. Other commentators have, however. Notably, Fred Exner and George

Waldbott,[18] Gladys Caldwell and Philip Zanfagna,[19] and Wendy Varney[20] have pointed fingers in that direction.

In 1949, one year before the U.S. Public Health Service endorsed fluoridation, the director of the Sugar Research Foundation, a lobby representing about 130 sugar interests, said that its research mission was "to find out how tooth decay may be controlled effectively without restriction of sugar intake."[21] For the sugar lobby, fluoride—delivered through the water supply— quickly became the magic bullet to achieve that goal. From the earliest days of fluoridation, considerable sums of money were paid to prominent fluoride researchers at leading American universities.[22]

One researcher at Harvard who gave the sugar lobby what it wanted was Dr. Frederick Stare. According to his obituary in the *Boston Globe* in 2002, Dr. Stare was the founder of the Harvard University Department of Nutrition. "During a nearly six-decade career, Dr. Stare attacked health food advocates as charlatans on national television and in his syndicated newspaper column, and *led boisterous campaigns to fluoridate public drinking water* and defend food additives like Alar" [emphasis added].[23]

According to Caldwell and Zanfagna in the book *Fluoridation and Truth Decay*, Dr. Stare held a position with the Sugar Research Foundation, for which he was "required to testify before congressional committees and to lecture to various groups on behalf of the cereal and sugar interests."[24] According to Wendy Varney, in a 1970 Senate hearing on consumer affairs "Stare was listed as a witness for at least six major trade organizations and food processing companies. These included National Biscuit Company, Kellogg Company and the Sugar Association."[25]

As far as those sugar interests were concerned, Stare provided good returns for their investment. According to Varney, he was quoted as saying, "There is no convincing evidence that in the average American diet decreasing the intake of sweets will lessen tooth decay" and describing ice cream, potato chips, cookies, and soft drinks as "nutritious snacks." Varney added that he even recommended "Coke as an after school teenage snack."[26] Caldwell reported that Stare called opponents of fluoridation "compulsive critics characterized as neurotics, driven by mystic, primitive, subconscious fears."[27]

According to Zanfagna, Stare was able to convince the Food and Nutrition Board to list fluoride as "essential" in 1958 and was quoted in the media in 1967 as saying that "fluoride deficiency, lack of fluoride, is probably the most prevalent nutritional deficiency in the country."[28]

Not only did Dr. Stare promote the notion that fluoride benefited the teeth, but he was also one of the early promoters of the idea that fluoride would strengthen bones. He was a coauthor of a study published in 1966 that purported to find a reduction in hip fractures in areas with high natural fluoride levels.[29] The methodology of this study was heavily criticized at the time,[30] but Stare was undaunted by the criticism, and the results of the study led him to state before the Senate's Select Committee on Nutrition and Health on September 8, 1969, "The fluoridation of water is more important for the health of the future elderly than the teeth of the children now."[31]

Stare was also one of the seven members of the board of directors of the industry-funded group ACSH, discussed above. In 1990, he was part of the effort by that group to restrain any federal agency from banning or seeking to reclassify fluoride from a non-carcinogen to a probable carcinogen. According to an article in *Food Chemical News*,[32] the ACSH threatened legal action if the EPA classified fluoride as a carcinogen in the wake of the publication of the National Toxicology Program's 1990 animal study reporting that there was "equivocal evidence" that fluoride caused osteosarcoma in rats (see chapter 18).

The article quotes Stare as saying, "Fluoridation is not dangerous and not expensive. It is absolutely safe for anyone of any age, either sex, and in any state of health." He also said, "It is one of the greatest advances of public health of all times. Those lucky enough to have access to fluoridated water from infancy through life will have 60 to 70 percent less tooth decay." He cited studies of other apparent benefits derived from fluoride use as a factor in preventing osteoporosis and as a possible deterrent to arteriosclerosis.[33]

As late as 1990, this renowned nutritionist and lobbyist for the sugar and food industries was still claiming that fluoride was a nutrient—and that its ingestion was beneficial to both teeth and bones.

The Aluminum Industry

Bryson documents the very prominent role that the aluminum industry (especially Alcoa) played in the early promotion of fluoridation.[34] Whether this support was generated by concerns about liabilities associated with fluoride pollution of the environment near its plants or fluoride poisoning of the workers inside the plants or whether the industry was eager to find ways to get rid of the huge quantities of fluoride waste generated by its operations is open to question. The latter issue has faded from the picture; as the availability of the mineral cryolite has been dramatically reduced, the aluminum industry today uses much of its waste fluoride to make synthetic cryolite. Regarding the former issue, however, aluminum industry executives may still be concerned about protecting the industry from lawsuits brought by workers whose health may have been damaged by fluoride. As long as fluoride is perceived as being safe enough to put into toothpaste and drinking water, it is difficult to convince juries that it is dangerous. See the cross-examination of Dr. Phyllis Mullenix by lawyers for the Reynolds Metals Company, as reported by Chris Bryson.[35]

The Phosphate Fertilizer Industry

In Florida, Cargill is among several giant companies that mine phosphate rock for the production of super-phosphate fertilizers and phosphoric acid. In the process, huge quantities of hexafluorosilicic acid are produced (see chapter 3). The willingness of communities to use this industrial-grade waste product in water fluoridation is a substantial financial benefit to the phosphate fertilizer industry. It turns what would otherwise be a costly disposal problem into a profitable business.

The Dental Products Industry

Nearly every dental product, from toothpicks to mouthwash to toothpaste to dental fillings, contains the "magic ingredient" fluoride. Were water fluoridation to cease, this industry would also take a hit. While sales of products that involve topical application might increase if fluoridation was stopped, the larger financial concern of dental product producers might be legal liability. If, or when, fluoride is proved to cause harm to a point that class-action lawyers are prepared to take the matter to court, there could be very large settlements. It should not be forgotten that the American Dental Association has its seal of approval on nearly all of those products and might also be found liable.

Summary

In short, fluoridation makes a lot of money and provides a lot of prestige and power for a relatively small number of people. Whether that makes them "true believers" in this matter despite the weak evidence of the practice's effectiveness and the growing evidence about health concerns is open to question. We like to think that for the vast majority of fluoridation promoters, it is more a matter of firm belief than a cause tainted with economic interest. However, it might take only a few people to be persuaded by larger economic considerations to influence the whole fluoridation-promoting apparatus. That is the danger and the power of the two chains of command, administered by the CDC and the ADA concurrently, discussed in chapter 23.

For those like ourselves who have studied water fluoridation it remains puzzling that rational people support this practice so vehemently. We will give the final word to Columbia University historian Jacques Barzun, who wrote this on the matter in 1964:

> In England, the Minister of Health has called the opponents of fluoridation cranks and fanatics; in this country, physicians who write on the subject to the newspapers fulminate against the unbelievers as if the Inquisition were back in our midst. To object to the plan is to be against science, that is to say a heretic. Scientific fact is of course irrelevant to the issue, which is purely civic, and which should be settled with the aid of simple questions, such as:
>
> Is it common sense to treat by universal dosing a small anonymous part of the population, without knowing how much or little of the treatment the intended beneficiaries will take?
>
> Is it economically wise to put medicine in the water supply, most of which will be used to wash streets, flush toilets, and make beer?
>
> And finally, is it right to subject everybody to a dosage of any kind without his consent?
>
> For there is no reason to stop at fluorides. The drinking water can carry tranquilizers, laxatives and aphrodisiacs, for the sake of giving chosen groups of the Children of Techne a happier life. One hopes behind the fluoride scheme there are politics and selfish business interests; the presence of solid ulterior motives would restore one's faith in common intelligence.[36]

Review and Conclusion

This book deals with fluoridation of the public water supply through the addition of a chemical compound yielding fluoride ions in the water to achieve a concentration of approximately 1 ppm, purportedly to fight tooth decay.

In part 1 (chapters 1–5) we examined the ethical and commonsense arguments against fluoridation and explained that most countries have rejected this practice. In part 2 (chapters 6–8) we examined the purported benefits and found the evidence for them very weak. In part 4 (chapters 11–19) we examined the risks. A reading of parts 2 and 4 should convince the independent observer that the risks far outweigh the benefits. Part 5 (chapters 20 and 21) puts the matter of risk into the context of a public policy decision. When exposing a whole population to a toxic substance—especially when the dose cannot be controlled—both decision makers and risk calculators have to be cautious, not cavalier. The decision to fluoridate does not provide an adequate margin of safety to protect everyone in the population, especially the most vulnerable. That is what the science tells us. This raises two questions: Why did this practice ever start? Why do a handful of countries, led by the United States, continue to promote this practice so relentlessly? We considered the early history in part 3 (chapters 9 and 10) and the politics of promotion in part 6 (chapters 22–26).

The following paragraphs contain some of the salient facts we have discussed that may increase the demand for an end to water fluoridation:

- *Fluoridation is a very bad medical practice.* Once fluoride has been added to the public water supply, there can be no control over the dose people receive or who receives it. There is no oversight of individual responses, and it is assumed that an individual may continue drinking the water over a lifetime.
- *Fluoridation defies medical ethics.* When communities fluoridate their water, they are doing to the whole community what an individual doctor is not allowed to do to anyone: prescribe medication without the individual's informed consent. There may be some situations where governments could reasonably claim the right to overrule that ethical principle, but this is clearly not one of them, since tooth decay is neither life threatening nor contagious at the community level.
- *Fluoridation defies common sense.* With leading proponents of fluorida-

tion admitting that the predominant benefit of fluoride is topical and not systemic, the practice of forcing people to ingest fluoride has become even more absurd.

- *None of the agencies of the U.S. Department of Health and Human Services, or any other U.S. federal agency, accepts responsibility for the safety of fluoridation.* Although many organizations promote and endorse fluoridation, including agencies of the U.S. Department of Health and Human Services, and over 180 million Americans drink fluoridated water every day, no U.S. federal agency (e.g., EPA, CDC, or FDA) accepts responsibility (liability) for the safety of the program or the chemicals used in it.
- *The FDA has never approved fluoride for ingestion.* The U.S. Food and Drug Agency has never approved fluoride for ingestion. It rates fluoride as an "unapproved drug." However, the FDA does require an acute-toxicity warning to be placed on fluoridated toothpaste. The designation "unapproved drug" puts into question the ethics and legality of school nurses and teachers administering fluoride pills and/or rinses to students in schools located in non-fluoridated areas.
- *Fluoride has never been subjected to rigorous, randomized clinical trials.* Fluoride has never undergone rigorous clinical trials for effectiveness by the FDA or any health authority in the world. Nor has any serious attempt been made to establish the long-term safety of fluoridation.
- *Fluoridation's benefits have been wildly exaggerated.* Even though the great majority of countries do not fluoridate their water, the tooth decay rates of children in those countries are no worse than the tooth decay rates of children in the countries that do. Very high rates of tooth decay in the United States occur in cities that have been fluoridated for years.
- *Bottle-fed babies are at risk.* The amount of fluoride added to the public water system, 1 ppm, is 25 to 250 times higher than the level of fluoride in mother's milk, so a bottle-fed baby (when the formula is made up with fluoridated tap water) will get far more fluoride than a breast-fed one.
- *U.S. children are being overexposed to fluoride.* Thirty-two percent of American children in fluoridated areas now have dental fluorosis—visible damage to the tooth enamel indicating that a child has swallowed too much fluoride before the permanent teeth have erupted.
- *There is no margin of safety.* There is no margin of safety from fluoride's harmful effects. In 2006, the National Research Council's review, *Fluoride in Drinking Water: A Review of EPA's Standards,* reported that

fluoride was associated with damage to the teeth, bone, brain, and endocrine system and possibly caused bone cancer. The review panel declared that the U.S. safe drinking water standard for fluoride (4 ppm) was not protective of health. Since the report was published, further evidence has emerged of lowered IQ associated with exposure to fluoride and of an increased incidence of osteosarcoma in boys who drink fluoridated water in the sixth to eighth years of life.

• *Fluoridation continues because its promoters have power and prestige.* Promoters get away with false or doubtful pronouncements on safety and efficacy not because they provide convincing scientific evidence to support their claims but rather because they use the "authority" of their office or position they hold.

• *Fluoridation started at a time when scientists and government officials held a very optimistic view about the safety of chemicals used in many products.* In 1950, when fluoridation began in the United States, DDT, PCBs, tetraethyl lead (a gasoline additive), asbestos, and fluoride were considered safe by scientists and government officials. Except for fluoride, all have since been banned.

• *There is some evidence that fluoridation was started for reasons of political and corporate financial expediency.* There was little solid scientific evidence to support fluoridation's effectiveness or its long-term safety when it was endorsed by the U.S. PHS in 1950.

• *Fluoridation was a huge gamble from the very beginning.* The only harm that promoters recognized in 1950 was that ingested fluoride caused dental fluorosis, and they were willing to take the gamble that while fluoride was interfering with the growing tooth cells, it was not interfering with any other cells in the body.

• *Absence of study does not mean absence of harm.* The only way fluoridating countries have been able to deny the adverse health effects of fluoridation is by not conducting relevant studies. Not only is the practice of fluoridation a giant experiment, but those who are conducting the experiment are not even collecting the data.

• *Any slight benefit from fluoridation must be judged against the risk of harm.* How much doubt regarding just one of the health concerns identified in this book is needed to override a benefit that, when quantified in the largest survey ever conducted in the United States, amounts to protecting less than one permanent tooth surface (out of 108) in a child's mouth?[1] This benefit has to be matched against the results of twenty-three studies that indicate a possible lowering of IQ at fluoride levels as low as 1.9 ppm—a level far too close to the 1 ppm used in artificial fluoridation to guarantee protection for every child drinking uncontrolled amounts of fluoridated water.

- *Bones are not protected from lifelong exposure.* About 50 percent of the fluoride we ingest each day concentrates in our bones and accumulates there. Governments promoting fluoridation have not done enough to demonstrate that such accumulation does not contribute to arthritic symptoms and bone fractures.

- *The precautionary principle should be applied.* A simple application of the precautionary principle, or indeed common sense, would show the practice of fluoridation to be indefensible. When exposing a whole population to a known toxic substance, decision makers should not wait until there is absolute proof of harm before acting. There is enough evidence of harm right now to stop this practice. This is perhaps the most fundamental point of difference between promoters and opponents of fluoridation.

- *Endorsements don't constitute scientific enquiry.* Instead of scientific enquiry, promoters of fluoridation use a long list of endorsements from associations and agencies that parrot one another and rarely present supporting data from the primary scientific literature.

- *Fluoridation is experimentation on humans without their informed consent.* With so many unanswered questions about fluoridation's safety, there is no question that the practice is experimental. Try as they may, fluoridation promoters cannot get around the fact that human experimentation without the individual's consent violates human rights treaties and conventions that most of the fluoridating countries have signed.

- *Governments are trying to protect their credibility.* Unfortunately, because U.S. government officials and officials in other fluoridating countries have put so much of their credibility on the line in defense of fluoridation, it is difficult for them to speak honestly and openly about the issue even if they wished to.

- *The 2006 NRC review is a beginning.* The restoration of scientific integrity to the issue of fluoride's toxicity begins with the 2006 review of fluoride in drinking water by the National Research Council. The chairman of the review panel, Dr. John Doull, is quoted in a 2008 article in *Scientific American* as follows:

What the committee found is that we've gone with the status quo regarding fluoride for many years—for too long, really—and now we need to take a fresh look . . . when we looked at the studies that have been done, we found that many of these [health] questions are unsettled and we have much less information than we should, considering how long this [fluoridation] has been going on.[2]

- *There are better ways to fight tooth decay.* As demonstrated in Europe, there are other ways of protecting teeth that do not force people to drink fluoridated water.

Conclusion

We have endeavored to show that water fluoridation has been propped up with poor science and poor ethical judgment for over fifty years. If we succeed in identifying and pulling those two cards away, then perhaps this house of cards may finally fall. As we have worked on this book, we have become more and more convinced about the short- and long-term health risks that fluoridation poses and increasingly disturbed about the willingness of so many qualified people to go along with the practice because of the authority of agencies and organizations that support it, rather than an objective assessment of the information available. This blind acceptance of authority is beneficial neither for science nor for the public's trust in government health policies.

So What Now?

Fluoridation is not going to disappear overnight. Change will require the pressure of public opinion. Here are a few things that we hope will happen:

1. We hope that this book will encourage many more scientists, doctors, dentists, health workers, environmentalists, and others to consider the issues raised and reach an informed opinion. The current attempts to extend fluoridation in the United States and elsewhere offer people an important opportunity to influence the course of events by talking to politicians and local and national media. We hope, too, that they will sign the Professionals' Statement to End Fluoridation. The number of signatories is already nearing three thousand from all parts of the world at the time of this writing and includes many distinguished physicians, dentists, scientists, politicians, and environmentalists. Their names can be viewed and signatures added online.[3]

2. Although we have not discussed alternative ways of reducing the incidence of tooth decay, it will be obvious to the reader that more needs to be done, particularly for poor and minority families who have the highest incidence. Education, not fluoridation, is the answer. We need education about better diets and better dental habits. In low-income areas there is clearly a need for free and accessible pediatric dental clinics. These might be combined with advice and counseling centers for pregnant mothers and their children and might also deal with the large and growing problem of obesity, as suggested by the work of Tavares and Chomitz.[4] The potential savings from reducing the incidence not only of tooth decay, but also of the various obesity-related illnesses such as diabetes, would more than justify the cost of such clinics.

3. Readers can also play an important part in informing the media, which have tended to be over-impressed by the apparent authority of the official line. We need everyone with an open mind to examine this issue more carefully. We need to enlist the involvement of teachers and students at universities, colleges, and high schools. We also need those environmental organizations that have so far stood on the sidelines of the debate to get involved. This is one environmental issue that is as easy to solve as turning off a tap, once we have the political will.

4. Everyone who is persuaded by the facts we have presented can contribute to informed political pressure at all levels. Those who have read this far will be well equipped to do that and to play a significant part in ending fluoridation.

Stopping fluoridation of the public water system may well be an uphill battle, but let's remember that great moments in history do not begin with everyone shouting yes, but with a few having the courage to say no.

APPENDIX 1

Fluoride and the Brain

Links to the references in the appendices and endnotes can be accessed at http://fluoridealert
.org/caseagainstfluoride.refs.html.

Twenty-three human studies that report an association of lowered IQ with fluoride exposure.
Y. Chen, F. Han, Z. Zhou, et al., "Research on the Intellectual Development of Children in
High Fluoride Areas," *Fluoride* 41, no. 2 (2008): 120–24, (originally published in 1991 in
Chinese Journal of Control of Endemic Diseases), http://www.fluorideresearch.org/412/files/
FJ2008_v41_n2_p120-124.pdf.

X. Guo, R. Wang, C. Cheng, et al., "A Preliminary Investigation of the IQs of 7–13 Year Old
Children from an Area with Coal Burning-Related Fluoride Poisoning," *Fluoride* 41, no. 2
(2008): 125–28 (originally published in 1991 in *Chinese Journal of Endemiology*), http://www.
fluorideresearch.org/412/files/FJ2008_v41_n2_p125-128.pdf.

F. Hong, Y. Cao, D. Yang, and H. Wang, "Research on the Effects of Fluoride on Child
Intellectual Development Under Different Environmental Conditions," *Fluoride* 41, no. 2
(2008): 156–60 (originally published in 2001 in *Chinese Primary Health Care*), http://www
.fluorideresearch.org/412/files/FJ2008_v41_n2_p156-160.pdf.

X. S. Li, J. L. Zhi, and R.O. Gao, "Effect of Fluoride Exposure on Intelligence in Children,"
Fluoride 28, no. 4 (1995): 189–92, http://fluoridealert.org/scher/li-1995.pdf.

Y. Li, X. Jing, D. Chen, L. Lin, and Z. Wang, "Effects of Endemic Fluoride Poisoning on the
Intellectual Development of Children in Baotou," *Fluoride* 41, no. 2 (2008): 161–64 (originally published in 2003 in *Chinese Journal of Public Health Management*), http://www
.fluorideresearch.org/412/files/FJ2008_v41_n2_p161-164.pdf.

F. F. Lin, Aihaiti, H. X. Zhao, et al., "The Relationship of a Low-Iodine and High-Fluoride
Environment to Subclinical Cretinism in Xinjiang," Xinjiang Institute for Endemic
Disease Control and Research; Office of Leading Group for Endemic Disease Control
of Hetian Prefectural Committee of the Communist Party of China; and County Health
and Epidemic Prevention Station, Yutian, Xinjiang, *Iodine Deficiency Disorder Newsletter* 7,
(1991): 3, http://fluoridealert.org/scher/lin-1991.pdf; also see http://www.fluoridealert.org/
IDD.htm.

S. Liu, Y. Lu, Z. Sun, et al., "Report on the Intellectual Ability of Children Living in High-
Fluoride Water Areas," *Fluoride* 41, no. 2 (2008): 144–47 (originally published in 2000 in
Chinese Journal of Control of Endemic Diseases), http://www.fluorideresearch.org/412/files/
FJ2008_v41_n2_p144-147.pdf.

Y. Lu, Z. R. Sun, L. N. Wu, et al., "Effect of High-Fluoride Water on Intelligence in
Children," *Fluoride* 33, no. 2 (2000): 74–78, http://www.fluorideresearch.org/332/files/
FJ2000_v33_n2_p74-78.pdf.

L. Qin, S. Huo, R. Chen, et al., "Using the Raven's Standard Progressive Matrices to
Determine the Effects of the Level of Fluoride in Drinking Water on the Intellectual
Ability of School-Age Children," *Fluoride* 41, no. 2 (2008): 115–19 (originally published in
1990 in *Chinese Journal of the Control of Endemic Disease*), http://www.fluorideresearch
.org/412/files/FJ2008_v41_n2_p115-119.pdf.

D. Ren, K. Li, and D. Liu, "A Study of the Intellectual Ability of 8–14 Year-Old Children in High Fluoride, Low Iodine Areas," *Fluoride* 41, no. 4 (2008): 319–20 (originally published in 1989 in Chinese *Journal of Control of Endemic Diseases*), http://www.fluorideresearch .org/414/files/FJ2008_v41_n4_p319-320.pdf.

D. Rocha-Amador, M. E. Navarro, L. Carrizales, et al., "Decreased Intelligence in Children and Exposure to Fluoride and Arsenic in Drinking Water," *Cadernos de Saúde Pública* 23, suppl. 4 (2007): S579–87.

B. Seraj, M. Shahrabi, M. Falahzade, et al., "Effect of High Fluoride Concentration in Drinking Water on Children's Intelligence," *Journal of Dental Medicine* 19, no. 2 (2007): 80–86. Note: English translation forwarded by lead author (B. Seraj, department of pediatric dentistry, faculty of dentistry, Tehran University of Medical Sciences), http://fluoridealert .org/scher/seraj-2007.trans.pdf.

M. H. Trivedi, R. J. Verma, N. J. Chinoy, et al., "Effect of High Fluoride Water on Intelligence of School Children in India," *Fluoride* 40, no. 3 (2007): 178–83, http://www.fluoride research.org/403/files/FJ2007_v40_n3_p178-183.pdf.

G. Wang, D. Yang, F. Jia, and H. Wang, "A Study of the IQ Levels of Four- to Seven-Year-Old Children in High Fluoride Areas," *Fluoride* 41, no. 4 (2008): 340–43 (originally published in 1996 in *Endemic Diseases Bulletin* [China]), http://www.fluorideresearch.org/414/files/ FJ2008_v41_n4_p340-343.pdf.

S. Wang, H. Zhang, W. Fan, et al., "The Effects of Endemic Fluoride Poisoning Caused by Coal Burning on the Physical Development and Intelligence of Children," *Fluoride* 41, no. 4 (2008): 344–48 (originally published in 2005 in *Journal of Applied Clinical Pediatrics* [China]), http://www.fluorideresearch.org/414/files/FJ2008_v41_n4_p344-348.pdf.

S. X. Wang, Z. H. Wang, X. T. Cheng, et al., "Arsenic and Fluoride Exposure in Drinking Water: Children's IQ and Growth in Shanyin County, Shanxi Province, China," *Environmental Health Perspectives* 115, no. 4 (2007): 643–47, http://www.ncbi.nlm.nih.gov/ pmc/articles/PMC1852689/.

Q. Xiang, Y. Liang, L. Chen, et al., "Effect of Fluoride in Drinking Water on Children's Intelligence," *Fluoride* 36, no. 2 (2003): 84–94, http://www.fluorideresearch.org/362/files/ FJ2003_v36_n2_p84-94.pdf. Also see Q. Xiang, Y. Liang, M. Zhou, and H. Zang, "Blood Lead of Children in Wamiao-Xinhuai Intelligence Study" (letter), *Fluoride* 36, no. 3 (2003): 198–99, http://www.fluorideresearch.org/363/files/FJ2003_v36_n3_p198-199.pdf.

L. B. Zhao, G. H. Liang, D. N. Zhang, and X. R. Wu, "Effect of High-Fluoride Water Supply on Children's Intelligence," *Fluoride* 29, no. 4 (1996): 190–92, http://fluoridealert.org/scher/ zhao-1996.pdf.

The following five Chinese I.Q. studies have not yet been translated:
J. A. An, S. Z. Mei, A. P. Liu, et al., "Effect of High Level of Fluoride on Children's Intelligence" (article in Chinese), *Zhong Guo Di Fang Bing Fang Zhi Za Zhi* 7, no. 2 (1992): 93–94.

Z. X. Fan, H. X. Dai, A. M. Bai, et al., "Effect of High Fluoride Exposure on Children's Intelligence" (article in Chinese), *Huan Jing Yu Jian Kang Za Zhi* 24, no. 10 (2007): 802–3.

Y. L. Xu, C. S. Lu, and X. N. Zhang, "Effect of Fluoride on Children's Intelligence" (article in Chinese), *Di Fang Bing Tong Bao* 9 (1994): 83–84.

L. M. Yao, Y. Deng, S. Y. Yang, et al., "Comparison of Children's Health and Intelligence Between the Fluorosis Area with Altering Water Source and Those without Altering Water Source" (article in Chinese), *Yu Fang Yi Xue Wen Xian Xin Xi* 3, no. 1 (1997): 42–43.

J. W. Zhang, H. Yao, and Y. Chen, "Effect of High Level of Fluoride and Arsenium on Children's Intelligence" (article in Chinese), *Zhong Guo Gong Gong Wei Sheng Xue Bao* 17, no. 2 (1998): 119.

Animal and biochemical studies in chronological order
(This is a list of some of the studies that have been published.)

1941

S. Ochoa, "'Coupling' of Phosphorylation with Oxidation of Pyruvic Acid in Brain," *The Journal of Biological Chemistry* 138 (1941): 751–73, http://www.jbc.org/content/138/2/751 .full.pdf+html.

1942

E. Racker and H. Kabat, "The Metabolism of the Central Nervous System in Experimental Poliomyelitis," *The Journal of Experimental Medicine* 76, no. 6 (1942): 579–85, http://www .ncbi.nlm.nih.gov/pmc/articles/PMC2135281/.

1943

D. Nachmansohn and A. L. Machado, "The Formation of Acetylcholine. A New Enzyme: 'Choline Acetylase,'" *Journal of Neurophysiology* 6 (1943): 397–403.

1966

G. Cimasoni, "Inhibition of Cholinesterases by Fluoride *In Vitro*," *The Biochemical Journal* 99, no. 1 (1966): 133–37, http://www.ncbi.nlm.nih.gov/pmc/articles/PMC1264967/.

1971

J. P. Perkins and M. M. Moore, "Adenyl Cyclase of Rat Cerebral Cortex. Activation of Sodium Fluoride and Detergents," *The Journal of Biological Chemistry* 246, no. 1 (1971): 62–68, http://www.jbc.org/content/246/1/62.long.

1973

R. A. Johnson and E. W. Sutherland, "Detergent-Dispersed Adenylate Cyclase from Rat Brain. Effects of Fluoride, Cations, and Chelators," *The Journal of Biological Chemistry* 248, no. 14 (1973): 5114–21, http://www.jbc.org/content/248/14/5114.long.

S. Katz and A. Tenenhouse, "The Relation of Adenyl Cyclase to the Activity of Other ATP Utilizing Enzymes and Phosphodiesterase in Preparations of Rat Brain; Mechanism of Stimulation of Cyclic AMP Accumulation by NaF," *British Journal of Pharmacology* 48, no. 3 (1973): 505–15, http://www.ncbi.nlm.nih.gov/pmc/articles/PMC1776132/pdf/ brjpharm00545-0143.pdf.

1974

K. Czechowicz, A. Osada, and B. Slesak, "Histochemical Studies on the Effect of Sodium Fluoride on Metabolism in Purkinje's Cells," *Folia Histochemica et Cytochemica (Krakow)* 12, no. 1 (1974): 37–44.

L. I. Popov, R. I. Filatova, and A. S. Shershever, "Aspects of Nervous System Affections in Occupational Fluorosis" (article in Russian), *Gigiena Truda I Professional'nye Zabolevaniia*, no. 5 (1974): 25–27.

1975

S. L. Manocha, H. Warner, and Z. L. Olkowski, "Cytochemical Response of Kidney, Liver and Nervous System to Fluoride Ions in Drinking Water," *Histochemical Journal* 7, no. 4 (1975): 343–55.

1977

C. O. Brostrom, M. A. Brostrom, and D. J. Wolff, "Calcium-Dependent Adenylate Cyclase from Rat Cerebral Cortex. Reversible Activation by Sodium Fluoride," *The Journal of Biological Chemistry* 252, no. 16 (1977): 5677–85, http://www.jbc.org/content/252/16/5677.long.

V. I. Tokar' and O. N. Savchenko, "Effect of Inorganic Fluorine Compounds on the Functional State of the Pituitary-Testis System" (article in Russian), *Problemy E'ndokrinologii (Mosk)* 23, no. 4 (1977): 104–7.

1978

M. Hebdon, H. Le Vine III, N. Sahyoun, et al., "Properties of the Interaction of Fluoride- and Guanylyl-5'-Imidodiphosphate-Regulatory Proteins with Adenylate Cyclase," *Proceedings of the National Academy of Sciences of the United States of America* 75, no. 8 (1978): 3693–97, http://www.ncbi.nlm.nih.gov/pmc/articles/PMC392852/pdf/pnas00020-0163.pdf.

1980

C. F. Hongslo, J. K. Hongslo, and R. I. Holland, "Fluoride Sensitivity of Cells from Different Organs," *Acta Pharmacologica et Toxicologica* 46, no. 1 (1980): 73–77.

M. M. Rasenick and M. W. Bitensky, "Partial Purification and Characterization of a Macromolecule which Enhances Fluoride Activation of Adenylate Cyclase," *Proceedings of the National Academy of Sciences of the United States of America* 77, no. 8 (1980): 4628–32, http://fluoridealert.org/re/rasenick-1980.pdf.

1981

T. Nanba, M. Ando, Y. Nagata, et al., "Distribution and Different Activation of Adenylate Cyclase by NaF and of Guanylate Cyclase by NaN3 in Neuronal and Glial Cells Separated from Rat Cerebral Cortex," *Brain Research* 218, no. 1–2 (1981): 267–77.

T. Tomomatsu, "Hygienic Study on Fluoride (4). Physiological Effects of Fluoride on Rat," *J Tokyo Med Coll.* 39, no. 3 (1981): 441–60.

1984

G. Janiszewska, L. Lachowicz, and R. Wojtkowiak, "Effect of Certain Agents on Subcellular cAMP Level in Different Areas of Rat Brain," *Acta Physiologica Polonica* 35, no. 3 (1984): 199–206.

M. G. Soni, M. S. Kachole, and S. S. Pawar, "Alterations in Drug Metabolising Enzymes and Lipid Peroxidation in Different Rat Tissues by Fluoride," *Toxicology Letters* 21, no. 2 (1984): 167–72.

1986

F. Geeraerts, G. Gijs, E. Finne, and R. Crokaert, "Kinetics of Fluoride Penetration in Liver and Brain," *Fluoride* 19, no. 3 (1986): 108–12.

Z. Z. Guan, "Morphology of the Brain of the Offspring of Rats with Chronic Fluorosis" (article in Chinese), *Zhonghua Bing Li Xue Za Zhi* 15, no. 4 (1986): 297–99.

A. R. Kay, R. Miles, and R. K. Wong, "Intracellular Fluoride Alters the Kinetic Properties of Calcium Currents Facilitating the Investigation of Synaptic Events in Hippocampal Neurons," *The Journal of Neuroscience* 6, no. 10 (1986): 2915–20, http://www.jneurosci.org/cgi/reprint/6/10/2915.

1987

I. Litosch, "Guanine Nucleotide and NaF Stimulation of Phospholipase C Activity in Rat Cerebral-Cortical Membranes. Studies on Substrate Specificity," *The Biochemical Journal* 244, no. 1 (1987): 35–40, http://www.biochemj.org/bj/244/0035/2440035.pdf.

1988

P. P. Godfrey and S. P. Watson, "Fluoride Inhibits Agonist-Induced Formation of Inositol Phosphates in Rat Cortex," *Biochemical and Biophysical Research Communications* 155, no. 2 (1988): 664–69.

R. S. Jope, "Modulation of Phosphoinositide Hydrolysis by NaF and Aluminum in Rat Cortical Slices," *Journal of Neurochemistry* 51, no. 6 (1988): 1731–36.

R. S. Jope and K. M. Lally, "Synaptosomal Calcium Influx is Activated by Sodium Fluoride," *Biochemical and Biophysical Research Communications* 151, no. 2 (1988): 774–80.

1989

W. X. Liu, "Experimental Study of Behavior and Cerebral Morphology of Rat Pups Generated by Fluorotic Female Rat" (article in Chinese), *Zhonghua Bing Li Xue Za Zhi* 18, no. 4 (1989): 290–92.

H. Machida, "The Rabbit Thermo-Regulatory System. Effects of High Dose of Sodium Fluoride" (article in Japanese), *Shikwa Gakuho* 89, no. 3 (1989): 607–26.

1990

E. Claro, M. A. Wallace, and J. N. Fain, "Dual Effect of Fluoride on Phosphoinositide Metabolism in Rat Brain Cortex. Stimulation of Phospholipase C and Inhibition of Polyphosphoinositide Synthesis," *The Biochemical Journal* 268, no. 3 (1990): 733–37, http://www.biochemj.org/bj/268/0733/2680733.pdf.

I. M. Gardiner and J. de Belleroche, "Modulation of Gamma-Aminobutyric Acid Release in Cerebral Cortex by Fluoride, Phorbol Ester, and Phosphodiesterase Inhibitors: Differential Sensitivity of Acetylcholine Release to Fluoride and K+ Channel Blockers," *Journal of Neurochemistry* 54, no. 4 (1990): 1130–35.

P. P. Li, D. Sibony, and J. J. Warsh, "Guanosine 5'-O-Thiotriphosphate and Sodium Fluoride Activate Polyphosphoinositide Hydrolysis in Rat Cortical Membranes by Distinct Mechanisms," *Journal of Neurochemistry* 54, no. 4 (1990): 1426–32.

G. Tiger, P. E. Björklund, G. Brannstrom, and C. J. Fowler, "Multiple Actions of Fluoride Ions Upon the Phosphoinositide Cycle in the Rat Brain," *Brain Research* 537, no. 1–2 (1990): 93–101.

G. Tiger, P. E. Björklund, R. F. Cowburn, et al., "Effect of Monovalent Ions upon G Proteins Coupling Muscarinic Receptors to Phosphoinositide Hydrolysis in the Rat Cerebral Cortex," *European Journal of Pharmacology* 188, no. 1 (1990): 51–62.

1991

S. J. Publicover, "Brief Exposure to the G-Protein Activator NaF/AlCl3 Induces Prolonged Enhancement of Synaptic Transmission in Area CA1 of Rat Hippocampal Slices," *Experimental Brain Research* 84, no. 3 (1991): 680–84.

S. D. Yuan, K. Q. Song, Q. W. Xie, and F. Y. Lu, "An Experimental Study of Inhibition on Lactation in Fluorosis Rats" (article in Chinese), *Sheng Li Xue Bao (Acta Physiologica Sinica)* 43, no. 5 (1991): 512–17.

1992

B. E. Hawes, J. E. Marzen, S. B. Waters, and P. M. Conn, "Sodium Fluoride Provokes Gonadotrope Desensitization to Gonadotropin-Releasing Hormone (GnRH) and Gonadotrope Sensitization to A23187: Evidence for Multiple G Proteins in GnRH Action," *Endocrinology* 130, no. 5 (1992): 2465–75.

A. Shashi, "Studies on Alterations in Brain Lipid Metabolism Following Experimental Fluorosis," *Fluoride* 25, no. 2 (1992): 77–84, http://fluoridealert.org/re/shashi-1992.pdf.

1993

T. J. Shafer, W. R. Mundy, and H. Tilson, "Aluminum Decreases Muscarinic, Adrenergic, and Metabotropic Receptor-Stimulated Phosphoinositide Hydrolysis in Hippocampal and Cortical Slices from Rat Brain," *Brain Research* 629, no. 1 (1993): 133–40.

B. M. Ross, M. McLaughlin, M. Roberts, et al., "Alterations in the Activity of Adenylate Cyclase and High Affinity GTPase in Alzheimer's Disease," *Brain Research* 622, no. 1–2 (1993): 35–42.

1994

A. Shashi, J. P. Singh, and S. P. Thapar, "Effect of Long-Term Administration of Fluoride on Levels of Protein, Free Amino Acids and RNA in Rabbit Brain," *Fluoride* 27, no. 3 (1994): 155–59, http://fluoridealert.org/re/shashi-1994.pdf.

X. L. Zhao, W. H. Gao, and Z. L. Zhao, "Effects of Sodium Fluoride on the Activity of Ca2+Mg(2+)-ATPase in Synaptic Membrane in Rat Brain" (article in Chinese), *Zhonghua Yu Fang Yi Xue Za Zhi* 28, no. 5 (1994): 264–66.

1995

N. A. Breakwell, T. Behnisch, S. J. Publicover, and K. G. Reymann, "Attenuation of High-Voltage-Activated Ca2+ Current Run-Down in Rat Hippocampal CA1 Pyramidal Cells by NaF," *Experimental Brain Research* 106, no. 3 (1995): 505–8.

P. J. Mullenix, P. K. Denbesten, A. Schunior, and W. J. Kernan, "Neurotoxicity of Sodium Fluoride in Rats," *Neurotoxicology and Teratology* 17, no. 2 (1995): 169–77.

T. Pushpalatha, M. Srinivas, and P. Sreenivasula Reddy, "Exposure to High Fluoride Concentration in Drinking Water will Affect Spermatogenesis and Steroidogenesis in Male Albino Rats," *Biometals* 18, no. 3 (1995): 207–12. Note: sodium fluoride administered orally to adult male rats at a dose level of 4.5 ppm and 9.0 ppm for 75 days caused significant decrease in the body weight, brain index, and testicular index.

1996

X. Li, L. Song, and R. S. Jope, "Cholinergic Stimulation of AP-1 and NF Kappa B Transcription Factors Is Differentially Sensitive to Oxidative Stress in SH-SY5Y Neuroblastoma: Relationship to Phosphoinositide Hydrolysis," *The Journal of Neuroscience* 16, no. 19 (1996): 5914–22.

1997

V. V. Frolkis, S. A. Tanin, and Y. N. Gorban, "Age-Related Changes in Axonal Transport," *Experimental Gerontology* 32, no. 4–5 (1997): 441–50.

Z. Z. Guan, Y. Wang, and K. Xiao, "Influence of Experimental Fluorosis on Phospholipid Content and Fatty Acid Composition in Rat Brain" (article in Chinese), *Zhonghua Yi Xue Za Zhi* 77, no. 8 (1997): 592–96.

R. L. Isaacson, J. A. Varner, and K. F. Jensen, "Toxin-Induced Blood Vessel Inclusions Caused by the Chronic Administration of Aluminum and Sodium Fluoride and Their Implications for Dementia," *Annals of the New York Academy of Sciences* 825 (1997): 152–66.

E. T. Koh and S. L. Clarke, "Effects of Fluoride and Aluminum Exposure to Dams Prior to and During Gestation on Mineral Compositions of Bone and Selected Soft Tissues of Female Mice Dams and Pups," *FASEB Journal* 11, no. 3 (1997): A406.

Y. Wang, Z. Guan, and K. Xiao, "Changes of Coenzyme Q Content in Brain Tissues of Rats with Fluorosis" (article in Chinese), *Zhonghua Yu Fang Yi Xue Za Zhi* 31, no. 6 (1997): 330–33.

1998

Z. Z. Guan, Y. N. Wang, K. Q. Xiao, et al., "Influence of Chronic Fluorosis on Membrane Lipids in Rat Brain," *Neurotoxicology and Teratology* 20, no. 5 (1998): 537–42.

V. Paul, P. Ekambaram, and A. R. Jayakumar, "Effects of Sodium Fluoride on Locomotor Behavior and a Few Biochemical Parameters in Rats," *Environmental Toxicology and Pharmacology* 6, no. 3 (1998): 187–91.

S. A. Plesneva, N. N. Nalivaeva, and I. A. Zhuravin, "Adenylate Cyclase System of the Rat Striatum: Regulatory Properties and the Effects of Gangliosides," *Neuroscience and Behavioral Physiology* 28, no. 4 (1998): 392–96.

J. A. Varner, K. F. Jensen, W. Horvath, and R. L. Isaacson, "Chronic Administration of Aluminum-Fluoride or Sodium-Fluoride to Rats in Drinking Water: Alterations in Neuronal and Cerebrovascular Integrity," *Brain Research* 784, no. 1–2 (1998): 284–98; extended excerpts at http://www.fluoride-journal.com/98-31-2/31291-95.htm.

X. L. Zhao and J. H. Wu, "Actions of Sodium Fluoride on Acetylcholinesterase Activities in Rats," *Biomedical and Environmental Sciences* 11, no. 1 (1998): 1–6.

1999

S. Bolea, E. Avignone, N. Berretta, et al., "Glutamate Controls the Induction of GABA-Mediated Giant Depolarizing Potentials Through AMPA Receptors in Neonatal Rat Hippocampal Slices," *Journal of Neurophysiology* 81, no. 5 (1999): 2095–102.

E. Sarri and E. Claro, "Fluoride-Induced Depletion of Polyphosphoinositides in Rat Brain Cortical Slices: A Rationale for the Inhibitory Effects on Phospholipase C," *International Journal of Developmental Neuroscience* 17, no. 4 (1999): 357–67.

G. B. van der Voet, O. Schijns, and F. A. de Wolff, "Fluoride Enhances the Effect of Aluminium Chloride on Interconnections Between Aggregates of Hippocampal Neurons," *Archives of Physiology and Biochemistry* 107, no. 1 (1999): 15–21.

C. Zhang, B. Ling, J. Liu, and G. Wang, "Effect of Fluoride-Arsenic Exposure on the Neurobehavioral Development of Rats Offspring" (article in Chinese), *Wei Sheng Yan Jiu* 28, no. 6 (1999): 337–38.

2000

J. Chen, X. Chen, and K. Yang, "Effects of Selenium and Zinc on the DNA Damage Caused by Fluoride in Pallium Neural Cells of Rats" (article in Chinese), *Wei Sheng Yan Jiu* 29, no. 4 (2000): 216–17.

X. H. Lu, G. S. Li, and B. Sun, "Study of the Mechanism of Neurone Apoptosis in Rats from the Chronic Fluorosis," *Chinese Journal of Endemiology* 19, no. 2 (2000): 96–98 (as abstracted in *Fluoride* 34, no. 1 (2001): 82).

Q. Shao, Y. Wang, and Z. Guan, "Influence of Free Radical Inducer on the Level of Oxidative Stress in Brain of Rats with Fluorosis" (article in Chinese), *Zhonghua Yu Fang Yi Xue Za Zhi* 34, no. 6 (2000): 330–32.

M. L. Vani and K. P. Reddy, "Effects of Fluoride Accumulation on Some Enzymes of Brain and Gastrocnemius Muscle of Mice," *Fluoride* 33, no. 1 (2000): 17–26, http://www.fluoride research.org/331/files/FJ2000_v33_n1_p17-26.pdf.

2001

Y. M. Shivarajashankara, A. R. Shivashankara, P. G. Bhat, et al., "Effect of Fluoride Intoxication on Lipid Peroxidation and Antitoxidant Systems in Rats," *Fluoride* 34, no. 2 (2001): 108–13, http://www.fluorideresearch.org/342/files/FJ2001_v34_n2_p108-113.pdf.

M. Trabelsi, F. Guermazi, and N. Najiba Zeghal, "Effect of Fluoride on Thyroid Function and Cerebellar Development in Mice," *Fluoride* 34, no. 3 (2001): 165–73, http://www.fluoride -journal.com/01-34-3/343-165.pdf.

Z. Zhang, X. Shen, and X. Xu, "Effects of Selenium on the Damage of Learning-Memory Ability of Mice Induced by Fluoride" (article in Chinese), *Wei Sheng Yan Jiu* 30, no. 3 (2001): 144–46.

2002

M. Bhatnagar, P. Rao, J. Sushma, and R. Bhatnagar, "Neurotoxicity of Fluoride: Neurodegeneration in Hippocampus of Female Mice," *Indian Journal of Experimental Biology* 40, no. 5 (2002): 546–54.

J. Chen, X. Chen, K. Yang, et al., "Studies on DNA Damage and Apoptosis in Rat Brain Induced by Fluoride" (article in Chinese), *Zhonghua Yu Fang Yi Xue Za Zhi* 36, no. 4 (2002): 222–24.

I. Ihnatovych, J. Novotny, R. Haugyicoya, et al., "Ontogenetic Development of the G Protein-Mediated Adenylyl Cyclase Signalling in Rat Brain," *Brain Research: Developmental Brain Research* 133, no. 1 (2002): 69–75.

Y. G. Long, Y. N. Wang, J. Chen, et al., "Chronic Fluoride Toxicity Decreases the Number of Nicotinic Acetylcholine Receptors in Rat Brain," *Neurotoxicology and Teratology* 24, no. 6 (2002): 751–57.

Y. M. Shivarajashankara, A. R. Shivashankara, and P. G. Bhat, et al., "Histological Changes in the Brain of Young Fluoride-Intoxicated Rats," *Fluoride* 35, no. 1 (2002): 12–21, http:// www.fluorideresearch.org/351/files/FJ2002_v35_n1_p12-21.pdf.

Y. M. Shivarajashankara, A. R. Shivashankara, P. G. Bhat, and S. H. Rao, "Brain Lipid Peroxidation and Antioxidant Systems of Young Rats in Chronic Fluoride Intoxication," *Fluoride* 35, no. 3 (2002): 197–203, http://www.fluoride-journal.com/02-35-3/353-197 .pdf.

2003

J. Chen, K. R. Shan, Y. G. Long, et al., "Selective Decreases of Nicotinic Acetylcholine Receptors in PC12 Cells Exposed to Fluoride," *Toxicology* 183, no. 1–3 (2003): 235–42.

I. Inkielewicz and J. Krechniak, "Fluoride Content in Soft Tissues and Urine of Rats Exposed to Sodium Fluoride in Drinking Water," *Fluoride* 36, no. 4 (2003): 263–66, http://www .fluoride-journal.com/03-36-4/364-263.pdf.

A. Shashi, "Histopathological Investigation of Fluoride-Induced Neurotoxicity in Rabbits," *Fluoride* 36, no. 2 (2003): 95–105, http://www.fluorideresearch.org/362/files/FJ2003_v36 _n2_p95-105.pdf.

J. X. Zhai, Z. Y. Guo, C. L. Hu, et al., "Studies on Fluoride Concentration and Cholinesterase Activity in Rat Hippocampus" (article in Chinese), *Zhonghua Lao Dong Wei Sheng Zhi Ye Bing Za Zhi* 21, no. 2 (2003): 102–4.

2004

P. G. Borasio, F. Cervellati, B. Pavan, and M. C. Pareschi, "'Low' Concentrations of Sodium Fluoride Inhibit Neurotransmitter Release from the Guinea-Pig Superior Cervical Ganglion," *Neuroscience Letters* 364, no. 2 (2004): 86–89.

A. Lubkowska, D. Chlubek, A. Machoy-Mokrzyńska, et al., "Concentrations of Fluorine, Aluminum and Magnesium in Some Structures of the Central Nervous System of Rats Exposed to Aluminum and Fluorine in Drinking Water" (article in Polish), *Annales Academiae Medicae Stetinensis* 50, suppl. 1 (2004): 73–76.

K. R. Shan, X.L. Qi, Y. G. Long, A. Nordberg, and Z. Z. Guan, "Decreased Nicotinic Receptors in PC12 Cells and Rat Brains Influenced by Fluoride Toxicity—a Mechanism Relating to a Damage at the Level in Post-Transcription of the Receptor Genes," *Toxicology* 200, no. 2–3 (2004): 169–77.

X. Shen, Z. Zhang, and X. Xu, "Influence of Combined Iodine and Fluoride on Phospholipid and Fatty Acid Composition in Brain Cells of Rats" (article in Chinese), *Wei Sheng Yan Jiu* 33, no. 2 (2004): 158–61.

2005

Y. Ge, H. Ning, S. Wang, and J. Wang, "Comet Assay of DNA Damage in Brain Cells of Adult Rats Exposed to High Fluoride and Low Iodine," *Fluoride* 38, no. 3 (2005): 209–14, http://www.fluorideresearch.org/383/files/383209-214.pdf.

J. Krechniak and I. Inkielewicz, "Correlations Between Fluoride Concentration and Free Radical Parameters in Soft Tissues of Rats," *Fluoride* 38, no. 4 (2005): 293–96, http://www.fluorideresearch.org/384/files/384293-296.pdf.

M. Tsunoda, Y. Aizawa, K. Nakano, et al., "Changes in Fluoride Levels in the Liver, Kidney, and Brain and in Neurotransmitters of Mice after Subacute Administration of Fluorides," *Fluoride* 38, no. 4 (2005): 284–92, http://www.fluorideresearch.org/384/files/384284-292.pdf.

2006

M. Bhatnagar, P. Rao, A. Saxena, et al., "Biochemical Changes in Brain and Other Tissues of Young Adult Female Mice from Fluoride in their Drinking Water," *Fluoride* 39, no. 4 (2006): 280–84, http://www.fluorideresearch.org/394/files/FJ2006_v39_n4_p280-284.pdf.

Y. Ge, H. Ning, C. Feng, et al., "Apoptosis in Brain Cells of Offspring Rats Exposed to High Fluoride and Low Iodine," *Fluoride* 39, no. 3 (2006): 173–78, http://www.fluorideresearch.org/393/files/FJ2006_v39_n3_p173-178.pdf.

2007

I. Bera, R. Sabatini, P. Auteri, et al., "Neurofunctional Effects of Developmental Sodium Fluoride Exposure in Rats," *European Review for Medical and Pharmacological Sciences* 11, no. 44 (2007): 211–24.

K. Chirumari and P. K. Reddy, "Dose-Dependent Effects of Fluoride on Neurochemical Milieu in the Hippocampus and Neocortex of Rat Brain," *Fluoride* 40, no. 2 (2007): 101–10, http://www.fluorideresearch.org/402/files/FJ2007_v40_n2_p101-110.pdf.

T. Xia, M. Zhang, W. H. He, et al., "Effects of Fluoride on Neural Cell Adhesion Molecules mRNA and Protein Expression Levels in Primary Rat Hippocampal Neurons" (article in Chinese), *Zhonghua Yu Fang Yi Xue Za Zhi* 41, no. 6 (2007): 475–78.

M. Zhang, A. Wang, W. He, et al., "Effects of Fluoride on the Expression of NCAM, Oxidative Stress, and Apoptosis in Primary Cultured Hippocampal Neurons," *Toxicology* 236, no. 3 (2007): 208–16.

2008

L. R. Chioca, I. M. Raupp, C. Da Cunha, et al., "Subchronic Fluoride Intake Induces Impairment in Habituation and Active Avoidance Tasks in Rats," *European Journal of Pharmacology* 579, no. 1–3 (2008): 196–201.

S. Chouhan and S. J. Flora, "Effects of Fluoride on the Tissue Oxidative Stress and Apoptosis in Rats: Biochemical Assays Supported by IR Spectroscopy Data," *Toxicology* 254, no. 1–2 (2008): 61–67.

Q. Gao, Y. J. Liu, and Z. Z. Guan, "Oxidative Stress Might Be a Mechanism Connected with the Decreased α7 Nicotinic Receptor Influenced by High-Concentration of Fluoride in SH-SY5Y Neuroblastoma Cells," *Toxicology in Vitro* 22, no. 4 (2008): 837–43. (Corrigendum in *Toxicology in Vitro* 22 [2008]: 1814. The concentrations of fluoride should have been given as mM, instead of μM.)

Y. Li, X. Li, and S. Wei, "Effects of High Fluoride Intake on Child Mental Work Capacity: Preliminary Investigation into Mechanisms Involved," *Fluoride* 41, no. 4 (2008): 331-5 (originally published in 1994 in *The Journal of West China University of Medical Sciences*), http://www.fluorideresearch.org/414/files/FJ2008_v41_n4_p331-335.pdf.

R. Niu, Z. Sun, J. Wang, Z. Cheng, and J. Wang, "Effects of Fluoride and Lead on Locomotor Behavior and Expression of Nissl Body in Brain of Adult Rats," *Fluoride* 41, no. 4 (2008): 276–82, http://www.fluorideresearch.org/414/files/FJ2008_v41_n4_p276-282.pdf.

Z. R. Sun, F. Liu, L. Wu, et al., "Effects of High Fluoride Drinking Water on the Cerebral Functions of Mice," *Fluoride* 41, no. 2 (2008): 148–51 (originally published in 2000 in the *Chinese Journal of Epidemiology*), http://www.fluorideresearch.org/412/files/FJ2008_v41_n2_p148-151.pdf.

N. Wu, Z. Zhao, W. Gao, and X. Li, "Behavioral Teratology in Rats exposed to Fluoride," *Fluoride* 41, no. 2 (2008): 129–133 (originally published in 1995 in *Chinese Journal of Control of Endemic Diseases*), http://www.fluorideresearch.org/412/files/FJ2008_v41_n2_p129-133.pdf.

M. Zhang, A. Wang, T. Xia, and P. He, "Effects of Fluoride on DNA Damage, S-phase Cell-cycle Arrest and the Expression of NF-KappaB in Primary Cultured Rat Hippocampal Neurons," *Toxicology Letters* 179, no. 1 (2008): 1–5.

Z. Zhang, X. Xu, X. Shen, and X. Xu, "Effect of Fluoride Exposure on Synaptic Structure of Brain Areas Related to Learning-memory in Mice," *Fluoride* 41, no. 2 (2008): 139–43 (originally published in 1999 in *Journal of Hygiene Research* [China]), http://www.fluorideresearch.org/412/files/FJ2008_v41_n2_p139-143.pdf.

2009

V. K. Bharti and R. S. Srivastava, "Fluoride-induced Oxidative Stress in Rat's Brain and Its Amelioration by Buffalo (Bubalus Bubalis) Pineal Proteins and Melatonin," *Biological Trace Element Research* 130, no. 2 (2009): 131–40.

S. J. Flora, M. Mittal, and D. Mishra, "Co-exposure to Arsenic and Fluoride on Oxidative Stress, Glutathione Linked Enzymes, Biogenic Amines and DNA Damage in Mouse Brain," *Journal of the Neurological Sciences* 285, no. 1–2 (2009): 198–205.

Q. Gao, Y. J. Liu, and Z. Z. Guan, "Decreased Learning and Memory Ability in Rats with Fluorosis: Increased Oxidative Stress and Reduced Cholinesterase Activity," *Fluoride* 42, no. 4 (2009): 277–85, http://www.fluorideresearch.org/424/files/FJ2009_v42_n4_p277-285.pdf.

E. A. García-Montalvo, H. Reyes-Pérez, and L. M. Del Razo, "Fluoride Exposure Impairs
Glucose Tolerance Via Decreased Insulin Expression and Oxidative Stress," *Toxicology*
263 (2009): 75–83. According to the authors, "Interestingly, values of F- in soft rat tissues
(kidney, liver, brain and testis) were similar to those in urine (312 μmoll⁻¹). According to
this information, urinary F- level is a good indicator of the F- concentration in soft tissues.
In cases of subchronic exposure, the level of F- in the plasma probably does not reflect the
levels of F- distributed in soft tissues."

T. Kaur, R. K. Bijarnia, and B. Nehru, "Effect of Concurrent Chronic Exposure of Fluoride
and Aluminum on Rat Brain," *Drug and Chemical Toxicology* 32, no. 3 (2009): 215–21.

N. Madhusudhan, P. M. Basha, S. Begum, and F. Ahmed, "Fluoride-induced Neuronal
Oxidative Stress Amelioration by Antioxidants in Developing Rats," *Fluoride* 42, no. 3
(2009): 179–87, http://www.fluorideresearch.org/423/files/FJ2009_v42_n3_p179-187
.pdf.

R. Niu, Z. Sun, Z. Cheng, Z. Li, and J. Wang, "Decreased Learning Ability and Low
Hippocampus Glutamate in Offspring Rats Exposed to Fluoride and Lead," *Environmental
Toxicology and Pharmacology* 28 (2009): 254–58.

M. Pereira, P. A. Dombrowski, E. M. Losso, et al., "Memory Impairment Induced by Sodium
Fluoride Is Associated with Changes in Brain Monoamine Levels, *Neurotoxicity Research*,
December 2009 (in press).

B. P. Wann, B. D'Anjou, T. M. Bah, et al., "Effect of Olfactory Bulbectomy on Adenylyl
Cyclase Activity in the Limbic System," *Brain Research Bulletin* 79, no. 1 (2009): 32–36.

G. M. Whitford, J. L. Whitford, and S. H. Hobbs, "Appetitive-based Learning in Rats:
Lack of Effect of Chronic Exposure to Fluoride," *Neurotoxicology and Teratology* 31, no.
4 (2009): 210–15. Note: This study reported "no significant effect on appetitive-based
learning."

2010

P. M. Basha and N. Madhusudhan, "Pre and Post Natal Exposure of Fluoride Induced
Oxidative Macromolecular Alterations in Developing Central Nervous System of Rat and
Amelioration by Antioxidants," *Neurochemical Research*, March 2010: 1017–28.

H. Bouaziz, I. Ben Amara, M. Essefi, F. Croute, and N. Zeghal, "Fluoride-Induced Brain
Damages in Suckling Mice," *Pesticide Biochemistry and Physiology* 96 (2010): 24–29.

S. Chouhan, V. Lomash, and S. J. Flora, "Fluoride-induced Changes in Haem Biosynthesis
Pathway, Neurological Variables and Tissue Histopathology of Rats," *Journal of Applied
Toxicology* 30, no. 1 (2010): 63–73.

Y. Ge, R. Niu, J. Zhang, and J. Wang, "Proteomic Analysis of Brain Proteins of Rats Exposed
to High Fluoride and Low Iodine," *Archives of Toxicology* (in press; online April 3, 2010).

C. Z. Gui, L. Y. Ran, J. Li, and Z. Z. Guan, "Changes of Learning and Memory Ability and
Brain Nicotinic Receptors of Rat Offspring with Coal Burning Fluorosis," *Neurotoxicology
and Teratology* (in press; available online April 8, 2010).

H. Kaoud and B. Kalifa, "Effect of Fluoride, Cadmium and Arsenic Intoxication on Brain and
Learning-Memory Ability in Rats," *Toxicology Letters* 196, suppl. 1 (2010): S53 (abstract
from the XII International Congress of Toxicology).

H. Li, H. Huang, Y. Xu, et al., "Toxic Effects of Fluoride on Rat Cerebral Cortex Astrocytes
in Vitro" (article in Chinese), *Wei Sheng Yan Jiu* 39, no. 1 (2010): 86–88.

Y. J. Liu, Q. Gao, C. X. Wu, and Z. Z. Guan, "Alterations of nAChRs and ERK1/2 in the
Brains of Rats with Chronic Fluorosis and Their Connections with the Decreased Capacity
of Learning and Memory," *Toxicology Letters* 192, no. 3 (2010): 324–29.

R. M. M. Sawan, G. A. S. Leite, M. C. P. Saraiva, et al., "Fluoride Increases Lead
   Concentrations in Whole Blood and in Calcified Tissues from Lead-Exposed Rats,"
   Toxicology 271, no. 1–2 (2010): 21–26.

J. Zhang, W. J. Zhu, X. H. Xu, and Z. G. Zhang, "Effect of Fluoride on Calcium Ion
   Concentration and Expression of Nuclear Transcription Factor Kappa-B Rho65 in Rat
   Hippocampus," *Experimental and Toxicologic Pathology* (in press; available online March 19,
   2010).

W. Zhu, J. Zhang, and Z. Zhang, "Effects of Fluoride on Synaptic Membrane Fluidity and
   PSD-95 Expression Level in Rat Hippocampus," *Biological Trace Element Research* (in press;
   available online March 9, 2010).

APPENDIX 2

Fluoride and Bone

Links to the references in the appendices and endnotes can be accessed at http://fluoridealert .org/caseagainstfluoride.refs.html.

Clinical trials on the treatment of osteoporosis with sodium fluoride

T. A. Bayley, J. E. Harrison, T. M. Murray, et al., "Fluoride-Induced Fractures: Relation to Osteogenic Effect," *Journal of Bone and Mineral Research* 5, suppl. 1 (1990): S217–22.

M. A. Dambacher, J. Ittner, and P. Ruegsegger, "Long-Term Fluoride Therapy of Postmenopausal Osteoporosis," *Bone* 7, no. 3 (1986): 199–205.

J. C. Gerster, S. A. Charhon, P. Jaeger, et al., "Bilateral Fractures of Femoral Neck in Patients with Moderate Renal Failure Receiving Fluoride for Spinal Osteoporosis," *British Medical Journal (Clinical Research Edition)* 287, no. 6394 (1983): 723–25.

D. H. Gutteridge, R. I. Price, G. N. Kent, et al., "Spontaneous Hip Fractures in Fluoride-Treated Patients: Potential Causative Factors," *Journal of Bone and Mineral Research* 5, suppl. 1 (1990): S205–15.

D. H. Gutteridge, G. O. Stewart, R. L. Prince, et al., "A Randomized Trial of Sodium Fluoride (60 mg) +/- Estrogen in Postmenopausal Osteoporotic Vertebral Fractures: Increased Vertebral Fractures and Peripheral Bone Loss with Sodium Fluoride; Concurrent Estrogen Prevents Peripheral Loss, but Not Vertebral Fractures," *Osteoporosis International* 13, no. 2 (2002): 158–70.

L. R. Hedlund and J. C. Gallagher, "Increased Incidence of Hip Fracture in Osteoporotic Women Treated with Sodium Fluoride," *Journal of Bone and Mineral Research* 4, no. 2 (1989): 223–25.

J. Inkovaara, R. Heikinheimo, K. Jarvinen, et al., "Prophylactic Fluoride Treatment and Aged Bones," *British Medical Journal* 3, no. 5975 (1975): 73–4.

J. D. O'Duffy, H. W. Wahner, W. M. O'Fallon, et al., "Mechanism of Acute Lower Extremity Pain Syndrome in Fluoride-Treated Osteoporotic Patients," *American Journal of Medicine* 80, no. 4 (1986): 561–66.

P. Orcel, M. C. de Vernejoul, A. Prier, et al., "Stress Fractures of the Lower Limbs in Osteoporotic Patients Treated with Fluoride," *Journal of Bone and Mineral Research* 5, suppl. 1 (1990): S191–94.

B. L. Riggs, S. F. Hodgson, W. M. O'Fallon, et al., "Effect of Fluoride Treatment on the Fracture Rate in Post-Menopausal Women with Osteoporosis," *New England Journal of Medicine* 322, no. 12 (1990): 802–9.

C. M. Schnitzler, J. R. Wing, K. A. Gear, and H. J. Robson, "Bone Fragility of the Peripheral Skeleton during Fluoride Therapy for Osteoporosis," *Clinical Orthopaedics* no. 261 (1990): 268–75.

Animal studies showing fluoride weakens bones

D. F. Beary, "The Effects of Fluoride and Low Calcium on the Physical Properties of the Rat Femur," *The Anatomical Record* 164, no. 3 (1969): 305–16.

A. Bohatyrewicz, "Bone Fluoride in Proximal Femur Fractures," *Fluoride* 34, no. 4 (2001): 227–35, http://www.fluorideresearch.org/344/files/FJ2001_v34_n4_p227-235.pdf.

A. Bohatyrewicz, "Effects of Fluoride on Mechanical Properties of Femoral Bone in Growing Rats," *Fluoride* 32, no. 2 (1999): 47–54, http://fluoridealert.org/re/bohatyrewicz-1999.pdf.

T. W. Burnell, E. R. Peo Jr., A. J. Lewis, and J. D. Crenshaw, "Effect of Dietary Fluorine on Growth, Blood and Bone Characteristics of Growing-Finishing Pigs," *Journal of Animal Science* 63, no. 6 (1986): 2053–67.

M. M. Chan, R. B. Rucker, F. Zeman, and R. S. Riggins, "Effect of Fluoride on Bone Formation and Strength in Japanese Quail," *Journal of Nutrition* 103, no. 10 (1973): 1431–40.

I. Gedalia, A. Frumkin, and H. Zukerman, "Effects of Estrogen on Bone Composition in Rats at Low and High Fluoride Intake," *Endocrinology* 75 (1964): 201–5.

M. H. Lafage, R. Balena, M. A. Battle, et al., "Comparison of Alendronate and Sodium Fluoride Effects on Cancellous and Cortical Bone in Minipigs. A One-Year Study," *The Journal of Clinical Investigation* 95, no. 5 (1995): 2127–33.

L. Mosekilde, J. Kragstrup, and A. Richards, "Compressive Strength, Ash Weight, and Volume of Vertebral Trabecular Bone in Experimental Fluorosis in Pigs," *Calcified Tissue International* 40, no. 6 (1987): 318–22.

R. S. Riggins, R. C. Rucker, M. M. Chan, et al., "The Effect of Fluoride Supplementation on the Strength of Osteopenic Bone," *Clinical Orthopaedics*, no. 114 (1976): 352–57.

R. S. Riggins, F. Zeman, and D. Moon, "The Effects of Sodium Fluoride on Bone Breaking Strength," *Calcified Tissue Research* 14, no. 4 (1974): 283–89.

J. C. Robin, B. Schepart, H. Calkins, et al., "Studies on Osteoporosis III. Effect of Estrogens and Fluoride," *Journal of Medicine* 11, no. 1 (1980): 1–14.

H. Roeckert, "X-ray Absorption and X-ray Fluorescence Micro-Analyses of Mineralized Tissue of Rats Which Have Ingested Fluoridated Water," *Acta Pathologica et Microbiologica Scandinavica* 59 (1963): 32–38.

H. Roeckert and H. Sunzel, "Skeletal Lesions Following Ingestion of Fluoridated Water," *Experientia* 15 (1960): 155–56.

C. H. Søgaard, L. Mosekilde, W. Schwartz, et al., "Effects of Fluoride on Rat Vertebral Body Biomechanical Competence and Bone Mass," *Bone* 16, no. 1 (1995): 163–9.

C. H. Turner, M. P. Akhter, and R. P. Heaney, "The Effects of Fluoridated Water on Bone Strength," *Journal of Orthopaedic Research* 10, no. 4 (1992): 581–87.

C. H. Turner and A. J. Dunipace, "On Fluoride and Bone Strength" (letter), *Calcified Tissue International* 53, no. 4 (1993): 289–90.

C. H. Turner, L. P. Garetto, A. J. Dunipace, et al., "Fluoride Treatment Increased Serum IGF-1, Bone Turnover, and Bone Mass, But Not Bone Strength, in Rabbits," *Calcified Tissue International* 61, no. 1 (1997): 77–83.

C. H. Turner, K. Hasegawa, W. Zhang, et al., "Fluoride Reduces Bone Strength in Older Rats," *Journal of Dental Research* 74, no. 8 (1995): 1475–81, http://jdr.sagepub.com/cgi/reprint/74/8/1475.

C. H. Turner, W. R. Hinckley, M. E. Wilson, et al., "Combined Effects of Diets with Reduced Calcium and Phosphate and Increased Fluoride Intake on Vertebral Bone Strength and Histology in Rats," *Calcified Tissue International* 69, no. 1 (2001): 51–57.

C. H. Turner, I. Owan, E. J. Brizendine, et al., "High Fluoride Intakes Cause Osteomalacia and Diminished Bone Strength in Rats with Renal Deficiency," *Bone* 19, no. 6 (1996): 595–601.

B. Uslu, "Effect of Fluoride on Collagen Synthesis in the Rat," *Research and Experimental Medicine* 182, no. 1 (1983): 7–12.

I. Wolinsky, A. Simkin, and K. Guggenheim, "Effects of Fluoride on Metabolism and Mechanical Properties of Rat Bone," *American Journal of Physiology* 223, no. 1 (1972): 46–50.

Nineteen studies on the possible association of hip fracture and fluoridated water published since 1990

Studies reporting an association between fluoridated water (1 ppm fluoride) and hip fracture

C. Cooper, C. Wickham, R. F. Lacey, and D. J. Barker, "Water Fluoride Concentration and Fracture of the Proximal Femur," *Journal of Epidemiology and Community Health* 44, no. 1 (1990): 17–19; and C. Cooper, C. A. Wickham, D. J. Barker, and S. J. Jacobsen, "Water Fluoridation and Hip Fracture" (letter, a reanalysis of data presented in 1990 paper), *Journal of the American Medical Association* 266, no. 4 (1990): 513–14.

C. Danielson, J. L. Lyon, M. Egger, and G. K. Goodenough, "Hip Fractures and Fluoridation in Utah's Elderly Population," *Journal of the American Medical Association* 268, no. 6 (1992): 746–48.

K. T. Hegmann et al., "The Effects of Fluoridation on Degenerative Joint Disease (DJD) and Hip Fractures," abstract no. 71 of the 33rd Annual Meeting of the Society for Epidemiological Research, June 15–17, 2000, published in a supplement of *American Journal of Epidemiology* (2000): P S18.

S. J. Jacobsen, J. Goldberg, C. Cooper, and S. A. Lockwood, "The Association Between Water Fluoridation and Hip Fracture Among White Women and Men Aged 65 Years and Older. A National Ecologic Study," *Annals of Epidemiology* 2, no. 5 (1992): 617–26.

S. J. Jacobsen, J. Goldberg, T. P. Miles, et al., "Regional Variation in the Incidence of Hip Fracture. US White Women Aged 65 Years and Older," *Journal of the American Medical Association* 264, no. 4 (1990): 500–502.

H. Jacqmin-Gadda, D. Commenges, and J. F. Dartigues, "Fluorine Concentration in Drinking Water and Fractures in the Elderly" (letter), *Journal of the American Medical Association* 273, no. 10 (1995): 775–76.

H. Jacqmin-Gadda, A. Fourrier, D. Commenges, and J. F. Dartigues, "Risk Factors for Fractures in the Elderly," *Epidemiology* 9, no. 4 (1998): 417–23. (An elaboration of the 1995 study referred to in the JAMA letter.)

C. Keller, "Fluorides in Drinking Water" (unpublished results), discussed in S. L. Gordon and S. B. Corbin "Summary of Workshop on Drinking Water Fluoride Influence on Hip Fracture on Bone Health," *Osteoporosis International* 2 (1992): 109–17.

P. Kurttio, N. Gustavsson, T. Vartiainen, and J. Pekkanen, "Exposure to Natural Fluoride in Well Water and Hip Fracture: A Cohort Analysis in Finland," *American Journal of Epidemiology* 150, no. 8 (1999): 817–24.

D. S. May and M. G. Wilson, "Hip Fractures in Relation to Water Fluoridation: An Ecologic Analysis (unpublished data), discussed in S. L. Gordon and S. B. Corbin "Summary of Workshop on Drinking Water Fluoride Influence on Hip Fracture on Bone Health," *Osteoporosis International* 2 (1992): 109–17.

Studies reporting an association between water-fluoride levels higher than that of fluoridated water (4 ppm+) and hip fracture

Y. Li, C. Liang, C. W. Slemenda, et al., "Effect of Long-Term Exposure to Fluoride in Drinking Water on Risks of Bone Fractures," *Journal of Bone and Mineral Research* 16, no. 5 (2001): 932–39.

M. F. Sowers, M. K. Clark, M. L. Jannausch, and R. B. Wallace, "A Prospective Study of Bone Mineral Content and Fracture in Communities with Differential Fluoride Exposure," *American Journal of Epidemiology* 133, no. 7 (1991): 649–60.

Studies reporting no association between water fluoride and hip fracture

Note that in four of these eight studies, an association was found between fluoride and some other form of fracture—e.g. wrist fracture. See notes and quotes below.

J. A. Cauley, P. A. Murphy, T. J. Riley, and A. M. Buhari, "Effects of Fluoridated Drinking Water on Bone Mass and Fractures: The Study of Osteoporotic Fractures," *Journal of Bone and Mineral Research* 10, no. 7 (1995): 1076–86.

D. Feskanich, W. Owusu, D. J. Hunter, et al., "Use of Toenail Fluoride Levels as an Indicator for the Risk of Hip and Forearm Fractures in Women," *Epidemiology* 9, no. 4 (1998): 412–16. Note: While this study didn't find an association between water fluoride and hip fracture, it did find an association—albeit not statistically significant 1.6 (0.8–3.1)—between fluoride exposure and elevated rates of forearm fracture.

S. Hillier, C. Cooper, S. Kellingray, et al., "Fluoride in Drinking Water and Risk of Hip Fracture in the UK: A Case Control Study," *The Lancet* 335, no. 9200 (2000): 265–69.

S. J. Jacobsen, W. M. O'Fallon, and L. J. Melton III, "Hip Fracture Incidence Before and After the Fluoridation of the Public Water Supply, Rochester, Minnesota," *American Journal of Public Health* 83, no. 5 (1993): 743–45, http://ajph.aphapublications.org/cgi/reprint/83/5/743.pdf.

M. R. Karagas, J. A. Baron, J. A. Barrett, and S. J. Jacobsen, "Patterns of Fracture Among the United States Elderly: Geographic and Fluoride Effects," *Annals of Epidemiology* 6, no. 3 (1996): 209–16. Note: As with Feskanich, et al. (1998), this study didn't find an association between fluoridation and hip fracture, but it did find an association between fluoridation and distal forearm fracture, as well as proximal humerus fracture. "Independent of geographic effects, men in fluoridated areas had modestly higher rates of fractures of the distal forearm and proximal humerus than did men in nonfluoridated areas."

R. Lehmann, M. Wapniarz, B. Hofmann, et al., "Drinking Water Fluoridation: Bone Mineral Density and Hip Fracture Incidence," *Bone* 22, no. 3 (1998): 273–78.

K. R. Phipps, E. S. Orwoll, J. D. Mason, and J. A Cauley, "Community Water Fluoridation, Bone Mineral Density and Fractures: Prospective Study of Effects in Older Women," *British Medical Journal* 321, no. 7265 (2000): 860–64. Note: As with Feskanich, et al. (1998) and Karagas, et al. (1996), this study didn't find an association between water fluoride and hip fracture, but it did find an association between water fluoride and other types of fracture—in this case, wrist fracture. "There was a non-significant trend toward an increased risk of wrist fracture."

M. E. Suarez-Almazor, G. Flowerdew, L. D. Saunders, et al., "The Fluoridation of Drinking Water and Hip Fracture Hospitalization Rates in Two Canadian Communities," *American Journal of Public Health* 83, no. 5 (1993): 689–93, http://www.ncbi.nlm.nih.gov/pmc/articles/PMC1694711/pdf/amjph00529-0067.pdf. Note: While the authors of this study conclude that there is no association between fluoridation and hip fracture, their own data reveals a statistically significant increase in hip fracture for men living in the fluoridated area. According to the authors, "Although a statistically significant increase in the risk of hip fracture was observed among Edmonton men, this increase was relatively small (RR=1.12)."

Endnotes

Links to the references in the endnotes and appendices can be accessed at http://fluoridealert
.org/caseagainstfluoride.refs.html.

Introduction

1. R. A. Freeze and J. A. Lehr, *The Fluoride Wars: How a Modest Public Health Measure Became America's Longest-Running Political Melodrama* (Hoboken, NJ: John Wiley, 2009).
2. E. D. Beltrán-Aguilar, B. F. Gooch, A. Kingman, et al., "Surveillance for Dental Caries, Dental Sealants, Tooth Retention, Edentulism, and Enamel Fluorosis—United States, 1988–1994 and 1999–2002," *Morbidity and Mortality Weekly Report* 54, no. 3 (August 26, 2005): 1–44, http://www.cdc.gov/mmwr/preview/mmwrhtml/ss5403a1.htm.
3. World Health Organization, "EURO incl. DMFT for 12-year-olds," WHO Oral Health Country/Area Profile Programme, WHO Headquarters Geneva, Oral Health Programme, Malmo University, Sweden, http://www.whocollab.od.mah.se/euro.html. Note: WHO has changed and updated its Web site several times over the last five years. The table on this page gives statistics by European country for DMFT (decayed/missing/filled teeth) for twelve-year-olds, as of March 3, 2010.
4. National Research Council of the National Academies, *Fluoride in Drinking Water: A Scientific Review of EPA's Standards* (Washington, DC: National Academies Press, 2006), http://books.nap.edu/openbook.php?record_id=11571.
5. Ibid.
6. Ibid.
7. R. J. Carton, "Review of the 2006 United States National Research Council Report: Fluoride in Drinking Water," *Fluoride* 39, no. 3 (2006): 163–72, http://www.fluoride alert.org/health/epa/nrc/carton-2006.pdf.
8. National Research Council, *Fluoride in Drinking Water*, 10 (n. 4 above).
9. Centers for Disease Control and Prevention, "Ten Great Public Health Achievements: United States, 1900–1999," *Morbidity and Mortality Weekly Report* 48, no. 12 (April 2, 1999): 241–43, http://www.cdc.gov/mmwr/preview/mmwrhtml/00056796.htm.
10. Centers for Disease Control and Prevention, "Achievements in Public Health, 1900–1999: Fluoridation of Drinking Water to Prevent Dental Caries," *Mortality and Morbidity Weekly Review* 48, no. 41 (October 22, 1999): 933–40, http://www.cdc.gov/ mmwr/preview/mmwrhtml/mm4841a1.htm. Note: The authors of this report were Scott Tomar and Susan Griffin, as cited in Tomar's curriculum vitae, paper number 27 on page 27, http://fluoridealert.org/re/tomar.scott.cv.ref.27.pdf.
11. M. W. Easley, "Community Fluoridation in America: The Unprincipled Opposition," 1999, posted on Dental Watch, http://www.dentalwatch.org/fl/opposition.pdf.
12. American Dental Association, *Fluoridation Facts*, an update commemorating the sixtieth anniversary of community water fluoridation, 2005, https://www.ada.org/sections/ professionalresources/pdfs/fluoridation_facts.pdf.
13. M. W. Easley, "Community Fluoridation in America: The Unprincipled Opposition," (n. 11 above).

Chapter 1

1. American Medical Association, "Patient Physician Relationship Topics: Informed Consent," http://www.ama-assn.org/ama/pub/physician-resources/legal-topics/patient -physician-relationship-topics/informed-consent.shtml.

2. U.S. Department of Health and Human Services, *Oral Health in America: A Report of the Surgeon General* (Rockville, MD: U.S. Department of Health and Human Services, National Institute of Dental and Craniofacial Research, National Institutes of Health, 2000), http://fluoridealert.org/teeth/surgeon.general-2000.pdf.

3. Institute of Medicine, *Dietary Reference Intakes for Calcium, Phosphorus, Magnesium, Vitamin D, and Fluoride* (Washington, DC: Standing Committee on the Scientific Evaluation of Dietary Reference Intakes, Food and Nutrition Board, National Academy Press, 1997), http://www.nap.edu/openbook.php?record_id=5776.

4. Letter coauthored by Bruce Alberts, president of the National Academy of Sciences, and Kenneth Shine, president of the Institute of Medicine, to Albert W. Burgstahler and others, November 20, 1998, http://www.fluoridation.com/fraud.htm.

5. Letter from Melinda K. Plaisier, FDA associate commissioner for legislation, to the Honorable Ken Calvert, chairman, Subcommittee on Energy and Environment, Committee on Science, U.S. House of Representatives, Washington, DC, December 21, 2000, http://www.fluoridealert.org/re/fda.letter.to.calvert.dec.2000.pdf.

6. At the Web site of the National Association of Pharmacy Regulatory Authorities, http://www.napra.org/, search the National Drug Schedules for "sodium fluoride" or "fluoride and its salts."

7. K. K. Cheng, I. Chalmers, and T. A. Sheldon, et al., "Adding Fluoride to Water Supplies," *British Medical Journal* 335, no. 7622 (2007): 699–702.

8. Centers for Disease Control and Prevention, "Recommendations for Using Fluoride to Prevent and Control Dental Caries in the United States," *Morbidity and Mortality Weekly Report* 50, no. RR14 (August 17, 2001): 1–42, http://www.cdc.gov/mmwr/preview/mmwrhtml/rr5014a1.htm.

9. American Dental Association, "Pediatric Journal Highlights Need for Translational Research, Medical-Dental Collaboration to Improve Children's Oral Health," 2009, http://www.ada.org/prof/resources/topics/science_pediatric_research.asp.

10. Letter from John V. Kelly, New Jersey assemblyman, 36th District, to Dr. David Kessler, commissioner of the Food and Drug Administration, June 3, 1993, http://www.fluoride alert.org/re/kelly.1993.pdf.

11. M. S. McDonagh, P. F. Whiting, P. M. Wilson, et al., "Systematic Review of Water Fluoridation," *British Medical Journal* 321, no. 7265 (2000): 855–59, http://www.bmj .com/cgi/content/full/321/7265/855. Note: The full report that this paper summarizes is commonly known as the York Review and is accessible at http://fluoridealert.org/re/york .review.2000.pdf.

12. E. Baldwin, video interview by Kevin Hurley, in "Professional Perspectives on Water Fluoridation," produced by Michael Connett for Fluoride Action Network, 2009, http://www.fluoridealert.org/prof.dvd.html.

13. Letter from Dr. Arvid Carlsson to the South Central Strategic Health Authority, UK, February 2009, http://www.fluoridealert.org/southhampton.html.

14. U.S. Environmental Protection Agency, "Pesticides and Food: Why Children May Be Especially Sensitive to Pesticides," 2008, http://www.epa.gov/pesticides/food/pest.htm.

15. U.S. Environmental Protection Agency, "National Primary Drinking Water Regulations: Fluoride. Final Rule," *Federal Register* 50, no. 220 (November 14, 1985), http://fluoride

alert.org/scher/epa-1985.pdf. Note: The MCL established on April 2, 1986 (51 FR 11396), finalizes regulations proposed in the *Federal Register* of May 14, 1985 (50 FR 20164), http://fluoridealert.org/scher/epa-1985.pdf.

16. Integrated Risk Information System, "Fluorine (Soluble Fluoride) (CASRN 7782–41–4)," Environmental Protection Agency, http://www.epa.gov/iris/subst/0053.htm.

17. National Research Council of the National Academies, *Fluoride in Drinking Water: A Scientific Review of EPA's Standards* (Washington, DC: National Academies Press, 2006), http://books.nap.edu/openbook.php?record_id=11571.

18. American Dental Association, "Interim Guidance on Reconstituted Infant Formula," ADA eGRAM, November 9, 2006, http://www.fluoridealert.org/scher/ada.egram-2006.pdf.

19. Centers for Disease Control and Prevention, "Statement on the 2006 National Research Council Report on Fluoride in Drinking Water," posted originally March 28, 2006, last updated August 24, 2009, http://www.cdc.gov/FLUORIDATION/safety/nrc_report.htm.

20. E. D. Beltrán-Aguilar, B. F. Gooch, A. Kingman, et al., "Surveillance for Dental Caries, Dental Sealants, Tooth Retention, Edentulism, and Enamel Fluorosis—United States, 1988–1994 and 1999–2002," *Morbidity and Mortality Weekly Report* 54, no. 3 (August 26, 2005): 1–44, http://www.cdc.gov/mmwr/preview/mmwrhtml/ss5403a1.htm.

21. S. Fisher, "Dangerous Fluoride?" Health Alert report, CBS-TV (Atlanta, Georgia), March 8, 2010. See also transcript "Fluoride: Friend or Foe?" by Stephany Fisher, http://www.cbsatlanta.com/health/22776266/detail.html.

22. "Ottawa Charter for Health Promotion," WHO/HPR/HEP/95.1, First International Conference on Health Promotion, Ottawa, cosponsored by the Canadian Public Health Association, Health and Welfare Canada, and the World Health Organization, November 21, 1986, http://www.who.int/healthpromotion/conferences/previous/ottawa/en/.

23. Council of Europe, "Convention for the Protection of Human Rights and Dignity of the Human Being with Regard to the Application of Biology and Medicine: Convention on Human Rights and Biomedicine," CETS no. 164 (1997), http://conventions.coe.int/Treaty/Commun/QueVoulezVous.asp?NT=164&CL=ENG.

Chapter 2

1. Centers for Disease Control and Prevention, "Achievements in Public Health, 1900–1999: Fluoridation of Drinking Water to Prevent Dental Caries," *Mortality and Morbidity Weekly Review* 48, no. 41 (October 22, 1999): 933–40, http://www.cdc.gov/mmwr/preview/mmwrhtml/mm4841a1.htm. Note: The authors of this report were Scott Tomar and Susan Griffin, as cited in Tomar's curriculam vitae, paper number 27 on page 27, http://fluoridealert.org/re/tomar.scott.cv.ref.27.pdf.

2. O. Fejerskov, A. Thylstrup, and M. J. Larsen, "Rational Use of Fluorides in Caries Prevention: A Concept Based on Possible Cariostatic Mechanisms," *Acta Odontologica Scandinavica* 39, no. 4 (1981): 241–49.

3. J. P. Carlos, "Comments on Fluoride," *Journal of Pedodontics* 7, no. 2 (1983): 135–36.

4. J. S. Wefel, "Effects of Fluoride on Caries Development and Progression Using Intra-Oral Models," *Journal of Dental Research* 69, special no. (1990): 626–33, 634–36.

5. D. H. Leverett, "Appropriate Uses of Systemic Fluoride: Considerations for the '90s," *Journal of Public Health Dentistry* 51, no. 1 (1991): 42–47.

6. D. T. Zero, R. F. Raubertas, J. Fu, et al., "Fluoride Concentrations in Plaque, Whole

Saliva, and Ductal Saliva after Application of Home-Use Topical Fluorides," *Journal of Dental Research* 71, no. 11 (1992): 1768–75, http://jdr.sagepub.com/cgi/reprint/71/11/1768.

7. J. Ekstrand, S. J. Fomon, E. E. Ziegler, and S. E. Nelson, "Fluoride Pharmacokinetics in Infancy," *Pediatric Research* 35, no. 2 (1994): 157–63.

8. J. D. B. Featherstone, "Prevention and Reversal of Dental Caries: Role of Low-Level Fluoride," *Community Dentistry and Oral Epidemiology* 27, no. 1 (1999): 31–40.

9. H. Limeback, "A Re-examination of the Pre-eruptive and Post-eruptive Mechanism of the Anti-Caries Effects of Fluoride: Is There Any Caries Benefit from Swallowing Fluoride?" *Community Dentistry and Oral Epidemiology* 27, no. 1 (1999): 62–71.

10. B. A. Burt, "The Case for Eliminating the Use of Dietary Fluoride Supplements for Young Children," *Journal of Public Health Dentistry* 59, no. 4 (1999): 260–74.

11. S. M. Adair, "Overview of the History and Current Status of Fluoride Supplementation Schedules," *Journal of Public Health Dentistry* 59, no. 4 (1999): 252–58.

12. D. Locker, *Benefits and Risks of Water Fluoridation: An Update of the 1996 Federal-Provincial Sub-committee Report,* prepared under contract for Public Health Branch, Ontario Ministry of Health First Nations and Inuit Health Branch, Health Canada (Ottawa: Ontario Ministry of Health and Long Term Care, 1999), http://fluoridealert.org/re/locker.1999.pdf.

13. Centers for Disease Control and Prevention, "Achievements in Public Health, 1900–1999" (n. 1 above).

14. M. S. McDonagh, P. F. Whiting, P. M. Wilson, et al., "Systematic Review of Water Fluoridation," *British Medical Journal* 321, no. 7265 (2000): 855–59, http://www.bmj.com/cgi/content/full/321/7265/855. Note: The full report that this paper summarizes is commonly known as the York Review and is accessible at http://fluoridealert.org/re/york.review.2000.pdf.

15. D. Carnall, "Water Fluoridation," *British Medical Journal* 321, no. 7265 (October 7, 2000): 904. Carnall's statement appeared on the *British Medical Journal* Web site on the day (October 7, 2000) the journal published a review of the York Report (n. 14 above), http://www.bmj.com/cgi/content/full/321/7265/904/a.

16. Michael Connett's video interview of Dr. Arvid Carlsson, October 2005. This interview is included on the DVD *Professional Perspectives on Water Fluoridation,* produced by Fluoride Action Network, http://fluoridealert.org/prof.dvd.html.

17. J. Colquhoun, "Education and Fluoridation in New Zealand: An Historical Study,'" Ph.D. diss., University of Auckland, New Zealand, 1987.

18. David L. Biles, "When It Comes to Fluoride, Education Is Better Than Medication," *Santa Cruz Sentinel* (California), March 7, 2010, http://www.santacruzsentinel.com/ci_14528191?source=most_emailed.

19. Ibid.

20. CNN-TV, "Diabetes Cases Could Double by 2034," news broadcast, November 27, 2009, http://transcripts.cnn.com/TRANSCRIPTS/0911/27/cnr.02.html.

Chapter 3

1. Florida Institute of Phosphate Research, "Public & Environmental Health," 2003–2004, http://www.fipr.state.fl.us/research-area-public-health.htm.

2. Letter from Rebecca Hanmer, deputy assistant administrator for water, U.S. Environmental Protection Agency, to Leslie A. Russell, D.M.D, March 30, 1983, http://fluoridealert.org/re/hanmer1983.pdf.

3. J. W. Hirzy testimony on behalf of the National Treasury Employees Union Chapter 280, before the Subcommittee on Wildlife, Fisheries and Drinking Water, U.S. Senate, Washington, DC, June 29, 2000. Video of testimony, "EPA Union Calls for Moratorium on Water Fluoridation," at http://video.google.com/videoplay?docid=8903910725020792574#; transcript of testimony at http://www.fluoridealert.org/testimony.htm.

4. Department of Human Services, *Water Fluoridation: Questions and Answers*, pamphlet distributed by the Department of Human Services, Victoria, Australia, February 2009, http://fluoridealert.org/re/australia.2009.victoria.pamphlet.pdf.

5. Letter from Stan Hazan, general manager, National Sanitation Foundation International's Drinking Water Additives Certification Program, to Ken Calvert, chairman, Subcommittee on Energy and the Environment, Committee on Science, U.S. House of Representatives, July 7, 2000, http://www.keepers-of-the-well.org/gov_resp _pdfs/NSF_response.pdf.

6. C. Wang, D. B. Smith, and G. M. Huntley, "Treatment Chemicals Contribute to Arsenic Levels," *Opflow* (a journal of the American Water Works Association), October 2000.

7. R. D. Masters and M. J. Coplan, "Water Treatment with Silicofluorides and Lead Toxicity," *International Journal of Environmental Studies* 56, no. 4 (1999): 435–49.

8. R. D. Masters, M. J. Coplan, B. T. Hone, and J. E. Dykes, "Association of Silicofluoride Treated Water with Elevated Blood Lead," *Neurotoxicology* 21, no. 6 (2000): 1091–99.

9. E. T. Urbansky and M. R. Schock, "Can Fluoridation Affect Lead (II) in Potable Water? Hexafluorosilicate and Fluoride Equilibria in Aqueous Solution," *International Journal of Environmental Studies* 57, no. 5 (2000): 597–637.

10. E. T. Urbansky, "Fate of Fluorosilicate Drinking Water Additives," *Chemical Reviews* 102, no. 8 (2002): 2837–54.

11. W. F. Finney, E. Wilson, A. Callender, et al., "Reexamination of Hexafluorosilicate Hydrolysis by Fluoride NMR and pH Measurement," *Environmental Science & Technology* 40, no. 8 (2006): 2572–77.

12. R. P. Maas, S. C. Patch, A. M. Christian, and M. J. Coplan, "Effects of Fluoridation and Disinfection Agent Combinations on Lead Leaching from Leaded-Brass Parts," *Neurotoxicology* 28, no. 5 (2007): 1023–31.

13. R. M. M. Sawan, G. A. S. Leite, M. C. P. Saraiva, et al., "Fluoride Increases Lead Concentrations in Whole Blood and in Calcified Tissues from Lead-Exposed Rats," *Toxicology* 271, no. 1–2 (2010): 21–66.

14. Ibid.

15. R. D. Masters and M. J. Coplan, "Water Treatment with Silicofluorides and Lead Toxicity" (n. 7 above).

16. R. D. Masters et al., "Association of Silicofluoride Treated Water with Elevated Blood Lead" (n. 8 above).

17. L. Hendricks, "Feds Note Fluoride Problems," *The Daily News* (Newburyport, Massachusetts), January 25, 2010, http://www.newburyportnews.com/punews/local _story_024222057.html#disqus_thread.

18. L. Hendricks, "Town Halts Use in Water Supply, Seeks Solutions," *The Daily News* (Newburyport, Massachusetts), January 19, 2010.

Chapter 4

1. Centers for Disease Control and Prevention, "Division of Oral Health," list of personnel, March 2008, http://www.fluoridealert.org/bailey3.html.

2. Agency for Toxic Substances and Disease Registry, *Toxicological Profile for Fluorides,*

Hydrogen Fluoride and Fluorine (Atlanta, GA: U.S. Department of Health and Human Services, Public Health Service, September 2003), http://www.atsdr.cdc.gov/toxprofiles/tp11.pdf.

3. National Research Council of the National Academies, *Fluoride in Drinking Water: A Scientific Review of EPA's Standards* (Washington, DC: National Academies Press, 2006), http://books.nap.edu/openbook.php?record_id=11571.

4. R. J. Carton, "Review of the 2006 United States National Research Council Report: Fluoride in Drinking Water," *Fluoride* 39, no. 3 (2006): 163–72, http://www.fluoridealert.org/health/epa/nrc/carton-2006.pdf.

5. The deposition of Stan Hazan was taken in a San Diego County Superior Court case titled *Macy v. City of Escondido*, case no. GIN015280, on March 9, 2004. The lawsuit sought to have the addition of hexafluorosilicic acid (HFSA) to the water declared unconstitutional under California law. The lawsuit was dismissed, and the dismissal was affirmed on appeal by the Fourth District Court of Appeals. The deposition is online at http://fluoridealert.org/re/hazan-2004.deposition.pdf.

6. NSF Joint Committee on Drinking Water Additives, *Drinking Water Treatment Chemicals—Health Effects*, NSF International Standard/American National Standard NSF/ANSI 60—2009 (Ann Arbor, MI: NSF International, 2009).

7. Ibid.

8. Ibid.

Chapter 5

1. National Health and Medical Research Council, *The Effectiveness of Water Fluoridation* (Canberra: Australian Government Publishing Service, 1991), 142.

2. National Research Council of the National Academies, *Fluoride in Drinking Water: A Scientific Review of EPA's Standards* (Washington, DC: National Academies Press, 2006), http://books.nap.edu/openbook.php?record_id=11571.

3. D. Fagin, "Second Thoughts on Fluoride," *Scientific American* 298, no. 1 (January 2008): 74–81; excerpts at http://www.fluoridealert.org/sc.am.jan.2008.html.

4. M. S. McDonagh, P. F. Whiting, P. M. Wilson, et al., "Systematic Review of Water Fluoridation," *British Medical Journal* 321, no. 7265 (2000): 855–59, http://www.bmj.com/cgi/content/full/321/7265/855. Note: The full report that this paper summarizes is commonly known as the York Review and is accessible at http://fluoridealert.org/re/york.review.2000.pdf.

5. Open letter from Professor Trevor Sheldon, DSc, FMedSci., of the Department of Health Sciences, University of York, Heslington, York, UK, January 3, 2001, http://www.appgaf.org.uk/archive/archive_letter_shel/.

6. "Regulations and Ethical Guidelines: Directives for Human Experimentation," Office of Human Subjects Research, National Institutes of Health, http://ohsr.od.nih.gov/guidelines/nuremberg.html. Reprinted from *Trials of War Criminals before the Nuremberg Military Tribunals under Control Council Law*, no. 10 (1949): 181–82.

7. UK Water Act, "The Drinking Water Inspectorate. Fluoridation of Water Supplies": "90 (2) The Secretary of State may also, with the consent of the Treasury, agree to indemnify any licensed water supplier in respect of liabilities which it may incur— (a) In supplying water to which fluoride has been added by a water undertaker by virtue of any such arrangements . . . " 2003, http://www.opsi.gov.uk/2003/37/section/58.

8. Letter from Dr. B. Havlik, DrSc, Ministerstvo Zdravotnictvi Ceske Republiky, to A. R.

Smith and C. A. Smith, England, October 14, 1999, http://www.fluoridealert.org/czech .jpeg.

9. World Health Organization, "EURO incl. DMFT for 12-year-olds," WHO Oral Health Country/Area Profile Programme, WHO Headquarters Geneva, Oral Health Programme (NPH), WHO Collaborating Centre, Malmo University, Sweden, http:// www.whocollab.od.mah.se/euro.html. Last update March 3, 2010. Note: WHO has changed and updated its Web site several times over the last five years. This online site gives statistics by European country for DMFT (decayed/missing/filled teeth) for twelve-year-olds; http://www.whocollab.od.mah.se/euro.html.

10. C. Neurath, "Tooth Decay Trends for 12 Year Olds in Nonfluoridated and Fluoridated Countries," graph in Fluoride & Tooth Decay (Caries) section at Fluoride Action Network Web site, 2004, http://www.fluoridealert.org/health/teeth/caries/.

11. L. Seppä, S. Kärkkäinen, and H. Hausen, "Caries Trends 1992–1998 in Two Low-Fluoride Finnish Towns Formerly with and without Fluoridation," *Caries Research* 34, no. 6 (2000): 462–68.

12. W. Künzel, T. Fischer, R. Lorenz, and S. Brühmann, "Decline in Caries Prevalence after the Cessation of Water Fluoridation in Former East Germany," *Community Dentistry and Oral Epidemiology* 28, no. 5 (2000): 382–89.

13. W. Künzel and T. Fischer, "Caries Prevalence after Cessation of Water Fluoridation in La Salud, Cuba," *Caries Research* 34, no. 1 (2000): 20–25.

14. G. Maupomé, D. C. Clark, S. M. Levy, and J. Berkowitz, "Patterns of Dental Caries Following the Cessation of Water Fluoridation," *Community Dentistry and Oral Epidemiology* 29, no. 1 (2001): 37–47.

15. American Dental Association, *Fluoridation Facts,* an update commemorating the sixtieth anniversary of community water fluoridation, 2005, https://www.ada.org/sections/ professionalresources/pdfs/fluoridation_facts.pdf.

Chapter 6

1. M. S. McDonagh, P. F. Whiting, P. M. Wilson, et al., "Systematic Review of Water Fluoridation," *British Medical Journal* 321, no. 7265 (2000): 855–59, http://www.bmj .com/cgi/content/full/321/7265/855. Note: The full report that this paper summarizes is commonly known as the York Review and is accessible at http://fluoridealert.org/re/york .review.2000.pdf.

2. H. T. Dean, F. A. Arnold Jr., and E. Elvove, "Domestic Water and Dental Caries. V. Additional Studies of the Relation of Fluoride Domestic Waters to Dental Caries Experience in 4425 White Children, age 12-14 years, of 13 Cities in 4 States," *Public Health Reports* 57, no. 32 (1942): 1155–79, http://www.ncbi.nlm.nih.gov/pmc/articles/ PMC1968063/pdf/pubhealthreporig01481-0001.pdf.

3. H. T. Dean, F. A. Arnold Jr., and E. Elvove, "Domestic Water and Dental Caries. II. A Study of 2,832 White Children, Aged 12 to 14 Years, of 8 Suburban Chicago Communities, Including *Lactobacillus Acidophilus* Studies of 1,761 Children," *Public Health Reports* 56 (1941): 761–92.

4. World Health Organization, "EURO incl. DMFT for 12-Year-Olds," WHO Oral Health Country/Area Profile Programme, Oral Health Programme (NPH), WHO Collaborating Centre, Malmo University, Sweden, http://www.whocollab.od.mah .se/euro.html. Last update March 3, 2010. Note: WHO has changed and updated its Web site several times over the last five years. This online site gives statistics by European country for DMFT (decayed/missing/filled teeth) for twelve-year-olds; http:// www.whocollab.od.mah.se/euro.html.

5. C. Neurath, "Tooth Decay Trends for 12 Year Olds in Nonfluoridated and Fluoridated Countries," graph in Fluoride & Tooth Decay (Caries) section at Fluoride Action Network Web site, 2004, http://www.fluoridealert.org/health/teeth/caries/.
6. K. K. Cheng, I. Chalmers, and T. A. Sheldon, "Adding Fluoride to Water Supplies," *British Medical Journal* 335, no. 7622 (2007): 699–702.
7. Centers for Disease Control and Prevention, "Ten Great Public Health Achievements: United States, 1900–1999," *Morbidity and Mortality Weekly Report* 48, no. 12 (April 2, 1999): 241–43, http://www.cdc.gov/mmwr/preview/mmwrhtml/00056796.htm.
8. C. Neurath, "Tooth Decay Trends for 12 Year Olds in Nonfluoridated and Fluoridated Countries," *Fluoride* 38, no. 4 (2005): 324–25, at http://fluoridealert.org/re/neurath-2005.pdf.
9. Centers for Disease Control and Prevention, "Achievements in Public Health, 1900–1999: Fluoridation of Drinking Water to Prevent Dental Caries," *Mortality and Morbidity Weekly Review* 48, no. 41 (October 22, 1999): 933–40, http://www.cdc.gov/mmwr/preview/mmwrhtml/mm4841a1.htm. Note: The authors of this report were Scott Tomar and Susan Griffin, as cited in Tomar's curriculum vitae, paper number 27 on page 27, http://fluoridealert.org/re/tomar.scott.cv.ref.27.pdf.
10. Ibid.
11. Centers for Disease Control and Prevention, "Achievements in Public Health, 1900–1999," 937 (n. 9 above).
12. U.S. Department of Health and Human Services, "The Oral Health of Children: A Portrait of States and the Nation 2005. Condition of Children's Teeth," based on data from the National Survey of Children's Health 2003, Health Resources and Services Administration, Maternal and Child Health Bureau, Rockville, Maryland, http://mchb.hrsa.gov/oralhealth/portrait/1cct.htm.
13. B. Osmunson, "Water Fluoridation Intervention: Dentistry's Crown Jewel or Dark Hour?" *Fluoride* 40, no. 4 (2007): 214–21, http://www.fluorideresearch.org/404/files/FJ2007_v40_n4_p214-221.pdf.
14. J. V. Kumar, D. L. Altshul, T. L. Cooke, and E. L. Green, "Oral Health Status of Third Grade Children: New York State Oral Health Surveillance System," December 15, 2005, http://fluoridealert.org/re/kumar-2005.nys.report.pdf.
15. Based on analysis performed by Michael Connett for Fluoride Action Network.
16. B. Osmunson, "Water Fluoridation Intervention" (n. 13 above).
17. Based on analysis performed by Michael Connett for Fluoride Action Network.
18. J. V. Kumar et al., "Oral Health Status of Third Grade Children: New York State Oral Health Surveillance System" (n. 14 above).
19. Based on analysis performed by Michael Connett for Fluoride Action Network.
20. J. V. Kumar et al., "Oral Health Status of Third Grade Children: New York State Oral Health Surveillance System" (n. 14 above).
21. M. Eisenstadt, "How Fluoride Makes a Difference in CNY; Cayuga County Lacks Fluoridation, and Has a Higher Rate of Cavities," *The Post-Standard* (Syracuse, New York), December 27, 2005, article begins on page A1.
22. J. Colquhoun, "Why I Changed My Mind About Fluoridation," *Perspectives in Biology and Medicine* 41 (1997): 29–44. Reprinted, with permission, in *Fluoride* 31, no. 2 (1998): 103–18, http://www.fluoride-journal.com/98-31-2/312103.htm.
23. American Dental Association, "Fluoridation Facts," an update commemorating the sixtieth anniversary of community water fluoridation, 2005, https://www.ada.org/sections/professionalresources/pdfs/fluoridation_facts.pdf.

24. D. H. Retief, E. L. Bradley, F. H. Barbakow, et al., "Relationships Among Fluoride Concentration in Enamel, Degree of Fluorosis and Caries Incidence in a Community Residing in a High Fluoride Area," *Journal of Oral Pathology* 8, no. 4 (1979): 224–36.

25. J. Mann, M. Tibi, and H. D. Sgan-Cohen, "Fluorosis and Caries Prevalence in a Community Drinking Above-Optimal Fluoridated Water," *Community Dentistry and Oral Epidemiology* 15, no. 5 (1987): 293–95.

26. J. Mann, W. Mahmoud, M. Ernest, et al., "Fluorosis and Dental Caries in 6-8-Year-Old Children in a 5 ppm Fluoride Area," *Community Dentistry and Oral Epidemiology* 18, no. 2 (1990): 77–79.

27. C. Steelink, "Fluoridation Controversy" (letter), *Chemical & Engineering News*, July 27, 1992, 2–3; C. Steelink et al., "Findings and Recommendations on Fluoridation," Citizen's Water Advisory Committee Report, Phoenix, Arizona, June 1992; Bob Carton, ed., *Fluoride Report* 2, no. 1 (1994): 7.

28. S. P. S. Teotia and M. Teotia, "Dental Caries: A Disorder of High Fluoride and Low Dietary Calcium Interactions (30 Years of Personal Research)," *Fluoride* 27, no. 2 (1994): 59–66, http://www.fluoridealert.org/re/teotia-1994.pdf.

29. S. R. Grobleri, A. J. Louw, and T. J. van Kotze, "Dental Fluorosis and Caries Experience in Relation to Three Different Drinking Water Fluoride Levels in South Africa," *International Journal of Paediatric Dentistry* 11, no. 5 (2001): 372–79.

30. A. K. Awadia, J. M. Birkeland, O. Haugejorden, and K. Bjorvatn, "Caries Experience and Caries Predictors—A Study of Tanzanian Children Consuming Drinking Water with Different Fluoride Concentrations," *Clinical Oral Investigations* 6, no. 2 (2002): 98–103.

31. L. Ekanayake and W. van der Hoek, "Dental Caries and Developmental Defects of Enamel in Relation to Fluoride Levels in Drinking Water in an Arid Area of Sri Lanka," *Caries Research* 36, no. 6 (2002): 398–404.

32. M. Diesendorf, "The Mystery of Declining Tooth Decay," *Nature* 322, no. 6075 (1986): 125–29.

33. R. Feltman and G. Kosel, "Prenatal and Postnatal Ingestion of Fluorides—Fourteen Years of Investigation. Final Report," *The Journal of Dental Medicine* 16 (1961): 190–99.

34. R. Leroy, K. Bogaerts, E. Lesaffre, and D. Declerck, "The Effect of Fluorides and Caries in Primary Teeth on Permanent Tooth Emergence," *Community Dentistry and Oral Epidemiology* 31, no. 6 (2003): 463–70.

35. A. Komárek, E. Lesaffre, T. Härkänen, et al., "A Bayesian Analysis of Multivariate Doubly-Interval-Censored Dental Data," *Biostatistics* 6, no. 1 (2005): 145–55.

36. Video of the debate on water fluoridation that took place between Professor Michael Lennon, chairman of the British Fluoridation Society, and Dr. Paul Connett, director of the Fluoride Action Network, Isle of Man, November 20, 2007, http://video.google.com/videoplay?docid=82194292805035136&hl=en.

37. M. Kelly and B. Bruerd, "The Prevalence of Baby Bottle Tooth Decay Among Two Native American Populations," *Journal of Public Health Dentistry* 47, no. 2 (1987): 94–97.

38. G. P. Barnes, W. A. Parker, T. C. Lyon Jr., et al., "Ethnicity, Location, Age, and Fluoridation Factors in Baby Bottle Tooth Decay and Caries Prevalence of Head Start Children," *Public Health Reports* 107, no. 2 (1992): 167–73, http://www.ncbi.nlm.nih.gov/pmc/articles/PMC1403626/pdf/pubhealthrep00074-0041.pdf.

39. P. Weinstein, P. Domoto, K. Wohlers, and M. Koday, "Mexican-American Parents with Children at Risk for Baby Bottle Tooth Decay: Pilot Study at Migrant Farmworkers Clinic," *ASDC Journal of Dentistry for Children* 59, no. 5 (1992): 376–83.

40. M. M. Von Burg, B. J. Sanders, and J. A. Weddell, "Baby Bottle Tooth Decay: A Concern for All Mothers," *Pediatric Nursing* 21, no. 6 (1995): 515–19.

41. C. Febres, E. A. Echeverri, and H. J. Keene, "Parental Awareness, Habits, and Social Factors and Their Relationship to Baby Bottle Tooth Decay," *Pediatric Dentistry* 19, no. 1 (1997): 22–27.

42. J. M. Tang, D. S. Altman, D. C. Robertson, et al., "Dental Caries Prevalence and Treatment Levels in Arizona Preschool Children," *Public Health Reports* 112, no. 4 (1997): 319–29, http://www.pubmedcentral.nih.gov/articlerender.fcgi?artid=1381972.

43. M. Blen, S. Narendran, and K. Jones, "Dental Caries in Children Under Age Three Attending a University Clinic," *Pediatric Dentistry* 21, no. 4 (1999): 261–64.

44. D. Kong, "City to Launch Battle Against Dental 'Crisis,'" *Boston Globe* (Massachusetts), November 11, 1999.

45. Centers for Disease Control and Prevention, "Achievements in Public Health, 1900–1999" (n. 8 above).

46. Centers for Disease Control and Prevention, "Recommendations for Using Fluoride to Prevent and Control Dental Caries in the United States," *Morbidity and Mortality Weekly Report* 50, no. RR14 (August 17, 2001): 1–42, http://www.cdc.gov/mmwr/preview/mmwrhtml/rr5014a1.htm.

47. V. C. Marinho, "Evidence-Based Effectiveness of Topical Fluorides," *Advances in Dental Research* 20, no. 1 (2008): 3–7.

48. M. S. McDonagh et al., "Systematic Review of Water Fluoridation" (n. 1 above).

49. K. A. Eaton and M. J. Carlile, "Toothbrushing Behavior in Europe: Opportunities for Dental Public Health," *International Dental Journal* 58, no. 5, suppl. 1 (2008): 287–93, http://www.unilever.com/images/sd_Tooth_brush_behaviour_in_Europe _opportunities_for_dental_public_health(International_Dental_Journal_2008) _tcm13-160710.pdf.

50. B. de Liefde, "The Decline of Caries in New Zealand over the Past 40 Years," *New Zealand Dental Journal* 94, no. 417 (1998): 109–13.

Chapter 7

1. H. T. Dean, F. A. Arnold Jr., and E. Elvove, "Domestic Water and Dental Caries. II. A Study of 2,832 White Children, Aged 12 to 14 Years, of 8 Suburban Chicago Communities, Including *Lactobacillus Acidophilus* Studies of 1,761 Children," *Public Health Reports* 56 (1941): 761–92.

2. H. T. Dean, F. A. Arnold Jr., and E. Elvove, "Domestic Water and Dental Caries. V. Additional Studies of the Relation of Fluoride Domestic Waters to Dental Caries Experience in 4425 White Children, Age 12-14 Years, of 13 Cities in 4 States," *Public Health Reports* 57, no. 32 (1942): 1155–79, http://www.ncbi.nlm.nih.gov/pmc/articles/PMC1968063/pdf/pubhealthreporig01481-0001.pdf.

3. B. C. Nesin, "A Water Supply Perspective of the Fluoridation Discussion," *Journal of the Maine Water Utilities Association* 32 (1956): 33–47.

4. Centers for Disease Control and Prevention, "Achievements in Public Health, 1900–1999: Fluoridation of Drinking Water to Prevent Dental Caries," *Mortality and Morbidity Weekly Review* 48, no. 41 (October 22, 1999): 933–40, http://www.cdc.gov/mmwr/preview/mmwrhtml/mm4841a1.htm. Note: The authors of this report were Scott Tomar and Susan Griffin, as cited in Tomar's curriculum vitae, paper number 27 on page 27, http://fluoridealert.org/re/tomar.scott.cv.ref.27.pdf.

5. H. T. Dean et al., "Domestic Water and Dental Caries. V" (n. 2 above).

6. F. B. Exner, "Analytical Commentary on the 1960 Testimony of Dr. H. Trendley Dean in the Suit to Enjoin Fluoridation of Chicago's Water, Part II," in *Fluoridation: Its Moral and Political Aspect; A New and Comprehensive Study* (New York), The Greater New York Committee Opposed to Fluoridation (undated).

7. R. Ziegelbecker, "Fluoridated Water and Teeth," *Fluoride* 14, no. 3 (1981): 123–28, http://fluoridealert.org/re/ziegelbecker-1981.pdf.

8. Ibid.

9. R. Ziegelbecker and R. C. Ziegelbecker, "WHO Data on Dental Caries and Natural Fluoride Levels," *Fluoride* 26, no. 4 (1993): 263–66, http://fluoridealert.org/re/ziegelbecker-1993.pdf.

10. R. Ziegelbecker, "Comments and Scientific Critique on the Report of the Working Group to Consider Section 3.1 Essential Composition in the Proposed Draft Revised Standard for Infant Formula at (Step 3)," submitted to Codex Alimentarius Commission FAO/WHO, Committee on Nutrition and Foods for Special Dietary Uses (CCNFSDU), March 30, 2003, http://fluoridealert.org/re/ziegelbecker.2003.codex.pdf.

11. R. Ziegelbecker, "Fluoridated Water and Teeth" (n. 7 above).

12. T. M. De Stefano, "The Fluoridation Research Studies and the General Practitioner," *Bulletin of Hudson County Dental Society,* February 1954.

13. P. R. N. Sutton, *Fluoridation: Errors and Omissions in Experimental Trials,* 1st ed. (Australia: Melbourne University Press, 1959). ·

14. P. R. N. Sutton, *Fluoridation: Errors and Omissions in Experimental Trials,* 2nd ed. (Australia: Melbourne University Press, 1960).

15. P. R. N. Sutton, *The Greatest Fraud: Fluoridation* (Lorne, Australia: A Factual Book, Kurunda Pty. Ltd., 1996).

16. R. Ziegelbecker, "A Critical Review on the Fluorine Caries Problem," *Fluoride* 3, no. 2 (1970): 71–79, http://fluoridealert.org/re/ziegelbecker-1970.pdf.

17. Letter from Hubert A. Arnold, PhD, University of California (Davis) to Dr. Ernest Newbrun, Medical Sciences Bldg. 653, San Francisco, California, May 28, 1980, http://www.fluoridealert.org/uc-davis.htm.

18. P. R. N. Sutton, *The Greatest Fraud: Fluoridation* (n. 15 above).

19. D. F. Radusch, "Variability of Diagnosis of Incidence of Dental Caries, *Journal of the American Dental Association* 28 (1941): 1959–61.

20. J. D. Boyd and N. E. Wessels, "Epidemiological Studies in Dental Caries. III. The Interpretation of Clinical Data Relating to Caries Advance," *American Journal of Public Health and the Nation's Health* 41, no. 8, pt. 1 (1951): 976–85, http://ajph.apha publications.org/cgi/reprint/41/8_Pt_1/976.

21. P. R. N. Sutton, *Fluoridation: Errors and Omissions in Experimental Trials,* 1st ed. (n. 13 above).

22. P. R. N. Sutton, *Fluoridation: Errors and Omissions in Experimental Trials,* 2nd ed. (n. 14 above).

23. P. R. N. Sutton, *The Greatest Fraud: Fluoridation* (n. 15 above).

24. Letter from John Forst, MD, New York State Education Department, to Dr. James Kerwin of the New Jersey Department of Health, October 26, 1954.

25. J. V. Kumar and E. L. Green, "Recommendations for Fluoride Use in Children. A Review," *The New York State Dental Journal* 64, no. 2 (1998): 40–47.

26. J. V. Kumar, P. H. Swango, L. L. Lininger, et al., "Changes in Dental Fluorosis and Dental Caries in Newburgh and Kingston, New York," *American Journal of Public Health* 88, no. 12 (1998): 1866–70, http://ajph.aphapublications.org/cgi/reprint/88/12/1866.

27. J. V. Kumar and E. L. Green, "Recommendations for Fluoride Use in Children. A Review" (n. 25 above.)

28. Ibid.

29. C. Bryson, *The Fluoride Deception* (New York: Seven Stories Press, 2004), 83–87.

30. J. Colquhoun and R. Mann, "The Hastings Fluoridation Experiment: Science or Swindle?" *The Ecologist* 16, no. 6 (1986): 243–48.

31. J. Colquhoun, "Education and Fluoridation in New Zealand: An Historical Study," Ph.D. diss., University of Auckland, New Zealand, 1987.

32. J. Colquhoun and B. Wilson, "The Lost Control and Other Mysteries: Further Revelations on New Zealand's Fluoridation Trial," *Accountability in Research* 6, no. 4 (1999): 373–94.

33. T. G. Ludwig, "The Hastings Fluoridation Project I. Dental Effects Between 1954 and 1957," *The New Zealand Dental Journal* 54 (1958): 165–72.

34. T. G. Ludwig, "The Hastings Fluoridation Project II. Dental Effects Between 1954 and 1959," *The New Zealand Dental Journal* 55 (1959): 176–79.

35. T. G. Ludwig, "The Hastings Fluoridation Project III. Dental Effects Between 1954 and 1961," *The New Zealand Dental Journal* 58 (1962): 22–24.

36. T. G. Ludwig, "The Hastings Fluoridation Project IV. Dental Effects Between 1954 and 1963," *The New Zealand Dental Journal* 59 (1963): 298–301.

37. T. G. Ludwig, "The Hastings Fluoridation Project V. Dental Effects Between 1954 and 1964," *The New Zealand Dental Journal* 61 (1965): 175–79.

38. T. G. Ludwig, "The Hastings Fluoridation Project VI. Dental Effects Between 1954 and 1970," *The New Zealand Dental Journal* 67 (1971): 155–60.

Chapter 8

1. Paul Connett's videotape interview with John Colquhoun in Auckland, New Zealand, 1997. Available from Paul Connett, 82 Judson Street, Canton, New York 13617.

2. J. Colquhoun, "New Evidence on Fluoridation," *Social Science & Medicine* 19, no. 11 (1984): 1239–46.

3. J. Colquhoun, "Influence of Social Class and Fluoridation on Child Dental Health," *Community Dentistry and Oral Epidemiology* 13, no. 1 (1985): 37–41.

4. J. Colquhoun, "Child Dental Health Differences in New Zealand," *Community Health Studies* 11, no. 2 (1987): 85–90.

5. J. Colquhoun, "Flawed Foundation: A Re-examination of the Scientific Basis for a Dental Benefit from Fluoridation," *Community Health Studies* 14, no. 3 (1990): 288–96.

6. J. Colquhoun, "Possible Explanations for Decline in Tooth Decay in New Zealand," *Community Dentistry and Oral Epidemiology* 20, no. 3 (1992): 161–66.

7. J. Colquhoun, "Dental Caries Among Children in New Zealand," *Community Dentistry and Oral Epidemiology* 23, no. 6 (1995): 381.

8. J. Colquhoun, "Education and Fluoridation in New Zealand: An Historical Study," Ph.D. diss., University of Auckland, New Zealand, 1987.

9. T. S. Kuhn, *The Structure of Scientific Revolutions* (Chicago and London: University of Chicago Press, 1962).

10. J. Colquhoun, "Why I Changed My Mind About Fluoridation," *Perspectives in Biology and Medicine* 41 (1997): 29–44. Reprinted, with permission, in *Fluoride* 31, no. 2 (1998): 103–18, http://www.fluoride-journal.com/98-31-2/312103.htm.

11. E. Newbrun and H. Horowitz, "Why We Have Not Changed Our Minds about the Safety and Efficacy of Water Fluoridation," *Perspectives in Biology and Medicine* 42, no. 4 (1999): 526–43.

12. D. H. Leverett, "Fluorides and the Changing Prevalence of Dental Caries," *Science* 217, no. 4554 (1982): 26–30.

13. Ibid., 27.

14. M. Diesendorf, "The Mystery of Declining Tooth Decay," *Nature* 322, no. 6075 (1986): 125–29.

15. Ibid.

16. Ibid.

17. Ibid.

18. M. Diesendorf, *Greenhouse Solutions with Sustainable Energy* (Sydney: University of New South Wales Press, 2007).

19. A. S. Gray, "Fluoridation: Time for a New Base Line?" *Journal of the Canadian Dental Association* 53, no. 10 (1987): 763–65.

20. Ibid.

21. J. A. Yiamouyiannis, "Water Fluoridation and Tooth Decay: Results from the 1986–87 National Survey of U.S. Schoolchildren," *Fluoride* 23, no. 2 (1990): 55–67, http://www .fluoridealert.org/health/teeth/caries/nidr-dmft.html.

22. J. A. Brunelle and J. P. Carlos, "Recent Trends in Dental Caries in U.S. Children and the Effect of Water Fluoridation," *Journal of Dental Research* 69 (1990): 723–27.

23. J. A. Yiamouyiannis, *Fluoride: The Aging Factor*, 3rd ed. (Delaware, Ohio: Health Action Press, 1993). Note: First edition published in 1983, and second edition in 1986.

24. J. A. Brunelle and J. P. Carlos, "Recent Trends in Dental Caries in U.S. Children and the Effect of Water Fluoridation" (n. 22 above).

25. J. A. Yiamouyiannis, "Water Fluoridation and Tooth Decay" (n. 21 above).

26. J. A. Brunelle and J. P. Carlos, "Recent Trends in Dental Caries in U.S. Children and the Effect of Water Fluoridation" (n. 22 above).

27. A. J. Spencer, G. D. Slade and M. Davies, "Water Fluoridation in Australia," *Community Dental Health* 13, suppl. 2 (1996): 27–37.

28. Ibid.

29. J. A. Brunelle and J. P. Carlos, "Recent Trends in Dental Caries in U.S. Children and the Effect of Water Fluoridation" (n. 22 above).

30. B. de Liefde, "The Decline of Caries in New Zealand over the Past 40 Years," *New Zealand Dental Journal* 94, no. 417 (1998): 109–13.

31. D. Locker, *Benefits and Risks of Water Fluoridation: An Update of the 1996 Federal-Provincial Sub-committee Report*, prepared under contract for Public Health Branch, Ontario Ministry of Health First Nations and Inuit Health Branch, Health Canada (Ottawa: Ontario Ministry of Health and Long Term Care, 1999), http://fluoridealert .org/re/locker.1999.pdf.

32. H. Cohen and D. Locker, "The Science and Ethics of Water Fluoridation," *Journal of the Canadian Dental Association* 67, no. 10 (2001): 578–80.

33. Ibid.

34. J. M. Armfield and A. J. Spencer, "Consumption of Nonpublic Water: Implications for Children's Caries Experience," *Community Dentistry and Oral Epidemiology* 32, no. 4 (2004): 283–96.

35. J. Spencer, "Dental Research on Fluoridation Misused," *Fluoride* 39, no. 4 (2006): 326–27, http://www.fluorideresearch.org/394/files/FJ2006_v39_n4_p326-330.pdf.

36. M. Diesendorf, "Response to John Spencer's Obfuscation of the Results of His Own Paper," *Fluoride* 39, no. 4 (2006): 327–30. Letter follows Spencer's at http://www.fluoride research.org/394/files/FJ2006_v39_n4_p326-330.pdf.

304 ENDNOTES

37. A. Komárek, E. Lesaffre, T. Härkänen, et al., "A Bayesian Analysis of Multivariate Doubly-Interval-Censored Dental Data," *Biostatistics* 6, no. 1 (2005): 145–55.
38. E. Lesaffre, "On the Spatial Distribution of Caries in Primary Teeth" (undated), http://www.stat.ucl.ac.be/ISpersonnel/lambert/biostat2000/lesaffre.html.
39. A. Komárek et al., "A Bayesian Analysis of Multivariate Doubly-Interval-Censored Dental Data" (n. 37 above).
40. Ibid.
41. Ibid.
42. J. Vanobbergen, L. Martens, E. Lesaffre, et al. 2001, "Assessing Risk Indicators for Dental Caries in the Primary Dentition," *Community Dentistry and Oral Epidemiology* 29, no. 6 (2001): 424–34.
43. A. Komárek et al., "A Bayesian Analysis of Multivariate Doubly-Interval-Censored Dental Data" (n. 37 above).
44. G. Pizzo, M. R. Piscopo, I. Pizzo, and G. Giuliana, "Community Water Fluoridation and Caries Prevention: A Critical Review," *Clinical Oral Investigations* 11, no. 3 (2007): 189–93.
45. J. J. Warren, S. M. Levy, B. Broffitt, et al., "Considerations on Optimal Fluoride Intake Using Dental Fluorosis and Dental Caries Outcomes—A Longitudinal Study," *Journal of Public Health Dentistry* 69, no. 2 (2009): 111–15.
46. E. Solvig, "Special Report: Cincinnati's Dental Crisis," *The Enquirer* (Cincinnati, Ohio), October 6, 2002, http://www.enquirer.com/editions/2002/10/06/loc_special_report.html.
47. D. Kong, "City to Launch Battle Against Dental 'Crisis,'" *Boston Globe* (Massachusetts), November 11, 1999.
48. R. Slate, "State Must Fund Plan to Provide Oral Health Care for the Poor," *New Haven Register* (Connecticut), May 5, 2005.
49. V. Law, "Sink Your Teeth into Health Care," *Pittsburgh Tribune-Review* (Pennsylvania), February 13, 2005, http://www.pittsburghlive.com/x/pittsburghtrib/s_303168.html.
50. S. Morse, "Bottled Water: Just Add Fluoride," *Washington Post*, March 5, 2002.
51. S. Voss, "Kentucky's Dental Disaster Begins Before Kindergarten," *Lexington Herald-Leader* (Kentucky), November 9, 2008, http://www.kentucky.com/181/story/585931.html.
52. U. Gerth, "Nothing to Smile About," *Fosters Daily Democrat* (Connecticut), May 22, 2005.
53. B. A. Burt, J. L. Kolker, A. M. Sandretto, et al., "Dietary Patterns Related to Caries in a Low-income Adult Population," *Caries Research* 40, no. 6 (2006): 473–80.
54. J. Kozol, *Savage Inequalities: Children in America's Schools* (New York: Crown Publishers, Inc., 1991).
55. E. Connett, "The Failure of the Fluoridation Experiment—Part 2. Oral Health Reports from the 50 States & District of Columbia," Fluoride Action Network, 2010, http://fluoridealert.org/teeth.state.reports.html.

Chapter 9
1. D. R. McNeil, *The Fight for Fluoridation* (New York: Oxford University Press, 1957).
2. R. R. Harris, *Dental Science in a New Age: A History of the National Institute of Dental Research* (Maryland: Montrose Press, 1989).
3. F. B. Exner and G. L. Waldbott, *The American Fluoridation Experiment* (New York: Devin-Adair, 1957).
4. C. Bryson, *The Fluoride Deception* (New York: Seven Stories Press, 2004).

5. H. Velu, "Dystrophie Dentaire des Mammifères des Zones Phosphatées (Darmous) et Fluorose Chronique," *Comptes Rendus des Séances de la Société de Biologie et de ses Filiales* 108 (1931): 750–52.

6. H. V. Churchill, "The Occurrence of Fluorides in Some Waters of the United States," *Industrial and Engineering Chemistry* 23, no. 9 (1931): 996–98. Reprinted in *The Journal of Dental Research* 12 (1932): 141–48, http://jdr.sagepub.com/cgi/reprint/12/1/141.

7. M. O. Smith, E. M. Lantz, and H. V. Smith, "The Cause of Mottled Enamel, a Defect of Human Teeth," *Technical Bulletin No. 32*, Agricultural Experiment Station, College of Agriculture, University of Arizona, June 10, 1931.

8. G. J. Cox, "New Knowledge of Fluorine in Relation to Dental Caries," *Journal of the American Waterworks Association* 31 (1939): 1926–30.

9. H. Cristiani, "Une Nouvelle Maladie. La Fluorose ou Cachexie Fluorique," *La Presse Médicale* 34, no. 30 (1926): 469–70. Reviewed in "Fluorine Poisoning," *Canadian Medical Association Journal* 16, no. 8 (1926): 970.

10. G. V. Black and F. S. McKay, "An Investigation of Mottled Teeth: An Endemic Developmental Imperfection of the Enamel of the Teeth, Heretofore Unknown in the Literature of Dentistry," *Dental Cosmos* 58 (1916): 129–56, 477–84, 627–44, 781–92, 894–904.

11. F. S. McKay, "The Relation of Mottled Enamel to Caries," *Journal of the American Dental Association* 15, no. 8 (1928): 1429–37.

12. H. Cristiani, "Alteration de la Glande Thyroide dans L'intoxication Fluorée," *Comptes Rendus des Séances de la Société de Biologie et de ses Filiales* 103 (1930): 554–56.

13. H. Cristiani, "Le Fluor des Os dans l'Intoxication Fluorique," *Annales d'Hygiène Publique* 8 (1930): 309–16.

14. H. Velu, "Dystrophie Dentaire des Mammifères des Zones Phosphatées (Darmous) et Fluorose Chronique" (n. 5 above).

15. H. V. Churchill, "The Occurrence of Fluorides in Some Waters of the United States" (n. 6 above).

16. M. O. Smith et al., "The Cause of Mottled Enamel, a Defect of Human Teeth" (n. 7 above).

17. C. Bryson, *The Fluoride Deception*, 39 (n. 4 above).

18. H. T. Dean, "Distribution of Mottled Enamel in the United States," *Public Health Reports* 48, no. 25 (1933): 703–34, http://www.ncbi.nlm.nih.gov/pmc/articles/PMC2016232/pdf/pubhealthreporig02047-0004.pdf.

19. P. F. Moeller and S. V. Gudjonsson, "Massive Fluorosis of Bones and Ligaments," *Acta Radiologica* 13 (1932): 269–94.

20. F. DeEds, "Chronic Fluorine Intoxication. A Review," *Medicine* (Baltimore) 12, no. 1 (1933): 1–60.

21. F. J. McClure, "A Review of Fluorine and Its Physiological Effects," *Physiological Reviews* 13, no. 3 (1933): 277–300.

22. K. Roholm, *Fluorine Intoxication: A Clinical-Hygienic Study, with a Review of the Literature and Some Experimental Investigations* (Copenhagen: Nyt Nordisk Forlag; London: H. K. Lewis and Co. Ltd., 1937), http://www.scribd.com/doc/11757791/Fluorine-Intoxication-Kaj-Roholm-1937-Copenhagen.

23. H. E. Shortt, G. R. McRobert, T. W. Barnard, and A. S. M. Nayar, "Endemic Fluorosis in the Madras Presidency," *Indian Journal of Medical Research* 25, no. 2 (1937): 553–68.

24. H. T. Dean, "A Review of *Fluorine Intoxication* by Kaj Roholm (1937)," *American Journal of Public Health* 28 (1938): 1008–9, http://www.ncbi.nlm.nih.gov/pmc/articles/PMC1527875/pdf/amjphnation01010-0110b.pdf.

25. D. G. Steyn, "Water Poisoning in Man and Animal, Together with a Discussion on Urinary Calculi," *Onderstepoort Journal of Veterinary Science and Animal Industry* 12 (1939): 167–230.

26. G. J. Cox, "New Knowledge of Fluorine in Relation to Dental Caries" (n. 8 above).

27. D. A. Greenwood, "Fluoride Intoxication," *Physiological Reviews* 20 (1940): 582–616.

28. C. G. Pandit, T. N. S. Raghavachari, D. S. Rao, and V. Krishnamurti, "Endemic Fluorosis in South India," *Indian Journal of Medical Research* 28, no. 2 (1940): 533–58.

29. H. T. Dean, F. A. Arnold Jr., and E. Elvove, "Domestic Water and Dental Caries. II. A Study of 2,832 White Children, Aged 12 to 14 Years, of 8 Suburban Chicago Communities, Including *Lactobacillus Acidophilus* Studies of 1,761 Children," *Public Health Reports* 56 (1941): 761–92.

30. H. T. Dean, F. A. Arnold Jr., and E. Elvove, "Domestic Water and Dental Caries. V. Additional Studies of the Relation of Fluoride Domestic Waters to Dental Caries Experience in 4,425 White Children, Aged 12 to 14 Years, of 13 Cities in 4 States," *Public Health Reports* 57, no. 32 (1942): 1155–79, http://www.ncbi.nlm.nih.gov/pmc/articles/PMC1968063/pdf/pubhealthreporig01481-0001.pdf.

31. F. J. McClure, "Fluoride Domestic Waters and Systemic Effects. I. Relation to Bone-Fracture Experience, Height, and Weight of High School Boys and Young Selectees of the Armed Forces of the United States," *Public Health Reports* 59, no. 48 (1944): 1543–58, http://www.ncbi.nlm.nih.gov/pmc/articles/PMC2017089/pdf/pubhealth reporig01549-0001.pdf.

32. F. J. McClure and C. A. Kinser, "Fluoride Domestic Waters and Systemic Effects. II. Fluorine Content of Urine in Relation to Fluorine in Drinking Water," *Public Health Reports* 59, no. 49 (1944): 1575–91, http://www.ncbi.nlm.nih.gov/pmc/articles/PMC2017101/pdf/pubhealthreporig01550-0001.pdf.

33. F. J. McClure, H. H. Mitchell, T. S. Hamilton, and C. A. Kinser, "Balances of Fluorine Ingested from Various Sources in Food and Water by Five Young Men. Excretion of Fluorine through the Skin," *The Journal of Industrial Hygiene and Toxicology* 27 (1945): 159.

34. C. Bryson, *The Fluoride Deception*, chapter 9 (n. 4 above).

35. F. B. Exner and G. L. Waldbott, *The American Fluoridation Experiment*, 8 (n. 3 above).

36. G. J. Cox and H. C. Hodge, "The Toxicity of Fluorides in Relation to Their Use in Dentistry," *Journal of the American Dental Association* 40 (1950): 440–51.

37. H. T. Dean and F. A. Arnold, "Dental Research and the National Institute of Health: I. Intramural Research," *Journal of the American Dental Association* 38, no. 1 (1949): 15–19.

38. H. Velu, "Dystrophie Dentaire des Mammifères des Zones Phosphatées (Darmous) et Fluorose Chronique" (n. 5 above).

39. H. V. Churchill, "The Occurrence of Fluorides in Some Waters of the United States" (n. 6 above).

40. M. O. Smith et al., "The Cause of Mottled Enamel, a Defect of Human Teeth" (n. 7 above).

41. H. T. Dean to Surgeon General, March 4, 1932. In the Ruth Roy Harris Papers, National Library of Medicine, History of Medicine Division, Bethesda, Maryland.

42. H. T. Dean, "Chronic Endemic Dental Fluorosis (Mottled Enamel)," *Journal of the American Medical Association* 107, no. 16 (1936): 1269–73.

43. C. H. Boissevain and W. F. Drea, "Spectroscopic Determination of Fluorine in Bones, Teeth, and Other Organs in Relation to Fluorine in Drinking Water," *Journal of Dental Research* 13, no. 6 (1933): 495–500, http://jdr.sagepub.com/cgi/reprint/13/6/495.

44. H. T. Dean and E. Elvove, "Some Epidemiological Aspects of Chronic Endemic Dental Fluorosis," *American Journal of Public Health* 26 (1936): 567–75, http://www.ncbi.nlm .nih.gov/pmc/articles/PMC1562676/pdf/amjphnation01063-0033.pdf.
45. H. Cristiani, "Le Fluor des Os dans l'Intoxication Fluorique" (n. 13 above).
46. H. T. Dean, "Chronic Endemic Dental Fluorosis (Mottled Enamel)" (n. 42 above).
47. Memorandum from H. T. Dean to Assistant Surgeon General L. R. Thompson, May 26, 1936. In the H. T. Dean Papers, National Library of Medicine, History of Medicine Division, Bethesda, Maryland.
48. F. DeEds, "Chronic Fluorine Intoxication. A Review" (n. 20 above).
49. F. DeEds, "Fluorine in Relation to Bone and Tooth Development," *Journal of the American Dental Association* 23 (1936): 568–74.
50. F. J. McClure, "A Review of Fluorine and Its Physiological Effects" (n. 21 above).
51. D. A. Greenwood, "Fluoride Intoxication" (n. 27 above).
52. P. F. Moeller and S. V. Gudjonsson, "Massive Fluorosis of Bones and Ligaments" (n. 19 above).
53. K. Roholm, *Fluorine Intoxication"* (n. 22 above).
54. H. E. Shortt et al., "Endemic Fluorosis in the Madras Presidency" (n. 23 above).
55. D. G. Steyn, "Water Poisoning in Man and Animal, Together with a Discussion on Urinary Calculi" (n. 25 above).
56. C. G. Pandit et al., "Endemic Fluorosis in South India" (n. 28 above).
57. G. Abbott, "Dangerous Water," *Journal of the American Dental Association* 27 (1939): 162. Reviewed in *Hygeia* 17 (1940): 899.
58. H. Cristiani, "Alteration de la Glande Thyroide dans L'intoxication Fluorée" (n. 12 above).
59. H. Cristiani, "Le Fluor des Os Dans l'Intoxication Fluorique" (n. 13 above).
60. G. von Mundy, "Ein neuer Weg zur Behandlung der Thyreotoxikose mit Fluorwasserstoffsäure," *Medizinische Klinik* 21 (1932): 717–19.
61. E. Spéder and A. Charnot, "Syndromes Osseux du Type Hyperparathyroidien et du Type Hypoparathyroidien, Provoqués par l'Intoxication par les Sivers Sels de Fluor et des Intoxications Minérales Associées," *La Presse Médicale* 90 (1936): 1754.
62. K. Kraft, "Beiträge zur Biochemie des Fluors I. Über den Antagonismus Zwischen Fluor und Thyroxin," *Hoppe-Seyler's Zeitschrift für Physiologische Chemie* 245 (1937): 58–65.
63. J. D. Hatfield, C. L. Shrewsbury, F. N. Andrews, and L. P. Doyle, "Iodine-Fluorine Relationship in Sheep Nutrition," *Journal of Animal Science* 3 (1944): 71–77.
64. P. H. Phillips and A. R. Lamb, "Histology of Certain Organs and Teeth in Chronic Toxicosis Due to Fluorine," *Archives of Pathology* 17 (1934): 169.
65. P. H. Phillips, H. E. English, and E. B. Hart, "The Influence of Sodium Fluoride upon the Basal Metabolism of the Rat under Several Experimental Conditions," *The American Journal of Physiology* 113 (1935): 441–49.
66. P. H. Phillips, H. English, and E. B. Hart, "The Augmentation of Fluorosis in the Chick by Feeding Desiccated Thyroid," *Journal of Nutrition* 10 (1935): 399–407, http:// jn.nutrition.org/cgi/reprint/10/4/399.
67. P. H. Phillips, "Further Studies on the Effects of NaF Administration upon the Basal Metabolic Rate of Experimental Animals," *The American Journal of Physiology* 117 (1936): 155–59, http://ajplegacy.physiology.org/cgi/pdf_extract/117/1/155.
68. L. Goldemberg, "Action Physiologique des Fluorures," *Comptes Rendus des Séances de la Société de Biologie et de ses Filiales* 95 (1926): 1169.
69. L. Goldemberg, "Traitement de la Maladie de Basedow et de l'Hyperthyroidisme par le Fluor," *La Presse Médicale* 102 (1930): 1751.

70. L. Goldemberg, "Comment Agiraient-ils Therapeutiquement les Fluorures dans le Goitre Exopthalmique et dans L'hyperthyroidisme," *La Semana Médica* 39 (1932): 1659.
71. W. May, "Antagonismus Zwischen Jod und Fluor im Organismus," *Klinische Wochenschrift* 14 (1935): 790–92.
72. W. May, "Behandlung der Hyperthyreosen Einschliesslich des Schweren Genuinen Morbus Basedow mit Fluor," *Klinische Wochenschrift* 16 (1937): 562–64.
73. W. Orlowski, "Sur la Valeur Therapeutique du Sang Animal du Bore et du Fluor dans la Maladie de Basedow," *La Presse Medicale* 42 (1932): 836–37.
74. D. G. Steyn, "Water Poisoning in Man and Animal, Together with a Discussion on Urinary Calculi" (n. 25 above).
75. D. G. Steyn, "Fluorine and Endemic Goiter," *South African Medical Journal* 22, no. 16 (1948): 525–26.
76. D. G. Steyn, J. Kieser, W. A. Odendaal, et al., "Endemic Goitre in the Union of South Africa and Some Neighbouring Territories" (Pretoria: Union of South Africa, Department of Nutrition, March 1955). Excerpts at http://www.slweb.org/south-africa.goitre.html.
77. R. H. Wilson and F. DeEds, "The Synergistic Action of Thyroid on Fluoride Toxicity," *Endocrinology* 26, no. 5 (1940): 851–56.
78. H. T. Dean, "A Review of *Fluorine Intoxication* by Kaj Roholm (1937)" (n. 24 above).
79. P. C. Hodges, O. J. Fareed, G. Ruggy, et al., "Skeletal Sclerosis in Chronic Sodium Fluoride Poisoning," *Journal of the American Medical Association* 117, no. 23 (1941): 1938.
80. Abstract of the proceedings of the meetings of the Technical Advisory Committee on the fluoridation of water supplies with the departmental working committee for the Newburgh–Kingston (NY) demonstration, April 24, 1944; in the H. T. Dean Papers, History of Medicine Division, National Library of Medicine, Bethesda, Maryland.
81. C. G. Pandit et al, "Endemic Fluorosis in South India" (n. 28 above).
82. American Medical Association, "Chronic Fluorine Intoxication" (editorial), *Journal of the American Medical Association* 123 (1943): 150.
83. Abstract of the proceedings of the meetings of the Technical Advisory Committee on the fluoridation of water supplies with the departmental working committee for the Newburgh–Kingston (NY) demonstration (n. 80 above).
84. N. C. Leone, M. B. Shimkin, F. A. Arnold, et al., "Medical Aspects of Excessive Fluoride in a Water Supply," *Public Health Reports* 69, no. 10 (1954): 925–36, http://www.ncbi.nlm.nih.gov/pmc/articles/PMC2024409/pdf/pubhealthreporig00178-0039.pdf.
85. N. C. Leone, F. A. Arnold Jr., E. R. Zimmermann, et al., "Review of the Bartlett-Cameron Survey: A Ten Year Fluoride Study," *Journal of the American Dental Association* 50, no. 3 (1955): 277–81.
86. N. C. Leone, C. A. Stevenson, T. F. Hilbish, and M. C. Sosman, "A Roentgenologic Study of a Human Population Exposed to High-Fluoride Domestic Water; a Ten-Year Study," *The American Journal of Roentgenology, Radium Therapy, and Nuclear Medicine* 74, no. 5 (1955): 874–85.
87. C. A. Stevenson and R. Watson, "Fluoride Osteosclerosis," *The American Journal of Roentgenology, Radium Therapy, and Nuclear Medicine* 78, no. 1 (1957): 13–18.
88. Abstract of the proceedings of the meetings of the Technical Advisory Committee on the fluoridation of water supplies with the departmental working committee for the Newburgh–Kingston (NY) demonstration (n. 80 above).
89. D. B. Ast, "Response on Receiving the John W. Knutson Distinguished Service Award in Dental Public Health," *Journal of Public Health Dentistry* 43, no. 2 (1983): 101–5.

90. Abstract of the proceedings of the meetings of the Technical Advisory Committee on the fluoridation of water supplies with the departmental working committee for the Newburgh–Kingston (NY) demonstration (n. 80 above).

91. Ibid.

92. Ibid.

93. American Dental Association, "The Effect of Fluorine on Dental Caries" (editorial), *Journal of the American Dental Association* 31 (1944): 1360–63.

94. D. B. Ast, "A Plan to Determine the Practicability, Efficacy, and Safety of Fluorinating a Communal Water-Supply, Deficient in Fluorine, to Control Dental Caries," in *Fluorine in Dental Public Health. A Symposium,* ed. W. J. Gies (New York City, 1945).

95. Letter from R. E. Dyer to E. S. Godfrey, November 20, 1944. In the H. T. Dean Papers, National Library of Medicine, History of Medicine Division, Bethesda, Maryland.

96. F. J. McClure, "Fluoride Domestic Waters and Systemic Effects. I" (n. 31 above).

97. F. B. Exner, "Fluoridation," *Northwest Medicine* 54 (1955). Note: The quotes we cite are in the section titled "McClure's Study of Bone Fragility."

98. F. J. McClure et al., "Balances of Fluorine Ingested from Various Sources in Food and Water by Five Young Men" (n. 33 above).

99. P. Wallace-Durbin, "The Metabolism of Fluorine in Rat using F^{18} as a Tracer," *Journal of Dental Research* 33, no. 6 (1954): 789–800, http://jdr.sagepub.com/cgi/reprint/33/6/789.

100. H. C. Hodge, "Safety Factors in Water Fluoridation Based on the Toxicology of Fluorides," *Proceedings of the Nutrition Society* 22 (1963): 111–17.

101. F. B. Exner, "Fluoridation" (n. 97 above).

102. F. R Moulton, *Dental Caries and Fluorine*, publication of the American Association for the Advancement of Science (Lancaster, Pennsylvania: The Science Press Printing Company, 1946).

103. Ibid., 74–92.

104. Ibid., foreword.

105. Ibid., 30.

106. Ibid., 33.

107. D. C. Wilson, "Fluorine in Aetiology of Endemic Goitre," *The Lancet* 240 (1941): 211–13.

108. C. D. M. Day, "Chronic Endemic Fluorosis in Northern India," *British Dental Journal* 68 (1940): 409.

109. F. R Moulton, *Dental Caries and Fluorine*, 34 (n. 102 above).

110. Ibid., 35.

111. C. Bryson, *The Fluoride Deception*, 81–87 (n. 4 above).

112. E. R. Schlesinger, D. E. Overton, and H. C. Chase, "Newburgh-Kingston Caries-Fluorine Study. II. Pediatric Aspects. Preliminary Report," *American Journal of Public Health* 40, no. 6 (1950): 725–27, http://www.ncbi.nlm.nih.gov/pmc/articles/PMC1528773/pdf/amjphnation01021-0070.pdf.

113. D. R. McNeil, *The Fight for Fluoridation,* chapters 3 and 4 (n. 1 above).

114. G. J. Cox and H. C. Hodge, "The Toxicity of Fluorides in Relation to Their Use in Dentistry" (n. 36 above).

115. C. Bryson, *The Fluoride Deception*, 40 (n. 4 above).

116. G. J. Cox, "New Knowledge of Fluorine in Relation to Dental Caries" (n. 8 above).

117. E. Welsome, *The Plutonium Files: America's Secret Medical Experiments in the Cold War* (New York: Delta, 1999).

118. C. Bryson, *The Fluoride Deception*, 66 (n. 4 above).

119. G. J. Cox and H. C. Hodge, "The Toxicity of Fluorides in Relation to Their Use in Dentistry" (n. 36 above).

120. F. J. McClure, "Fluoride Domestic Waters and Systemic Effects. I" (n. 31 above).

121. R. J. Evans, P. H. Phillips, and E. B. Hart, "Fluoride Storage in Cattle Bones," *Journal of Dairy Science* 21, no. 2 (1938): 81–84.

122. G. J. Cox and H. C. Hodge, "The Toxicity of Fluorides in Relation to Their Use in Dentistry" (n. 36 above).

123. R. J. Evans and P. H. Phillips, "The Fluorine Content of the Thyroid Gland in Cases of Hyperthyroidism," *Journal of the American Medical Association* 111, no. 4 (1938): 300–302.

124. P. H. Phillips and A. R. Lamb, "Histology of Certain Organs and Teeth in Chronic Toxicosis Due to Fluorine" (n. 64 above).

125. P. H. Phillips et al., "The Influence of Sodium Fluoride upon the Basal Metabolism of the Rat under Several Experimental Conditions" (n. 65 above).

126. P. H. Phillips et al., "The Augmentation of Fluorosis in the Chick by Feeding Desiccated Thyroid" (n. 66 above).

127. P. H. Phillips, "Further Studies on the Effects of NaF Administration upon the Basal Metabolic Rate of Experimental Animals" (n. 67 above).

128. H. Cristiani, "Alteration de la Glande Thyroide dans L'intoxication Fluorée" (n. 12 above).

129. H. Cristiani, "Le Fluor des Os Dans l'Intoxication Fluorique" (n. 13 above).

130. G. von Mundy, "Ein neuer Weg zur Behandlung der Thyreotoxikose mit Fluorwasserstoffsäure" (n. 60 above).

131. E. Spéder and A. Charnot, "Syndromes Osseux du Type Hyperparathyroidien et du Type Hypoparathyroidien, Provoqués par l'Intoxication par les Sivers Sels de Fluor et des Intoxications Minérales Associées" (n. 61 above).

132. K. Kraft, "Beiträge zur Biochemie des Fluors I. Über den Antagonismus Zwischen Fluor und Thyroxin" (n. 62 above).

133. J. D. Hatfield et al., "Iodine-Fluorine Relationship in Sheep Nutrition" (n. 63 above).

134. L. Goldemberg, "Action Physiologique des Fluorures" (n. 68 above).

135. L. Goldemberg, "Traitement de la Maladie de Basedow et de l'Hyperthyroidisme par le Fluor" (n. 69 above).

136. L. Goldemberg, "Comment Agiraient-ils Therapeutiquement les Fluorures dans le Goitre Exopthalmique et dans L'hyperthyroidisme" (n. 70 above).

137. W. May, "Antagonismus Zwischen Jod und Fluor im Organismus" (n. 71 above).

138. W. May, "Behandlung der Hyperthyreosen Einschliesslich des Schweren Genuinen Morbus Basedow mit Fluor" (n. 72 above).

139. W. Orlowski, "Sur la Valeur Therapeutique du Sang Animal du Bore et du Fluor dans la Maladie de Basedow" (n. 73 above).

140. D. G. Steyn, "Water Poisoning in Man and Animal, Together with a Discussion on Urinary Calculi" (n. 25 above).

141. D. G. Steyn, "Fluorine and Endemic Goiter" (n. 75 above).

142. R. H. Wilson and F. DeEds, "The Synergistic Action of Thyroid on Fluoride Toxicity" (n. 77 above).

143. American Medical Association, "Chronic Fluorine Intoxication" (n. 82 above).

144. American Dental Association, "The Effect of Fluorine on Dental Caries" (n. 93 above).

145. F. J. McClure, "Fluoride Domestic Waters and Systemic Effects. I" (n. 31 above).

146. F. J. McClure et al., "Balances of Fluorine Ingested from Various Sources in Food and Water by Five Young Men. Excretion of Fluorine through the Skin" (n. 33 above).

147. Cox and Hodge, "The Toxicity of Fluorides in Relation to their Use in Dentistry" (n. 36 above).

148. Abstract of the proceedings of the meetings of the Technical Advisory Committee on the fluoridation of water supplies with the departmental working committee for the Newburgh-Kingston (NY) demonstration (n. 80 above).

149. E. R. Schlesinger et al., "Newburgh-Kingston Caries-Fluorine Study. II" (n. 112 above).

150. American Dental Association, "U.S. Public Health Service Recommends Fluoridation of Communal Water Supplies as Caries Control Measure," *ADA Newsletter* 3, no. 11 (June 1, 1950).

151. D. R. McNeil, *The Fight for Fluoridation,* 73 and 74 (n. 1 above).

152. C. Bryson, *The Fluoride Deception*, chapter 9 (n. 4 above).

153. Ibid., 39.

154. Ibid., 40–41.

155. Ibid., 185–86.

156. F. B. Exner and G. L. Waldbott, *The American Fluoridation Experiment*, 8 (n. 3 above).

157. C. Bryson, *The Fluoride Deception*, 81–87 (n. 4 above).

158. Ibid, 92–93.

159. E. Welsome, *The Plutonium Files* (n. 117 above).

160. American Dental Association, "This First Half Century," *Journal of the American Dental Association* 40, no. 6 (1950): 643.

161. American Dental Association, "U.S. Public Health Service Recommends Fluoridation of Communal Water Supplies as Caries Control Measure" (n. 150 above).

162. American Dental Association, "USPHS Recommends Public Water Fluoridation," *Journal of the American Dental Association* 41, no. 1 (1950): 93–94.

163. American Dental Association, "Dental Health of the Nation's Children Furthered by Actions of House of Delegates," *Journal of the American Dental Association* 41, no. 6 (1950). 722–23.

Chapter 10

1. F. B. Exner and G. L. Waldbott, *The American Fluoridation Experiment* (New York: Devin-Adair Publishing Company, 1957).

2. U.S. Public Health Service, "Proceeding. Fourth Annual Conference of State Dental Directors with the Public Health Service and the Children's Bureau," Washington, DC, June 6–8, 1951, page 20, http://fluoridealert.org/re/StateDental Directors-1.pdf.

3. Ibid., 22.

4. Ibid., 23.

5. Ibid., 19.

6. J. W. Knutson, "The Case for Water Fluoridation," *New England Journal of Medicine* 246, no. 19 (1952): 737–43.

7. Ibid., 737.

8. Ibid., 738.

9. Ibid.

10. Ibid., 739.

11. Ibid., 741.

12. National Research Council, *Report of Ad Hoc Committee on Fluoridation of Water Supplies* (Washington, DC: Division of Medical Sciences, November 1951).

13. J. W. Knutson, "The Case for Water Fluoridation," 742 (n. 6 above).

14. R. F. Sognnaes, F. A. Arnold, H. C. Hodge, and O. L. Kline, "The Problem of Providing Optimum Fluoride Intake for Prevention of Dental Caries." A report of the Committee on Dental Health of the Food and Nutrition Board prepared by the Subcommittee on Optimum Fluoride Levels, Division of Biology and Agriculture, National Research Council, Publication 294, November 1953.

15. N. C. Leone, M. B. Shimkin, F. A. Arnold, et al., "Medical Aspects of Excessive Fluoride in a Water Supply. A Ten Year Study," 110–29. In *Fluoridation as a Public Health Measure*, ed. J. H. Shaw, (Washington, DC: American Association for the Advancement of Science, 1954).

16. N. C. Leone, M. B. Shimkin, F. A. Arnold, et al., "Medical Aspects of Excessive Fluoride in a Water Supply," *Public Health Reports* 69, no. 10 (1954): 925–36, http://www.ncbi .nlm.nih.gov/pmc/articles/PMC2024409/pdf/pubhealthreporig00178-0039.pdf.

17. Short biography of Nicholas Charles Leone in: "Fluoridation of Water," Hearings before the Committee on Interstate and Foreign Commerce, House of Representatives, Second Session of H.R.2341, "A Bill to Protect the Public Health from the Dangers of Fluorination of Water," May 25, 26, and 27, 1954, page 392.

18. N. C. Leone et al., "Medical Aspects of Excessive Fluoride in a Water Supply" (n. 16 above).

19. Ibid.

20. Ibid.

21. R. F. Sognnaes et al., "The Problem of Providing Optimum Fluoride Intake for Prevention of Dental Caries" (n. 14 above).

22. F. B. Exner and G. L. Waldbott, *The American Fluoridation Experiment*, 73–75 (n. 1 above).

23. Ibid., 73–75.

24. Ibid.

25. Ibid.

26. Ibid.

27. N. C. Leone et al., "Medical Aspects of Excessive Fluoride in a Water Supply" (n. 16 above).

28. K. Roholm, *Fluorine Intoxication: A Clinical-Hygienic Study, with a Review of the Literature and Some Experimental Investigations* (Copenhagen: Nyt Nordisk Forlag; London: H. K. Lewis and Co. Ltd., 1937), http://www.scribd.com/doc/11757791/ Fluorine-Intoxication-Kaj-Roholm-1937-Copenhagen.

29. H. E. Shortt, G. R. McRobert, T. W. Barnard, and A. S. M. Nayar, "Endemic Fluorosis in the Madras Presidency," *Indian Journal of Medical Research* 25, no. 2 (1937): 553–68.

30. C. G. Pandit, T. N. S. Raghavachari, D. S. Rao, and V. Krishnamurti, "Endemic Fluorosis in South India," *Indian Journal of Medical Research* 28, no. 2 (1940): 533–58.

31. National Research Council of the National Academies, *Fluoride in Drinking Water: A Scientific Review of EPA's Standards* (Washington, DC: National Academies Press, 2006), 170–71, http://www.nap.edu/openbook.php?record_id=11571&page=170; and http://www.nap.edu/openbook.php?record_id=11571&page=171.

32. F. B. Exner and G. L. Waldbott, *The American Fluoridation Experiment*, 66 (n. 1 above).

33. C. Bryson, *The Fluoride Deception* (New York: Seven Stories Press, 2004), 178–79.

34. Ibid., 180.

35. Ibid., 40–42.

36. H. L. Needleman, "Clair Patterson and Robert Kehoe: Two Views of Lead Toxicity," *Environmental Research* 78, no. 2 (1998): 79–85.

37. C. Bryson, *The Fluoride Deception*, 106–7 (n. 33 above).

38. I. R. Campbell, *The Role of Fluoride in Public Health: The Soundness of Fluoridation of Communal Water Supplies. A Selected Bibliography*, supported by Research Grant DE-01493 (Formerly D-1493) from the National Institute of Dental Research, Public Health Service, U.S. Department of Health, Education, and Welfare, 1963.

39. D. B. Ast, D. J. Smith, B. Wachs, and K. T. Cantwell, "Newburgh-Kingston Caries-Fluorine Study. XIV. Combined Clinical and Roentgenographic Dental Findings After Ten Years of Fluoride Experience," *Journal of the American Dental Association* 52, no. 3 (1956): 314–25.

40. E. R. Schlesinger, D. E. Overton, H. C. Chase, and B. A. Cantwell, "Newburgh-Kingston Caries-Fluorine Study. XIII. Pediatric Findings After Ten Years," *Journal of the American Dental Association* 52, no. 3 (1956): 296–306.

41. Ibid., 304.

42. N. C. Leone et al., "Medical Aspects of Excessive Fluoride in a Water Supply" (n. 16 above).

43. E. R. Schlesinger, "The Medical Aspects of Water Fluoridation," *Pediatrics* 19, no. 1 (1957): 156–61.

44. Ibid., 158 and 160.

45. Ibid., 158.

46. Ibid., 157.

47. C. G. Pandit et al., "Endemic Fluorosis in South India" (n. 30 above).

48. E. R. Schlesinger, "The Medical Aspects of Water Fluoridation," 160 (n. 43 above).

49. Ibid., 157.

50. C. Bryson, *The Fluoride Deception*, 83–87 (n. 33 above).

51. Committee to Protect Our Children's Teeth, Inc., *Our Children's Teeth*. A digest of expert opinion based on studies of the use of fluorides in public water supplies, submitted to the Mayor and the Board of Estimate of the City of New York, March 6, 1957.

52. C. Bryson, *The Fluoride Deception*, 162 (n. 33 above).

53. Committee to Protect Our Children's Teeth, Inc., *Our Children's Teeth*, 2 (n. 51 above).

54. Ibid.

55. American Dental Association, *Dental Caries, Findings and Conclusions on Its Causes and Control*, Advisory Committee on Research in Dental Caries (New York: Lancaster Press Inc., 1939). Cited by P. C. Baehni and B. Guggenheim, "Potential of Diagnostic Microbiology for Treatment and Prognosis of Dental Caries and Periodontal Disease," *Critical Reviews in Oral Biology and Medicine* 7, no. 3 (1996): 259–77.

56. Committee to Protect Our Children's Teeth, Inc., *Our Children's Teeth*, 5 (n. 51 above).

57. A P. Black, "Facts in Refutation of Claims by Opponents of Fluoridation," *Journal of the American Dental Association* 50, no. 6 (1955): 655–64.

58. G. L. Waldbott, A. W. Burgstahler, and H. L. McKinney, *Fluoridation: The Great Dilemma* (Lawrence, Kansas: Coronado Press, 1978), 311.

59. C. Bryson, *The Fluoride Deception*, 163–65 (n. 33 above).

60. Ibid., 161.

61. Ibid.

62. G. J. Cox and H. C. Hodge, "The Toxicity of Fluorides in Relation to Their Use in Dentistry," *Journal of the American Dental Association* 40 (1950): 440–51.

63. "Professional Perspectives on Water Fluoridation," a DVD produced by Michael Connett for Fluoride Action Network, 2009, http://www.fluoridealert.org/prof.dvd.html.

64. E. Welsome, *The Plutonium Files: America's Secret Medical Experiments in the Cold War* (New York: Delta, 1999).

65. H. C. Hodge and F. A. Smith, "Some Public Health Aspects of Water Fluoridation," *Fluoridation as a Public Health Measure,* ed. J. H. Shaw (Washington, DC: American Association for the Advancement of Science, 1954).

66. F. A. Smith, D. E. Gardner, and H. C. Hodge, "Investigations on the Metabolism of Fluoride. III. Effect of Acute Renal Tubular Injury in Urinary Excretion of Fluoride by the Rabbit," *A.M.A. Archives of Industrial Health* 11, no. 1 (1955): 2–10.

67. H. C. Hodge, "Fluoride Metabolism: Its Significance in Water Fluoridation," *Journal of the American Dental Association* 52, no. 3 (1956): 307–14.

68. H. C. Hodge, "Notes on the Effects of Fluoride Deposition on Body Tissues," *A.M.A. Archives of Industrial Health* 21 (1960): 350–52.

69. H. C. Hodge, "Safety Factors in Water Fluoridation Based on the Toxicology of Fluorides," *Proceedings of the Nutrition Society* 22 (1963): 111–17, http://journals .cambridge.org/action/displayFulltext?type=1&fid=784060&jid=PNS&volumeId =22&issueId=01&aid=784052.

70. H. C. Hodge and F. A. Smith, "Biological Effects of Inorganic Fluorides," in: *Fluorine Chemistry,* ed. J. H. Simons (New York: Academic Press, 1963).

71. H. C. Hodge and F. A. Smith, *Fluorine Chemistry,* vol. 4 (New York and London: Academic Press, 1965).

72. H. C. Hodge and F. A. Smith, "Air Quality Criteria for the Effects of Fluorides on Man," *Journal of the Air Pollution Control Association* 20 (1970): 226–32.

73. H. C. Hodge and F. A. Smith, "Occupational Fluoride Exposure," *Journal of Occupational Medicine* 19, no. 1 (1977): 12–39.

74. H. C. Hodge, "The Safety of Fluoride Tablets or Drops," 253–74, in: *Continuing Evaluation of the Use of Fluorides,* ed. E. Johansen, D. R. Taves, and T. O. Olsen, American Association for the Advancement of Science, Selected Symposium (Boulder, Colorado: Westview Press, 1979).

75. H. C. Hodge, "Safety Factors in Water Fluoridation Based on the Toxicology of Fluorides," 113 (n. 69 above).

76. National Research Council, *Fluoride in Drinking Water,* 9, 30, 292 (n. 31 above).

77. H. C. Hodge, "Fluoride Metabolism: Its Significance in Water Fluoridation" (n. 67 above).

78. "Examples of Acute Poisoning from Water Fluoridation." A list of fluoridation accidents, Fluoride Action Network, http://www.fluoridealert.org/health/accidents/fluoridation .html.

79. H. C. Hodge, "Safety Factors in Water Fluoridation Based on the Toxicology of Fluorides," 112–13 (n. 69 above).

80. C. M. McCay, W. F. Ramseyer, and C. A. Smith, "Effect of Sodium Fluoride Administration on Body Changes in Old Rats," *Journal of Gerontology* 12, no. 1 (1957): 14–19.

81. A. H. Siddiqui, "Fluorosis in Nalgonda District, Hyderabad-Deccan," *British Medical Journal* 2, no. 4953 (1955): 1408–13.

82. J. A. Varner, K. F. Jensen, W. Horvath, and R. L. Isaacson, "Chronic Administration of Aluminum-Fluoride and Sodium-Fluoride to Rats in Drinking Water: Alterations in Neuronal and Cerebrovascular Integrity," *Brain Research* 784, no. 1–2 (1998): 284–98. Extended excerpts at http://www.fluoride-journal.com/98-31-2/31291-95.htm.

83. J. L. Borke and G. M. Whitford, "Chronic Fluoride Ingestion Decreases 45Ca Uptake by Rat Kidney Membranes," *Journal of Nutrition* 129 (1999): 1209–13, http://jn.nutrition .org/cgi/content/full/129/6/1209.

84. J. A. Varner et al., "Chronic Administration of Aluminum-Fluoride and Sodium-Fluoride to Rats in Drinking Water" (n. 82 above).

85. J. L. Borke and G. M. Whitford, "Chronic Fluoride Ingestion Decreases 45Ca Uptake by Rat Kidney Membranes" (n. 83 above).

86. Ibid.

87. H. C. Hodge, "Safety Factors in Water Fluoridation Based on the Toxicology of Fluorides," 113 (n. 69 above).

88. P. Galletti and G. Joyet, "Effect of Fluorine on Thyroidal Iodine Metabolism in Hyperthyroidism," *Journal of Clinical Endocrinology* 18, no. 10 (1958): 1102–10.

89. P. P. Bachinskii, O. A. Gutsalenko, N. D. Naryzhniuk et al., "Action of Fluoride on the Function of the Pituitary-thyroid System of Healthy Persons and Patients with Thyroid Disorders," *Problemy Endokrinologii (Mosk)* 31, no. 6 (1985): 25–9. Article in Russian; English translation at http://www.fluoridealert.org/bachinskii.1985.pdf.

90. F. F. Lin, Aihaiti, H. X. Zhao, et al., "The Relationship of a Low-Iodine and High-Fluoride Environment to Subclinical Cretinism in Xinjiang," Xinjiang Institute for Endemic Disease Control and Research; Office of Leading Group for Endemic Disease Control of Hetian Prefectural Committee of the Communist Party of China; and County Health and Epidemic Prevention Station, Yutian, Xinjiang, *Iodine Deficiency Disorder Newsletter* 7 (1991): 3, http://fluoridealert.org/scher/lin-1991.pdf; also see http://www.fluoridealert.org/IDD.htm.

91. H. C. Hodge, "Safety Factors in Water Fluoridation Based on the Toxicology of Fluorides," 114 (n. 69 above).

92. H. C. Hodge and F. A. Smith, "Some Public Health Aspects of Water Fluoridation," (n. 65 above).

93. C. Bryson, *The Fluoride Deception,* 125 (n. 33 above).

94. A. H. Siddiqui, "Fluorosis in Nalgonda District, Hyderabad-Deccan" (n. 81 above).

95. H. C. Hodge, "Safety Factors in Water Fluoridation Based on the Toxicology of Fluorides," 115 (n. 69 above).

96. H. C. Hodge, "Notes on the Effects of Fluoride Deposition on Body Tissues," *A.M.A. Archives of Industrial Health* 21 (1960): 350–52.

97. National Research Council, *Fluorides* (Washington, DC: Committee on Biologic Effects of Atmospheric Pollutants, National Academy of Science, 1971).

98. H. C. Hodge, "The Safety of Fluoride Tablets or Drops" (n. 74 above).

99. National Research Council, *Health Effects of Ingested Fluoride,* 89 (Washington, DC: National Academy Press, 1993), http://www.nap.edu/openbook.php?isbn=030904975X.

100. Institute of Medicine, *Dietary Reference Intakes for Calcium, Phosphorus, Magnesium, Vitamin D, and Fluoride* (Washington, DC: Standing Committee on the Scientific Evaluation of Dietary Reference Intakes, Food and Nutrition Board, 1997), http://www.nap.edu/openbook.php?record_id=5776.

101. U.S. Environmental Protection Agency, "National Primary Drinking Water Regulations; Fluoride. Final Rule," *Federal Register,* 40 CM Part 104 [WH-FRL-2913-8(b)], November 14, 1985. Note: The MCL established on April 2, 1986 [51 FR 11396], finalizes regulations proposed in the Federal Register of May 14, 1985 (50 FR 20164)]; http://fluoridealert.org/scher/epa-1985.pdf.

102. National Research Council, *Fluoride in Drinking Water* (n. 31 above).

103. E. R. Schlesinger et al., "Newburgh-Kingston Caries-Fluorine Study XIII. Pediatric Findings after Ten Years" (n. 40 above).

104. E. R. Schlesinger, "The Medical Aspects of Water Fluoridation" (n. 43 above).

105. H. C. Hodge, "Safety Factors in Water Fluoridation Based on the Toxicology of Fluorides," 105 (n. 69 above).
106. Ibid., 116.
107. G. L. Waldbott, *A Struggle with Titans: Forces Behind Fluoridation,* chapter 12 (New York: Carlton Press, 1965).
108. C. Bryson, *The Fluoride Deception,* chapter 2 (n. 33 above).

Chapter 11

1. M.O. Smith, E. M. Lantz, and H.V. Smith, "The Cause of Mottled Enamel, a Defect of Human Teeth," Technical Bulletin No. 32, Agricultural Experiment Station, College of Agriculture, University of Arizona, June 10, 1931.
2. H. V. Churchill, "The Occurrence of Fluorides in Some Waters of the United States," *Industrial and Engineering Chemistry* 23 no. 9: 996–8. Reprinted in *The Journal of Dental Research* 12 (1932): 141–48, http://jdr.sagepub.com/cgi/reprint/12/1/141.
3. H. Velu, "Dystrophie Dentaire des Mammifères des Zones Phosphatées (Darmous) et Fluorose Chronique," *Comptes Rendus des Séances de la Société de Biologie et de ses Filiales* 108 (1931): 750–52.
4. C. Bryson, *The Fluoride Deception* (New York: Seven Stories Press, 2004), 39.
5. H. T. Dean, "Classification of Mottled Enamel Diagnosis," *Journal of the American Dental Association* 49, no. 1 (1934): 1421–26.
6. H. T. Dean, F. S. McKay, and E. Elvove, "Mottled Enamel Survey of Bauxite, Ark., 10 Years After a Change in the Common Water Supply," *Public Health Reports* 53 (1938): 1736–48; article begins on page 1736 at http://www.ncbi.nlm.nih.gov/pmc/articles/PMC2110835/pdf/pubhealthreporig00982-0004.pdf.
7. H. T. Dean and E. Elvove, "Some Epidemiological Aspects of Chronic Endemic Dental Fluorosis," *American Journal of Public* 26 (1936): 567–75, http://www.ncbi.nlm.nih.gov/pmc/articles/PMC1562676/pdf/amjphnation01063-0033.pdf.
8. H. T. Dean, "Endemic Fluorosis and Its Relation to Dental Caries," *Public Health Reports* 53, no. 33 (1938): 1443–52, http://www.ncbi.nlm.nih.gov/pmc/articles/PMC2110810/pdf/pubhealthreporig00976-0004.pdf.
9. H T. Dean, P. Jay, F. A. Arnold Jr., and E. Elvove, "Domestic Water and Dental Caries. II. A Study of 2,832 White Children, Ages 12-14 years, of 8 Suburban Chicago Communities, Including *Lactobacillus Acidophilus* Studies of 1, 761 Children," *Public Health Reports* 56 (1941): 761–92.
10. H. T. Dean, F. A. Arnold Jr., and E. Elvove, "Domestic Water and Dental Caries, V. Additional Studies of the Relation of Fluoride Domestic Waters to Dental Caries Experience in 4425 White Children, Age 12–14 Years, of 13 Cities in 4 States," *Public Health Reports* 57 (1942): 1155–79, http://www.ncbi.nlm.nih.gov/pmc/articles/PMC1968063/pdf/pubhealthreporig01481-0001.pdf.
11. H. T. Dean in: Testimony of Isadore Zipkin, Ph.D., National Institutes of Health, Bethesda, Md., in *Chemicals in Foods and Cosmetics: Hearings Before the House Select Committee to Investigate the Use of Chemicals in Foods and Cosmetics, House of Representatives, 82nd Congress* (Washington, DC: U.S. Government Printing Office, 1952), 1652.
12. Ibid.
13. K. E. Heller, S. A. Eklund, and B. A. Burt, "Dental Caries and Dental Fluorosis at Varying Water Fluoride Concentrations," *Journal of Public Health Dentistry* 57, no. 3 (1997): 136–43.

14. Ibid.
15. Ibid.
16. M. S. McDonagh, P. F. Whiting, P. M. Wilson, et al., "Systematic Review of Water Fluoridation," *British Medical Journal* 321, no. 7265 (2000): 855–59, http://www.bmj .com/cgi/content/full/321/7265/855. Note: The full report that this paper summarizes is commonly known as the York Review and is accessible at http://fluoridealert.org/re/york .review.2000.pdf.
17. E. Helleret al., "Dental Caries and Dental Fluorosis at Varying Water Fluoride Concentrations" (n. 13 above.)
18. Ibid.
19. E. D. Beltrán-Aguilar, B. F. Gooch, A. Kingman, et al., "Surveillance for Dental Caries, Dental Sealants, Tooth Retention, Edentulism, and Enamel Fluorosis—United States, 1988–1994 and 1999–2002," *Morbidity and Mortality Weekly Report* 54, no. 3 (August 26, 2005): 1–44, http://www.cdc.gov/mmwr/preview/mmwrhtml/ss5403a1.htm.
20. Ibid.
21. E. Dincer, "Why Do I Have White Spots on My Front Teeth," *New York State Dental Journal* 74, no. 1 (2008): 58–60, http://www.nysdental.org/img/current-pdf/JrnlJan2008 .pdf.
22. T. Aoba and O. Fejerskov, "Dental Fluorosis: Chemistry and Biology," *Critical Reviews in Oral Biology* 13, no. 2 (2002): 155–70.
23. P. K. DenBesten, "Effects of Fluoride on Protein Secretion and Removal During Enamel Development in the Rat," *Journal of Dental Research* 65, no. 10 (1986): 1272–7, http://jdr .sagepub.com/cgi/reprint/65/10/1272.
24. P. K. DenBesten and H. Thariani, "Biological Mechanisms of Fluorosis and Level and Timing of Systemic Exposure to Fluoride with Respect to Fluorosis," *Journal of Dental Research* 71, no. 5 (1992): 1238–43, http://jdr.sagepub.com/cgi/reprint/71/5/1238.
25. P. K. DenBesten, "Biological Mechanism of Dental Fluorosis Relevant to the Use of Fluoride Supplements," *Community Dentistry and Oral Epidemiology* 27, no. 1 (1999): 41–47.
26. S. Matsuo, K. Kiyomiya, and M. Kurebe, "Mechanism of Toxic Action of Fluoride in Dental Fluorosis: Whether Trimeric G Proteins Participate in the Disturbance of Intracellular Transport of Secretory Ameloblast Exposed to Fluoride," *Archives of Toxicology* 72, no. 12 (1998): 798–806.
27. A. Schuld, "Is Dental Fluorosis Caused by Thyroid Hormonal Disturbances?" *Fluoride* 38, no. 2 (2005): 91–94, http://www.fluorideresearch.org/382/files/38291-94.pdf.
28. U.S. Public Health Service, "Proceeding. Fourth Annual Conference of State Dental Directors with the Public Health Service and the Children's Bureau," page 15, Washington, DC, June 6–8, 1951, http://fluoridealert.org/re/StateDentalDirectors-1.pdf.
29. Video of the presentation by Dr. Peter Cooney, Chief Dental Officer of Canada, on the case for fluoridation of drinking water in Dryden, Ontario, Canada, April 1, 2008, http:// video.google.com/videoplay?docid=4888471756915953833&hl=en.

Chapter 12

1. The quote from Nobel laureate Dr. James Sumner, who was the director of enzyme chemistry in the department of biochemistry and nutrition at Cornell University, was circulated in the booklet "When Doctors Disagree," ninth printing, March 1965. No citation is given for Sumner's quote. As Sumner's reservations about water fluoridation were well known at the time, we do not doubt its authenticity. Publishers of the

booklet: Greater New York Committee Opposed to Fluoridation, Inc., New Jersey Council Opposing Fluoridation, Massachusetts Citizens Rights Association, Inc., and Fluoridation Evaluation Committee (Connecticut).

2. J. Emsley, D. J. Jones, J. M. Miller, et al., "An Unexpectedly Strong Hydrogen Bond: AB Initio Calculations and Spectroscopic Studies of Amide-Fluoride Systems," *Journal of the American Chemical Society* 103, no. 1 (1981): 24–28.

3. K. R. Mahaffey and C. L. Stone, "Effect of High Fluorine (F) Intake on Tissue Lead (Pb) Concentrations," *Federation Proceedings* 35 (1976): 256.

4. P. Allain, F. Gauchard, and N. Krari, "Enhancement of Aluminum Digestive Absorption by Fluoride in Rats," *Research Communications in Molecular Pathology and Pharmacology* 91, no. 2 (1996): 225–31.

5. J. A. Varner, K. F. Jensen, W. Horvath, and R. L. Isaacson, "Chronic Administration of Aluminum-Fluoride and Sodium-Fluoride to Rats in Drinking Water: Alterations in Neuronal and Cerebrovascular Integrity," *Brain Research* 784, no. 1–2 (1998): 284–98. Extended excerpts at http://www.fluoride-journal.com/98-31-2/31291-95.htm.

6. R. M. M. Sawan, G. A. S. Leite, M. C. P. Saraiva, et al., "Fluoride Increases Lead Concentrations in Whole Blood and in Calcified Tissues from Lead-Exposed Rats," *Toxicology* 271, no. 1–2 (2010): 21–26.

7. J. Bigay, P. Deterre, C. Pfister, and M. Chabre, "Fluoroaluminates Activate Transducin-GDP by Mimicking the Gamma-Phosphate of GTP in Its Binding Site," *FEBS Letters* 191, no. 2 (1985): 181–85.

8. J. Bigay, P. Deterre, C. Pfister, and M. Chabre, "Fluoride Complexes of Aluminium or Beryllium Act on G-Proteins as Reversibly Bound Analogues of the Gamma Phosphate of GTP," *EMBO Journal* 6, no. 10 (1987)): 2907–13.

9. A. Strunecka and J. Patocka, "Pharmacological and Toxicological Effects of Aluminofluoride Complexes," *Fluoride* 32, no. 4 (1999): 230–42.

10. L. Li, "The Biochemistry and Physiology of Metallic Fluoride: Action, Mechanism, and Implications," *Critical Reviews of Oral Biology and Medicine* 14, no. 2 (2003): 100–114.

11. K. L. Kirk, *Biochemistry of the Elemental Halogens and Inorganic Halides* (New York: Plenum Press, 1991).

12. J. Zhang, W. J. Zhu, X. H. Xu, and Z. G. Zhang, "Effect of Fluoride on Calcium Ion Concentration and Expression of Nuclear Transcription Factor Kappa-B Rho65 in Rat Hippocampus," *Experimental and Toxicologic Pathology*, March 2010 (in press).

13. E. Gazzano, L. Bergandi, C. Riganti, et al., "Fluoride Effects: The Two Faces of Janus," *Current Medicinal Chemistry*, May 24, 2010 (in press).

14. National Research Council of the National Academies, *Fluoride in Drinking Water: A Scientific Review of EPA's Standards*, page 36 (Washington, DC: National Academies Press, 2006), http://www.nap.edu/openbook.php?record_id=11571&page=36.

15. Ibid. TABLE 2-6 "Summary of Typical Fluoride Concentrations of Selected Food and Beverages in the United States," page 40. Note: levels of fluoride in breast milk from a fluoridated area (1 mg/L) measured at 0.007-0.01 mg/L and levels of fluoride in breast milk from a nonfluoridated area measured at 0.004 mg/L, http://books.nap.edu/openbook.php?isbn=030910128X&page=40.

16. O. B. Dirks, J. M. Jongeling-Eijndhoven, T. D. Flissebaalje, and I. Gedalia, "Total and Free Ionic Fluoride in Human and Cow's Milk as Determined by Gas-Liquid Chromatography and the Fluoride Electrode," *Caries Research* 8, no. 2 (1974): 181–86.

17. R. W. Dabeka, K. F. Karpinski, A. D. McKenzie, and C. D. Bajdik, "Survey of Lead, Cadmium and Fluoride in Human Milk and Correlation of Levels with Environmental and Food Factors," *Food & Chemical Toxicology* 24, no. 9 (1986): 913–21.

18. E. Koparal, F. Ertugrul, and K. Oztekin, "Fluoride Levels in Breast Milk and Infant Foods," *Journal of Clinical Pediatric Dentistry* 24, no. 4 (2000): 299–302.

19. S. Chuckpaiwong, S. Nakornchai, R. Surarit, and S. Soo-ampon, "Fluoride Analysis of Human Milk in Remote Areas of Thailand," *Southeast Asian Journal of Tropical Medicine & Public Health* 31, no. 3 (2000): 583–86.

20. C. J. Spak, L. I. Hardell, and P. De Chateau, "Fluoride in Human Milk," *Acta Paediatrica Scandinavica* 72, no. 5 (1983): 699–701.

21. R. W. Dabeka et al., "Survey of Lead, Cadmium and Fluoride in Human Milk and Correlation of Levels with Environmental and Food Factors" (n. 17 above).

22. R. Latifah and R. Duguid, "Measurements of Ionic Fluoride in Milk," *Annals of the Academy of Medicine, Singapore* 15, no. 3 (1986): 299–304.

23. C. J. Spak et al., "Fluoride in Human Milk" (n. 20 above).

24. G. N. Opinya, N. Bwibo, J. Valderhaug, et al., "Intake of Fluoride and Excretion in Mothers' Milk in a High Fluoride (9 ppm) Area in Kenya," *European Journal of Clinical Nutrition* 45, no. 1 (1991): 37–41.

25. Ibid.

26. J. Ekstrand, L.O. Boreus, and P. de Chateau, "No Evidence of Transfer of Fluoride from Plasma to Breast Milk," *British Medical Journal* 283, no. 6294 (1981): 761–62.

27. J. Ekstrand, C. J. Spak, J. Falch, et al., "Distribution of Fluoride to Human Breast Milk Following Intake of High Doses of Fluoride," *Caries Research* 18, no. 1 (1984): 93–95.

28. A. Carlsson, "Current Problems Relating to the Pharmacology and Toxicology of Fluorides," *Lakartidningen* 25 (1978): 1388–92.

29. I. Inkielewicz and J. Krechniak, "Fluoride Content in Soft Tissues and Urine of Rats Exposed to Sodium Fluoride in Drinking Water," *Fluoride* 36, no. 4 (2003): 263–66, http://www.fluoride-journal.com/03-36-4/364-263.pdf.

30. J. Luke, "The Effect of Fluoride on the Physiology of the Pineal Gland," PhD thesis, University of Surrey, Guildford, UK, 1997. Thesis online, with permission of author, at http://fluoridealert.org/luke-1997.pdf.

31. J. Luke, "Fluoride Deposition in the Aged Human Pineal Gland," *Caries Research* 35, no. 2 (2001): 125–28.

32. National Research Council, *Fluoride in Drinking Water*, 92 (n. 14 above).

33. Ibid.

34. C. Justus and L. P. Krook, "Allergy in Horses from Artificially Fluoridated Water," *Fluoride* 39, no. 2 (2006): 89–94, http://www.fluorideresearch.org/392/files/39289-94.pdf.

35. David Kennedy, DDS, produced the DVD *Poisoned Horses* for the International Academy of Oral Medicine and Toxicology, 2008. Excerpts are available at http://www.youtube.com/watch?v=t9RXfOuylWo.

36. C. Justus and L. P. Krook, "Allergy in Horses from Artificially Fluoridated Water" (n. 34 above).

37. O. Naidenko, "Dog Food Comparison Shows High Fluoride Levels," Environmental Working Group, June 2009, http://www.ewg.org/pets/fluorideindogfood.

Chapter 13

1. B. Spittle, *Fluoride Fatigue: Is Fluoride in Your Drinking Water—and from Other Sources—Making You Sick?* (Dunedin, New Zealand: Paua Press, 2008), http://www.pauapress.com/fluoride/files/1418.pdf.

2. G. L. Waldbott, *Health Effects of Environmental Pollutants,* 2nd ed. (St. Louis: C. V. Mosby Company, 1978).

3. G. L. Waldbott, "Chronic Fluorine Intoxication from Drinking Water," *International Archives of Allergy and Applied Immunology* 7, no. 2 (1955): 70–74.

4. H. T. Petraborg, "Chronic Fluoride Intoxication from Drinking Water (Preliminary Report)," *Fluoride* 7, no. 1 (1974): 47–52.

5. J. J. Shea, S. M. Gillespie, and G. L. Waldbott, "Allergy to Fluoride," *Annals of Allergy* 25 (1967): 388–91.

6. H. T. Petraborg, "Hydrofluorosis in the Fluoridated Milwaukee Area," *Fluoride* 10, no. 4 (1977): 165–69.

7. B. Spittle, *Fluoride Fatigue* (n. 1 above).

8. D. M. Green, "Pre-Existing Conditions. Placebo Reactions and 'Side Effects,'" *Annals of Internal Medicine* 60 (1964): 255–65 (as cited by D. R. Taves, 1979 [see n. 9 below]).

9. D. R. Taves, "Claims of Harm from Fluoridation," in: *Continuing Evaluation of the Use of Fluorides,* ed. E. Johansen, D. R. Taves, and T. O. Olsen, AAAS Selected Symposium, (Boulder, Colorado: Westview Press, 1979), 295–321.

10. G. W. Grimbergen, "A Double Blind Test for Determination of Intolerance to Fluoridated Water (Preliminary Report)," *Fluoride* 7, no. 3 (1974): 146–52, http://fluoridealert.org/re/grimbergen-1974.pdf.

11. G. L. Waldbott, "Facts About Fluoridation," Seminar, Rice University, Houston, Texas, October 16, 1974. Cited by Phillip Sutton in *Fluoridation, 1979: Scientific Criticisms and Fluoride Dangers,* submission to the Commission of Inquiry into the Fluoridation of Victorian Water Supplies, published with an appendix in January 1980.

12. J. D. Shulman and L. M. Wells, "Acute Fluoride Toxicity from Ingesting Home-Use Dental Products in Children, Birth to 6 Years of Age," *Journal of Public Health Dentistry* 57, no. 3 (1997): 150–58.

13. R. Feltman, "Prenatal and Postnatal Ingestion of Fluoride Salts: A Progress Report," *Dental Digest* 62 (1956): 353–57.

14. J. Rorty: see appendix 1 in: *The American Fluoridation Experiment* by F. B. Exner and G. L. Waldbott (New York: Devin-Adair Company, 1957), 229–41.

15. R. Feltman and G. Kosel, "Prenatal and Postnatal Ingestion of Fluorides—Fourteen Years of Investigation—Final Report," *The Journal of Dental Medicine* 16 (1961): 190–99.

16. G. L. Waldbott, A. W. Burgstahler, and H. L. McKinney, *Fluoridation: The Great Dilemma* (Lawrence, Kansas: Coronado Press, 1978).

17. G. L. Waldbott, *A Struggle with Titans: Forces Behind Fluoridation* (New York: Carlton Press, 1965).

18. J. J. Shea et al., "Allergy to Fluoride" (n. 5 above).

19. T. E. Douglas, "Fluoride Dentifrice and Stomatitis," *Northwest Medicine* 56, no. 9 (1957): 1037–39.

20. M. A. Saunders, "Fluoride Toothpaste: A Cause of Acne-Like Eruptions" (letter), *Archives of Dermatology* 111 (1975): 793.

21. M. A. Saunders, "Fluoride Toothpaste as a Cause of Acne-Like Eruptions" (letter in reply to Ervin Epstein's letter), *Archives of Dermatology* 112 (1976): 1033–34.

22. J. R. Mellette, J. L. Aeling, and D. D. Nuss, "Fluoride Tooth Paste: A Cause of Perioral Dermatitis" (letter), *Archives of Dermatology* 112, no. 5 (1976): 730–31.

23. J. R. Mellette, J. L. Aeling, and D. D. Nuss, "Perioral Dermatitis," *Journal of the Association of Military Dermatologists* 9 (1983): 3–8.

24. T. E. Douglas, "Fluoride Dentifrice and Stomatitis" (n. 19 above).

25. B. L. Riggs, E. Seeman, S. F. Hodgson, et al., "Effect of the Fluoride/Calcium Regimen on Vertebral Fracture Occurrence in Postmenopausal Osteoporosis. Comparison with Conventional Therapy," *New England Journal of Medicine* 306, no. 8 (1982): 446–50.

26. A. Singh, S. S. Jolly, and B. C. Bansal, "Skeletal Fluorosis and Its Neurological Complications," *The Lancet* 1 (1961): 197–200.

27. J. L. Shupe, "Fluorine Toxicosis and Industry," *American Industrial Hygiene Association Journal* 31, no. 2 (1970): 240–47.

28. J. J. Franke, F. Rath, H. Runge, et al., "Industrial Fluorosis," *Fluoride* 8, no. 2 (1975): 61–83, http://www.fluoridealert.org/re/franke-1975.pdf.

29. Y. Wang, Y. Yin, L. A. Gilula, and A. J. Wilson, "Endemic Fluorosis of the Skeleton: Radiographic Features in 127 Patients," *American Journal of Roentgenology* 162, no. 1 (1994): 93–98.

30. L. I. Popov, R. I. Filatova, and A. S. Shershever, "Aspects of Nervous System Affections in Occupational Fluorosis" (article in Russian), *Gigiena Truda I Professional'nye Zabolevaniia* 5 (1974): 25–27.

31. K. Czechowicz, A. Osada, and B. Slesak, "Histochemical Studies on the Effect of Sodium Fluoride on Metabolism in Purkinje's Cells," *Folia Histochemica et Cytochemica* 12, no. 1 (1974): 37–44.

32. G. L. Waldbott et al., *Fluoridation: The Great Dilemma,* 161 (n. 16 above).

33. J. Routt Reigart and J. R. Roberts, *Recognition and Management of Pesticide Poisonings,* 5th ed., U.S. Environmental Protection Agency, Office of Prevention, Pesticides and Toxic Substances, EPA 735-R-98-003, 1999.

34. J. D. Shulman and L. M. Wells, "Acute Fluoride Toxicity from Ingesting Home-Use Dental Products in Children, Birth to 6 Years of Age" (n. 12 above).

35. C. J. Spak, S. Sjöstedt, L. Eleborg, et al., "Studies of Human Gastric Mucosa after Application of 0.42% Fluoride Gel," *Journal of Dental Research* 69, no. 2 (1990): 426–29, http://jdr.sagepub.com/cgi/reprint/69/2/426.

36. B. L. Riggs, "Treatment of Osteoporosis with Sodium Fluoride: an Appraisal," *Bone and Mineral Research* 2 (1983): 366–93.

37. A. B. Hodsman and D. J. Drost, "The Response of Vertebral Bone Mineral Density during the Treatment of Osteoporosis with Sodium Fluoride," *Journal of Clinical Endocrinology and Metabolism* 69, no. 5 (1989): 932–38.

38. A. K. Susheela, A. Kumar, M. Bhatnagar, et al., "Prevalence of Endemic Fluorosis with Gastrointestinal Manifestations in People Living in Some North-Indian Villages," *Fluoride* 26, no. 2 (1993): 97–104, http://www.fluoridealert.org/re/susheela-1993.pdf.

39. S. Dasarathy, T. K. Das, I. P. Gupta, et al., "Gastroduodenal Manifestations in Patients with Skeletal Fluorosis," *Journal of Gastroenterology* 31, no. 3 (1996): 333–37.

40. K. F. Austen, M. Dworetzky, R. S. Farr, et al., "Editorial: American Academy of Allergy Statement on the Question of Allergy to Fluoride as Used in the Fluoridation of Community Water Supplies," *The Journal of Allergy* 47, no. 6 (1971): 347–48.

41. G. L. Waldbott, *A Struggle with Titans: Forces Behind Fluoridation* (n. 17 above).

42. G. L. Waldbott et al., *Fluoridation: The Great Dilemma,* 287–88 (n. 16 above).

43. Royal College of Physicians of London, *Fluoride, Teeth and Health,* (Kent, UK: Pitman Medical Publishing Co. Ltd., 1976), 64.

44. D. M. Myers, V. D. Plueckhahn, and A. L. G. Rees, *Report of the Committee of Inquiry into the Fluoridation of Victorian Water Supplies for 1979–80,* no. 14, (Melbourne: F.D. Atkinson, Government Printer, 1980), 114.

45. National Health and Medical Research Council, *Report of the Working Party on Fluorides*

in the Control of Dental Caries, as Adopted at 100th Session (Canberra: Australian
Government Publishing Service, 1985), 109.

46. National Health and Medical Research Council, *The Effectiveness of Water Fluoridation* (Canberra: Australian Government Publishing Service, 1991), 109.

47. World Health Organization, *Appropriate Use of Fluoride for Human Health*, page 87, Geneva, 1986, ISBN 92 4 154203 9. Note: This report is online in two parts. Page 87 is in the second part at http://whqlibdoc.who.int/publications/1986/9241542039_(part2) .pdf. The first part is at http://whqlibdoc.who.int/publications/1986/9241542039 _(part1).pdf.

48. U.S. Department of Health and Human Services, *Review of Fluoride: Benefits and Risks*, page 69, Public Health Service, Washington, DC, February 1991, http://health.gov/ environment/ReviewofFluoride/.

49. Public Health Commission, *Water Fluoridation in New Zealand. An Analysis and Monitoring Report*, Wellington, New Zealand, July 1994, ISBN 0-478-08524-9.

50. National Research Council, *Health Effects of Ingested Fluoride* (Washington, DC: National Academy Press, 1993), 89, http://www.nap.edu/openbook .php?isbn=030904975X.

51. M. Prival, "Fluoride and Human Health," Center for Science in the Public Interest, 1972. Excerpts at http://www.fluoridealert.org/health/allergy/prival-1972.html.

52. D. R. Taves, "Claims of Harm from Fluoridation," 299–300 (n. 9 above).

53. M. Prival, "Fluoride and Human Health" (n. 51 above).

54. D. R. Taves, "Claims of Harm from Fluoridation," 299–300 (n. 9 above).

55. National Health and Medical Research Council, *The Effectiveness of Water Fluoridation*, 142 (n. 46 above).

56. P. Robertson, personal communication to Paul Connett, 2008.

57. Ibid.

58. M. Kuza and W. Kazimierczak, "On the Mechanism of Histamine Release from Sodium Fluoride-Activated Mouse Mast Cells," *Agents Actions* 12, no. 3 (1982): 289–94.

59. P. E. Alm, "Sodium Fluoride Evoked Histamine Release from Mast Cells. A Study of Cyclic AMP Levels and Effects of Catecholamines," *Agents Actions* 13, no. 2–3 (1983): 132–37.

Chapter 14

1. National Research Council of the National Academies, *Fluoride in Drinking Water: A Scientific Review of EPA's Standards* (Washington, DC: National Academies Press, 2006), http://books.nap.edu/openbook.php?record_id=11571.

2. Presentation by Joyce Donahue, PhD, toxicologist, Office of Science and Technology, U.S. EPA Office of Drinking Water, to National Academies' National Research Council Committee: Toxicologic Risk of Fluoride in Drinking Water [BEST-K-02-05-A], August 12, 2003, http://www.fluoridealert.org/pesticides/nrc.aug.2003.epa.html.

3. National Research Council, *Health Effects of Ingested Fluoride* (Washington, DC: National Academy Press, 1993), 89, http://www.nap.edu/openbook .php?isbn=030904975X.

4. National Research Council, *Fluoride in Drinking Water*, 2 (n. 1 above).

5. American Dental Association, "Statement on Fluoride in Drinking Water: A Scientific Review of EPA's Standards [the NRC 2006 report]," news release, March 22, 2006.

6. Centers for Disease Control and Prevention, "Statement on the 2006 National Research Council Report, Fluoride in Drinking Water: A Scientific Review of EPA's Standards,"

Division of Oral Health. Posted originally on March 28, 2006. Date last updated: August 24, 2009, http://www.cdc.gov/FLUORIDATION/safety/nrc_report.htm.

7. National Health and Medical Research Council, *A Systematic Review of the Efficacy and Safety of Fluoridation,* reference no. EH41, Australian Government, December 27, 2007, http://www.nhmrc.gov.au/publications/synopses/eh41syn.htm.

8. Bazian Ltd., "Critical Appraisal of 'Fluoride in Drinking Water: A Scientific Review of EPA's standards.'" A report for South Central Strategic Health Authority, UK, delivery date: February 11, 2009, http://fluoridealert.org/sha.basian.nrc.feb09.pdf.

9. F. F. Lin, Aihaiti, H. X. Zhao, et al., "The Relationship of a Low-Iodine and High-Fluoride Environment to Subclinical Cretinism in Xinjiang," Xinjiang Institute for Endemic Disease Control and Research; Office of Leading Group for Endemic Disease Control of Hetian Prefectural Committee of the Communist Party of China; and County Health and Epidemic Prevention Station, Yutian, Xinjiang, *Iodine Deficiency Disorder Newsletter* 7 (1991): 3, http://fluoridealert.org/scher/lin-1991.pdf; also see http://www.fluoridealert.org/IDD.htm.

10. Y. Li, C. Liang, C. W. Slemenda, et al., "Effect of Long-Term Exposure to Fluoride in Drinking Water on Risks of Bone Fractures," *Journal of Bone and Mineral Research* 16, no. 5 (2001): 932–39.

11. M. T. Alarcón-Herrera, I. R. Martín-Domínguez, R. Trejo-Vázquez, et al., "Well Water Fluoride, Dental Fluorosis, Bone Fractures in the Guadiana Valley of Mexico," *Fluoride* 34, no. 2 (2001): 139–49, http://www.fluoride-journal.com/01-34-2/342-139.pdf.

12. Q. Xiang, Y. Liang, L. Chen, et al., "Effect of Fluoride in Drinking Water on Children's Intelligence," *Fluoride* 36, no. 2 (2003): 84–94, http://www.fluorideresearch.org/362/files/FJ2003_v36_n2_p84-94.pdf.

13. Q. Xiang, Y. Liang, M. Zhou, and H. Zang, "Blood Lead of Children in Wamiao-Xinhuai Intelligence Study" (letter), *Fluoride* 36, no. 3 (2003): 198–99, http://www.fluorideresearch.org/363/files/FJ2003_v36_n3_p198-199.pdf.

14. J. A. Varner, K. F. Jensen, W. Horvath, and R. L. Isaacson, "Chronic Administration of Aluminum-Fluoride and Sodium-Fluoride to Rats in Drinking Water: Alterations in Neuronal and Cerebrovascular Integrity," *Brain Research* 784, no. 1–2 (1998): 284–98. Extended excerpts at http://www.fluoride-journal.com/98-31-2/31291-95.htm.

15. P. Connett and M. Connett. Invited presentation to the National Research Council of the National Academies committee reviewing the safety of the U.S. Environmental Protection Agency's maximum contaminant level (MCL) for fluoride in drinking water, 2003. This PowerPoint presentation is at http://www.fluoridealert.org/nrc-final.ppt, and the paper supporting this presentation at http://www.fluoridealert.org/nrc-paper.pdf. See table 2, page 9.

16. M. S. McDonagh, P. F. Whiting, P. M. Wilson, et al., "Systematic Review of Water Fluoridation," *British Medical Journal* 321, no. 7265 (2000): 855–59, http://www.bmj.com/cgi/content/full/321/7265/855. Note: The full report that this paper summarizes is commonly known as the York Review and is accessible at http://fluoridealert.org/re/york.review.2000.pdf.

17. National Health and Medical Research Council, *A Systematic Review of the Efficacy and Safety of Fluoridation* (n. 7 above).

18. Integrated Risk Information System on Fluorine (soluble fluoride) (CASRN 7782-41-4), U.S. Environmental Protection Agency, http://www.epa.gov/iris/subst/0053.htm.

19. National Research Council, *Fluoride in Drinking Water,* 170–71 (n. 1 above), http://www

.nap.edu/openbook.php?isbn=030910128X&page=170 and http://www.nap.edu/
openbook.php?isbn=030910128X&page=171.

20. Ibid., 3, http://www.nap.edu/openbook.php?isbn=030910128X&page=3.

21. Ibid., 2, http://www.nap.edu/openbook.php?record_id=11571&page=2.

22. R. J. Carton, "Review of the 2006 National Research Council Report: Fluoride in
Drinking Water," *Fluoride* 39, no. 3 (2006): 163–72, http://www.fluorideresearch
.org/393/files/FJ2006_v39_n3_p163-172.pdf.

23. American Dental Association, "Statement on Fluoride in Drinking Water" (n. 5 above).

24. Centers for Disease Control and Prevention, "Statement on the 2006 National Research
Council Report, Fluoride in Drinking Water" (n. 6 above).

25. National Health and Medical Research Council, *A Systematic Review of the Efficacy and
Safety of Fluoridation"* (n. 7 above).

26. Bazian Ltd., "Critical Appraisal of 'Fluoride in Drinking Water'" (n. 8 above).

27. Presentations by Barry Cockcroft, chief dental officer for England, at "Question Time on
Fluoridation" held on October 20, November 18, and December 3, 2008. Organized by
the South Central Strategic Health Authority Southampton, UK.

28. Bazian Ltd., "Critical Appraisal of 'Fluoride in Drinking Water'" (n. 8 above).

29. J. Newton, "Water Fluoridation—The Scientific Evidence." Report by Professor John
Newton, Regional Director of Public Health, South Central Strategic Health Authority,
UK, February 20, 2009, http://fluoridealert.org/sha.sc.evidence.feb09.pdf.

30. Bazian Ltd., "Critical Appraisal of 'Fluoride in Drinking Water'" (n. 8 above).

31. Integrated Risk Information System on Fluorine (soluble fluoride) (n. 18 above).

32. Y. Li et al., "Effect of Long-Term Exposure to Fluoride in Drinking Water on Risks of
Bone Fractures" (n. 10 above).

33. P. P. Bachinskii, O. A. Gutsalenko, N. D. Naryzhniuk, et al., "Action of Fluoride on the
Function of the Pituitary-thyroid System of Healthy Persons and Patients with Thyroid
Disorders" (article in Russian), *Problemy Endokrinologii (Mosk)* 31, no. 6 (1985): 25–29.
English translation at http://www.fluoridealert.org/bachinskii.1985.pdf.

34. K. M. Thiessen, "Water Fluoridation: Suggested Issues for Consideration," December
13, 2006, http://www.fluoridealert.org/thiessen-statement.pdf.

35. K. M. Thiessen, "Comments on: Prioritization of Chemicals for Carcinogen
Identification Committee Review. Proposed Chemicals for Committee Consideration
and Consultation. Proposition 65 Implementation, Office of Environmental Health
Hazard Assessment, California Environmental Protection Agency," May 5, 2009, http://
fluoridealert.org/ca/thiessen-2009.pdf.

36. K. M. Thiessen, "Water Fluoridation: Suggested Issues for Consideration" (n. 34 above).

37. K. M. Thiessen, "Comments on: Prioritization of Chemicals for Carcinogen
Identification Committee Review" (n. 35 above).

38. K. M. Thiessen, "Water Fluoridation: Suggested Issues for Consideration" (n. 34 above).

39. E. B. Bassin, D. Wypij, R. B. Davis, and M. A. Mittleman, "Age-specific Fluoride
Exposure in Drinking Water and Osteosarcoma (United States)," *Cancer Causes and
Control* 17, no. 4 (May 2006): 421–28.

Chapter 15

1. C. Bryson, *The Fluoride Deception* (New York: Seven Stories Press, 2004), 27.

2. B. Spittle, "Psychopharmacology of Fluoride: A Review," *International Clinical
Psychopharmacology* 9, no. 2 (1994): 79–82.

3. C. Bryson, *The Fluoride Deception,* 23–24 (n. 1 above).

4. P. J. Mullenix, P. K. Denbesten, A. Schunior, and W. J. Kernan, "Neurotoxicity of Sodium Fluoride in Rats," *Neurotoxicology and Teratology* 17, no. 2 (1995): 169–77.

5. P. J. Mullenix, personal communication with Paul Connett, October 24, 1996.

6. H. C. Hodge and F. A. Smith, *Fluorine Chemistry*, vol. 4 (New York and London: Academic Press, 1965).

7. B. Spittle, "Psychopharmacology of Fluoride: A Review" (n. 2 above).

8. G. L. Waldbott, A. W. Burgstahler, and H. L. McKinney, *Fluoridation: The Great Dilemma* (Lawrence, Kansas: Coronado Press, 1978).

9. X. S. Li, J. L. Zhi, and R.O. Gao, "Effect of Fluoride Exposure on Intelligence in Children," *Fluoride* 28, no. 4 (1995): 189–92, http://fluoridealert.org/scher/li-1995.pdf.

10. L. B. Zhao, G. H. Liang, D. N. Zhang, and X. R. Wu, "Effect of High-Fluoride Water Supply on Children's Intelligence," *Fluoride* 29, no. 4 (1996): 190–92, http://fluoridealert .org/scher/zhao-1996.pdf.

11. P. J. Mullenix et al., "Neurotoxicity of Sodium Fluoride in Rats" (n. 4 above).

12. G. M. Whitford, "The Metabolism and Toxicity of Fluoride," in: *Monographs in Oral Science*, vol. 16, 2nd rev. ed. (New York: Karger, 1996).

13. J. X. Zhai, Z. Y. Guo, C. L. Hu, et al., "Studies on Fluoride Concentration and Cholinesterase Activity in Rat Hippocampus" (article in Chinese), *Zhonghua Lao Dong Wei Sheng Zhi Ye Bing Za Zhi* 21, no. 2 (2003): 102–4.

14. I. Inkielewicz and J. Krechniak, "Fluoride Content in Soft Tissues and Urine of Rats Exposed to Sodium Fluoride in Drinking Water," *Fluoride* 36, no. 4 (2003): 263–66, http://www.fluoride-journal.com/03-36-4/364-263.pdf.

15. M. L. Vani and K. P. Reddy, "Effects of Fluoride Accumulation on Some Enzymes of Brain and Gastrocnemius Muscle of Mice," *Fluoride* 33, no. 1 (2000): 17–26, http:// www.fluorideresearch.org/331/files/FJ2000_v33_n1_p17-26.pdf.

16. K. Chirumari and P. K. Reddy, "Dose-Dependent Effects of Fluoride on Neurochemical Milieu in the Hippocampus and Neocortex of Rat Brain," *Fluoride* 40, no. 2 (2007): 101–10, http://www.fluorideresearch.org/402/files/FJ2007_v40_n2 _p101-110.pdf.

17. J. A. Varner, K. F. Jensen, W. Horvath, and R. L. Isaacson, "Chronic Administration of Aluminum-Fluoride or Sodium-Fluoride to Rats in Drinking Water: Alterations in Neuronal and Cerebrovascular Integrity," *Brain Research* 784, no. 1–2 (1998): 284–98. Excerpts at http://www.fluoride-journal.com/98-31-2/31291-95.htm.

18. A. Lubkowska, D. Chlubek, A. Machoy-Mokrzyska, et al., "Concentrations of Fluorine, Aluminum and Magnesium in some Structures of the Central Nervous System of Rats Exposed to Aluminum and Fluorine in Drinking Water" (article in Polish), *Annales Academiae Medicae Stetinensis* 50, suppl. 1 (2004): 73–76.

19. Y. M. Shivarajashankara, A. R. Shivashankara, and P. G. Bhat, et al., "Histological Changes in the Brain of Young Fluoride-Intoxicated Rats," *Fluoride* 35, no. 1 (2002): 12–21, http://www.fluorideresearch.org/351/files/FJ2002_v35_n1_p12-21.pdf.

20. Letter from Gary M. Whitford, PhD, DMD, Medical College of Georgia, to David M. Apanian, PE, Centers for Disease Control, Division of Oral Health, Chamblee, GA, March 28, 1997. Letter begins, "As requested, I have reviewed the paper by Mullenix et al. (*Neurotoxicology and Teratology* 17: 169–177) and offer the following critique . . ."

21. P. J. Mullenix, "Central Nervous System Damage from Fluorides," September 14, 1998, http://www.fluoridation.com/brain2.htm.

22. R. M. M. Sawan, G. A. S. Leite, M. C. P. Saraiva, et al., "Fluoride Increases Lead Concentrations in Whole Blood and in Calcified Tissues from Lead-Exposed Rats," *Toxicology* 271, no. 1–2 (2010): 21–26.

23. Z. Z. Guan, Y. N. Wang, K. Q. Xiao, et al., "Influence of Chronic Fluorosis on Membrane Lipids in Rat Brain," *Neurotoxicology and Teratology* 20, no. 5 (1998): 537–42.

24. Q. Gao, Y. J. Liu, and Z. Z. Guan, "Decreased Learning and Memory Ability in Rats with Fluorosis: Increased Oxidative Stress and Reduced Cholinesterase Activity," *Fluoride* 42, no. 4 (2009): 277–85, http://www.fluorideresearch.org/424/files/FJ2009 _v42_n4_p277-285.pdf.

25. Y. J. Liu, Q. Gao, C. X. Wu, and Z. Z. Guan, "Alterations of nAChRs and ERK1/2 in the Brains of Rats with Chronic Fluorosis and Their Connections with the Decreased Capacity of Learning and Memory," *Toxicology Letters* 192, no. 3 (2010): 324–29.

26. J. X. Zhai et al., "Studies on Fluoride Concentration and Cholinesterase Activity in Rat Hippocampus" (n. 13 above).

27. I. Inkielewicz and J. Krechniak, "Fluoride Content in Soft Tissues and Urine of Rats Exposed to Sodium Fluoride in Drinking Water" (n. 14 above).

28. J. A. Varner et al., "Chronic Administration of Aluminum-Fluoride or Sodium-Fluoride to Rats in Drinking Water" (n. 17 above).

29. M. Bhatnagar, P. Rao, J. Sushma, and R. Bhatnagar, "Neurotoxicity of Fluoride: Neurodegeneration in Hippocampus of Female Mice," *Indian Journal of Experimental Biology* 40, no. 5 (2002): 546–54.

30. Z. Zhang, X. Shen, and X. Xu, "Effects of Selenium on the Damage of Learning-Memory Ability of Mice Induced by Fluoride" (article in Chinese), *Wei Sheng Yan Jiu* 30, no. 3 (2001): 144-46.

31. G. B. van der Voet, O. Schijns, and F. A. de Wolff, "Fluoride Enhances the Effect of Aluminium Chloride on Interconnections Between Aggregates of Hippocampal Neurons," *Archives of Physiology and Biochemistry* 107, no. 1 (1999): 15–21.

32. A. R. Kay, R. Miles, and R. K. Wong, "Intracellular Fluoride Alters the Kinetic Properties of Calcium Currents Facilitating the Investigation of Synaptic Events in Hippocampal Neurons," *The Journal of Neuroscience* 6, no. 10 (1986): 2915–20, http:// www.jneurosci.org/cgi/reprint/6/10/2915.

33. Z. Zhang, X. Xu, X. Shen, and X. Xu, "Effect of Fluoride Exposure on Synaptic Structure of Brain Areas Related to Learning-memory in Mice," *Fluoride* 41, no. 2 (2008): 139–43 (originally published in 1999 in *Journal of Hygiene Research* [China]), http://www.fluorideresearch.org/412/files/FJ2008_v41_n2_p139-143.pdf.

34. W. Zhu, J. Zhang, and Z. Zhang, "Effects of Fluoride on Synaptic Membrane Fluidity and PSD-95 Expression Level in Rat Hippocampus," *Biological Trace Element Research,* March 2010 (in press).

35. M. Pereira, P. A. Dombrowski, E. M. Losso, et al., "Memory Impairment Induced by Sodium Fluoride Is Associated with Changes in Brain Monoamine Levels," *Neurotoxicity Research,* December 2009 (in press).

36. M. Zhang, A. Wang, T. Xia, and P. He, "Effects of Fluoride on DNA Damage, S-phase Cell-cycle Arrest and the Expression of NF-KappaB in Primary Cultured Rat Hippocampal Neurons," *Toxicology Letters* 179, no. 1 (2008): 1–5.

37. T. Xia, M. Zhang, W. H. He, et al., "Effects of Fluoride on Neural Cell Adhesion Molecules mRNA and Protein Expression Levels in Primary Rat Hippocampal Neurons" (article in Chinese), *Zhonghua Yu Fang Yi Xue Za Zhi* 41, no. 6 (2007): 475–78.

38. M. Zhang, A. Wang, W. He, et al., "Effects of Fluoride on the Expression of NCAM, Oxidative Stress, and Apoptosis in Primary Cultured Hippocampal Neurons," *Toxicology* 236, no. 3 (2007): 208–16.

39. R. L. Isaacson, J. A. Varner, and K. F. Jensen, "Toxin-Induced Blood Vessel Inclusions Caused by the Chronic Administration of Aluminum and Sodium Fluoride and Their Implications for Dementia," *Annals of the New York Academy of Sciences* 825 (1997): 152–66.

40. J. A. Varner et al., "Chronic Administration of Aluminum-Fluoride or Sodium-Fluoride to Rats in Drinking Water" (n. 17 above).

41. National Research Council of the National Academies, *Fluoride in Drinking Water: A Scientific Review of EPA's Standards,* chapter 7 (Washington, DC: National Academies Press, 2006), http://books.nap.edu/openbook.php?record_id=11571.

42. Ibid., 222, http://books.nap.edu/openbook.php?record_id=11571&page=222#.

43. Ibid., 223, http://books.nap.edu/openbook.php?record_id=11571&page=223.

44. Ibid.

45. Ibid., 8, http://books.nap.edu/openbook.php?record_id=11571&page=8.

46. Ibid.

47. Q. Xiang, Y. Liang, L. Chen, et al., "Effect of Fluoride in Drinking Water on Children's Intelligence," *Fluoride* 36, no. 2 (2003): 84–94, http://www.fluorideresearch.org/362/files/FJ2003_v36_n2_p84-94.pdf.

48. Q. Xiang, Y. Liang, M. Zhou, and H. Zang, "Blood Lead of Children in Wamiao-Xinhuai Intelligence Study" (letter), *Fluoride* 36, no. 3 (2003): 198–9, http://www.fluorideresearch.org/363/files/FJ2003_v36_n3_p198-199.pdf.

49. F. F. Lin, Aihaiti, H. X. Zhao, et al., "The Relationship of a Low-Iodine and High-Fluoride Environment to Subclinical Cretinism in Xinjiang," Xinjiang Institute for Endemic Disease Control and Research; Office of Leading Group for Endemic Disease Control of Hetian Prefectural Committee of the Communist Party of China; and County Health and Epidemic Prevention Station, Yutian, Xinjiang, *Iodine Deficiency Disorder Newsletter* 7 (1991): 3, http://fluoridealert.org/scher/lin-1991.pdf; also see http://www.fluoridealert.org/IDD.htm.

50. Q. Xiang et al., "Blood Lead of Children in Wamiao-Xinhuai Intelligence Study" (n. 48 above).

51. Q. Xiang et al., "Effect of Fluoride in Drinking Water on Children's Intelligence" (n. 47 above).

52. H. F. Pollick, "Water Fluoridation and the Environment: Current Perspective in the United States," *International Journal of Occupational Environmental Health* 10 (2004): 343–50.

53. P. Connett, "Scientific Evidence Fails to Support Fluoridation of Public Water Supplies" (letter), *International Journal of Occupational Environmental Health* 11 (2005): 215–16.

54. H. F. Pollick, "Scientific Evidence Continues to Support Fluoridation of Public Water Supplies" (letter), *International Journal of Occupational Environmental Health* 11 (2005): 322–26.

55. P. Connett, "Water Fluoridation—A Public Health Hazard" (letter), *International Journal of Occupational Environmental Health* 12 (2006): 88–90.

56. H. F. Pollick, "Concerns about Water Fluoridation, IQ, and Osteosarcoma Lack Credible Evidence" (letter), *International Journal of Occupational Environmental Health* 12 (2006): 91–94.

57. F. T. Shannon, D. M. Fergusson, and L. J. Horwood, "Exposure to Fluoridated Water Supplies and Child Behaviour," *New Zealand Medical Journal* 99, no. 803 (1986): 416–18.

58. Y. Yu, W. Yang, Z. Dong, et al., "Neurotransmitter and Receptor Changes in the Brains of Fetuses from Areas of Endemic Fluorosis," *Fluoride* 41, no. 2 (2008): 134–38 (originally

published in 1996 in *Chinese Journal of Endemiology*), http://www.fluorideresearch
.org/412/files/FJ2008_v41_n2_p134-138.pdf.

59. L. Du, C. Wan, X. Cao, and J. Liu, "The Effect of Fluorine on the Developing
Human Brain," *Fluoride* 41, no. 4 (2008): 327–30 (originally published in 1992 in
Chinese Journal of Pathology), http://www.fluorideresearch.org/414/files/FJ2008_v41_
n4_p327-330.pdf.

60. H. He, Z. Cheng, and W. Q. Liu, "Effects of Fluorine on the Human Fetus," *Fluoride*
41, no. 4 (2008): 321–26 (originally published in 1989 in *Chinese Journal of Control of
Endemic Diseases*), http://www.fluorideresearch.org/414/files/FJ2008_v41_n4_p321-326
.pdf.

61. L. Du et al., "The Effect of Fluorine on the Developing Human Brain" (n. 59 above).

62. Z. Guo, Y. He, and Q. Zhu, "Research on the Neurobehavioural Function of Workers
Occupationally Exposed to Fluoride," *Fluoride* 41, no. 2 (2008): 152–55 (originally
published in 2001 in *Industrial Health and Occupational Disease* [China]), http://www
.fluorideresearch.org/412/files/FJ2008_v41_n2_p152-155.pdf.

63. J. Li , L. Yao, Q. L. Shao, and C. Y. Wu, "Effects of High Fluoride on Neonatal
Neurobehavioral Development," *Fluoride* 41, no. 2 (2008): 165–70 (originally published
in 2004 in *Chinese Journal of Endemiology*), http://www.fluorideresearch.org/412/files/
FJ2008_v41_n2_p165-170.pdf.

64. B. Spittle, "Psychopharmacology of Fluoride: A Review" (n. 2 above).

65. P. J. Mullenix et al., "Neurotoxicity of Sodium Fluoride in Rats" (n. 4 above).

66. Z. Z. Guan et al., "Influence of Chronic Fluorosis on Membrane Lipids in Rat Brain" (n.
23 above).

67. X. S. Li et al., "Effect of Fluoride Exposure on Intelligence in Children" (n. 9 above).

68. L. B. Zhao et al., "Effect of High-Fluoride Water Supply on Children's Intelligence" (n.
10 above).

69. Medical Research Council, *Water Fluoridation and Health*, Working Group Report, UK,
September 2002, http://fluoridealert.org/re/mrc-2002.pdf.

70. L. Morgan, E. Allred, M. Tavares, et al., "Investigation of the Possible Associations
Between Fluorosis, Fluoride Exposure, and Childhood Behavior Problems," *Pediatric
Dentistry* 20, no. 4 (1998): 244–52.

71. F. T. Shannon et al., "Exposure to Fluoridated Water Supplies and Child Behaviour" (n.
57 above).

72. T. Schettler, J. Stein, F. Reich, et al., *In Harm's Way: Toxic Threats to Child Development.*
A report by the Greater Boston Physicians for Social Responsibility, prepared for a joint
project with Clean Water Fund, May 2000. Excerpts at http://www.fluoridealert.org/
health/brain/psr.html.

73. P. J. Mullenix et al., "Neurotoxicity of Sodium Fluoride in Rats" (n. 4 above).

74. X. L. Zhao and J. H. Wu, "Actions of Sodium Fluoride on Acetylcholinesterase
Activities in Rats," *Biomedical and Environmental Sciences* 11, no. 1 (1998): 1–6.

75. X. S. Li et al., "Effect of Fluoride Exposure on Intelligence in Children" (n. 9 above).

76. L. B. Zhao et al., "Effect of High-Fluoride Water Supply on Children's Intelligence" (n.
10 above).

77. T. Schettler et al., *In Harm's Way*, 92 (n. 72 above).

78. P. Grandjean and P. J. Landrigan, "Developmental Neurotoxicity of Industrial
Chemicals," *The Lancet* 368, no. 9553 (2006): 2167–78.

79. R. D. Masters and M. J. Coplan, "Water Treatment with Silicofluorides and Lead
Toxicity," *International Journal of Environmental Studies* 56, no. 4 (1999): 435–49.

80. R. D. Masters, M. J. Coplan, B. T. Hone, and J. E. Dykes, "Association of Silicofluoride Treated Water with Elevated Blood Lead," *Neurotoxicology* 21, no. 6 (2000): 1091–99.
81. R. M. M. Sawan et al., "Fluoride Increases Lead Concentrations in Whole Blood and in Calcified Tissues from Lead-exposed Rats" (n. 22 above).
82. Bazian Ltd., "Independent Critical Appraisal of Selected Studies Reporting an Association between Fluoride in Drinking Water and IQ." A report for South Central Strategic Health Authority, UK, delivery date: February 11, 2009, http://fluoridealert .org/iq.bazian.feb09.pdf.
83. Q. Xiang et al., "Effect of Fluoride in Drinking Water on Children's Intelligence" (n. 47 above).
84. J. Newton, "Water Fluoridation—The Scientific Evidence." Report by Professor John Newton, Regional Director of Public Health, South Central Strategic Health Authority, UK, February 20, 2009, http://fluoridealert.org/sha.sc.evidence.feb09.pdf.

Chapter 16

1. *Forum on Fluoridation* (Dublin, Ireland: Stationery Office, 2002), http://fluoridealert.org/ re/fluoridation.forum.2002.pdf.
2. Medical Research Council, *Water Fluoridation and Health,* Working Group Report, UK, September 2002, http://fluoridealert.org/re/mrc-2002.pdf.
3. J. Fawell, K. Bailey, J. Chilton, et al., *Fluoride in Drinking-Water,* World Health Organization (London and Seattle: IWA Publishing, 2006).
4. National Health and Medical Research Council, *A Systematic Review of the Efficacy and Safety of Fluoridation,* reference no. EH41, Australian Government, December 27, 2007, http://www.nhmrc.gov.au/publications/synopses/eh41syn.htm.
5. Health Canada, "Findings and Recommendations of the Fluoride Expert Panel (January 2007)," April 2008, http://fluoridealert.org/re/canada.fluoride.expert.panel.2007.pdf.
6. National Research Council of the National Academies, *Fluoride in Drinking Water: A Scientific Review of EPA's Standards* (Washington, DC: National Academies Press, 2006), 266, http://www.nap.edu/openbook.php?isbn=030910128X&page=266.
7. E. Maumené, "Expérience pour Déterminer L'action des Florures sur L'économie Animale," *Comptes Rendus Hebdomadaires des Séances de l'Académie des Sciences* 39 (1854): 538.
8. Parents of Fluoride Poisoned Children, "Thyroid History. History of the Fluoride/Iodine Antagonism," http://www.bruha.com/pfpc/html/thyroid_history.html.
9. D. G. Steyn, "Fluorine and Endemic Goitre," *South African Medical Journal* 22, no. 16 (1948): 525–26.
10. D. G. Steyn et al., "Endemic Goitre in the Union of South Africa and Some Neighbouring Territories," Union of South Africa, Department of Nutrition, 1955.
11. D. C. Wilson, "Fluorine in Aetiology of Endemic Goiter," *The Lancet* 237, no. 6129 (1941): 211–12.
12. T. K. Day and P. R. Powell-Jackson, "Fluoride, Water Hardness, and Endemic Goiter," *The Lancet* 1, no. 7761 (1972): 1135–38.
13. A. O. Obel, "Goitre and Fluorosis in Kenya," *East African Medical Journal* 59, no. 6 (1982): 363–65.
14. V. K. Desai, D. M. Solanki, and R. K. Bansal, "Epidemiological Study of Goitre in Endemic Fluorosis District of Gujarat," *Fluoride* 26, no. 3 (1993): 187–90.
15. P. L. Jooste, M. J. Weight, J. A. Kriek, and A. J. Louw, "Endemic Goitre in the Absence

of Iodine Deficiency in Schoolchildren of the Northern Cape Province of South Africa," *European Journal of Clinical Nutrition* 53, no. 1 (1999): 8–12.

16. H. Bürgi, L. Siebenhüner, and E. Miloni, "Fluorine and Thyroid Gland Function: A Review of the Literature," *Klinische Wochenschrift* 62, no. 12 (1984): 564–69.

17. L. Goldemberg, "Action Physiologique des Fluorures," *Comptes Rendus des Séances de la Société de Biologie et de ses Filiales* (Paris) 95 (1926): 1169.

18. L. Goldemberg, "Traitement de la Maladie de Basedow et de l'Hyperthyroidisme par le Fluor," *La Presse Médicale* 102 (1930): 1751.

19. L. Goldemberg, "Comment Agiraient-ils Therapeutiquement les Fluoers dans le Goitre Exopthalmique et dans L'Hyperthyroidisme," *La Semana Médica* 39 (1932): 1659.

20. W. May, "Antagonismus Zwischen Jod und Fluor im Organismus," *Klinische Wochenschrift* 14 (1935): 790–92.

21. W. May, "Behandlung the Hyperthyreosen Einschliesslich des Schweren Genuinen Morbus Basedow mit Fluor," *Klinische Wochenschrift* 16 (1937): 562–64.

22. W. Orlowski, "Sur la Valeur Therapeutique du Sang Animal du Bore et du Fluor dans la Maladie de Basedow," *La Presse Medicale* 42 (1932): 836–37.

23. P. Galletti and G. Joyet, "Effect of Fluorine on Thyroidal Iodine Metabolism in Hyperthyroidism," *Journal of Clinical Endocrinology* 18, no. 10 (1958): 1102–10.

24. Ibid.

25. U.S. Department of Health and Human Services, *Review of Fluoride: Benefits and Risks,* table 11, page 17, Public Health Service, Washington, DC, February 1991, http://health. gov/environment/ReviewofFluoride/.

26. P. P. Bachinskii, O. A. Gutsalenko, N. D. Naryzhniuk, et al., "Action of Fluoride on the Function of the Pituitary-thyroid System of Healthy Persons and Patients with Thyroid Disorders" (article in Russian), *Problemy Endokrinologii (Mosk)* 31, no. 6 (1985): 25–29. English translation at http://www.fluoridealert.org/bachinskii.1985.pdf.

27. N. D. Mikhailets, M. I. Balabolkin, V. A. Rakitin, and I. P. Danilov, "Thyroid Function During Prolonged Exposure to Fluorides" (article in Russian), *Problemy Endokrinologii (Mosk)* 42, no. 1 (1996): 6–9.

28. Ibid.

29. National Research Council, *Fluoride in Drinking Water*, 263 (n. 6 above).

30. M. Li, G. Ma, S. C. Boyages, and C. J. Eastman, "Re-emergence of Iodine Deficiency in Australia," *Asia Pacific Journal of Clinical Nutrition* 10, no. 3 (2001): 200–203.

31. F. F. Lin, Aihaiti, H. X. Zhao, et al., "The Relationship of a Low-Iodine and High-Fluoride Environment to Subclinical Cretinism in Xinjiang," Xinjiang Institute for Endemic Disease Control and Research; Office of Leading Group for Endemic Disease Control of Hetian Prefectural Committee of the Communist Party of China; and County Health and Epidemic Prevention Station, Yutian, Xinjiang, *Iodine Deficiency Disorder Newsletter* 7 (1991): 3, http://fluoridealert.org/scher/lin-1991.pdf; also see http://www.fluoridealert.org/IDD.htm.

32. National Research Council, *Fluoride in Drinking Water,* chapter 8 (n. 6 above).

33. Ibid., 234, http://www.nap.edu/openbook.php?record_id=11571&page=234.

34. Ibid., 262, http://books.nap.edu/openbook.php?record_id=11571&page=262.

35. Ibid., 263, http://books.nap.edu/openbook.php?record_id=11571&page=263.

36. Centers for Disease Control and Prevention, "Iodine Level, United States, 2000," National Center for Health Statistics, 2002, http://www.cdc.gov/nchs/data/hestat/iodine.htm.

37. P. R. Larsen and T. F. Davies, in: *Williams Textbook of Endocrinology*, 10th ed., ed. Larsen et al., (Philadelphia: Saunders, 2002).

38. D. Fagin, "Second Thoughts on Fluoride," *Scientific American* 298, no. 1 (January 2008): 74–81. Excerpts at http://www.fluoridealert.org/sc.am.jan.2008.html.

39. M. J. Schneider, S. N. Fiering, S. E. Pallud, et al., "Targeted Disruption of the Type 2 Selenodeiodinase Gene (DIO2) Results in a Phenotype of Pituitary Resistance to T4," *Molecular Endocrinology* 15, no. 12 (2001): 2137–48.

40. F. F. Lin et al., "The Relationship of a Low-Iodine and High-Fluoride Environment to Subclinical Cretinism in Xinjiang" (n. 31 above).

41. A. K. Susheela, M. Bhatnagar, K. Vig, and N. K. Mondal, "Excess Fluoride Ingestion and Thyroid Hormone Derangements in Children Living in Delhi, India," *Fluoride* 38, no. 2 (2005): 98–108, http://www.fluorideresearch.org/382/files/38298-108.pdf.

42. D. L. St. Germain, V. A. Galton, and A. Hernandez, "Minireview: Defining the Roles of the Iodothyronine Deiodinases: Current Concepts and Challenges," *Endocrinology* 150, no. 3 (2009): 1097–107.

43. C. Clinch, "Fluoride Interactions with Iodine and Iodide: Implications for Breast Health," *Fluoride* 42, no. 2 (2009): 75–87, http://www.fluorideresearch.org/422/files/FJ2009_v42_n2_p075-087.pdf.

44. N. D. Mikhailets et al., "Thyroid Function During Prolonged Exposure to Fluorides" (n. 27 above).

45. S. Tezelman, A. E. Siperstein, Q. Y. Duh, et al., "Desensitization of Adenylate Cyclase in Chinese Hamster Ovary Cells Transfected with Human Thyroid-stimulating Hormone Receptor," *Endocrinology* 134, no. 3 (1994): 1561–69.

46. "British Fluoridation Society Statement (January 2006) on the Absence of an Association between Water Fluoridation and Thyroid Disorders," available online as of May 2, 2010, http://www.bfsweb.org/facts/sof_effects/statementofflo.htm.

47. M. S. McDonagh, P. F. Whiting, P. M. Wilson, et al., "Systematic Review of Water Fluoridation," *British Medical Journal* 321, no. 7265 (2000): 855–59, http://www.bmj.com/cgi/content/full/321/7265/855. Note: The full report that this paper summarizes is commonly known as the York Review and is accessible at http://fluoridealert.org/re/york.review.2000.pdf.)

48. World Health Organization, *Fluorides,* Environmental Health Criteria 227, International Programme on Chemical Safety, Geneva, Switzerland, 2002, http://www.inchem.org/documents/ehc/ehc/ehc227.htm.

49. Royal College of Physicians of London, *Fluoride, Teeth and Health* (Kent, UK: Pitman Medical Publishing Co. Ltd., 1976).

50. American Dental Association, "Fluoridation Facts," page 34, an update commemorating the sixtieth anniversary of community water fluoridation, 2005, https://www.ada.org/sections/professionalResources/pdfs/fluoridation_facts.pdf.48.

51. N. C. Leone, E. C. Leatherwood, I. M. Petrie, and L. Lieberman, "Effect of Fluoride on Thyroid Gland: Clinical Study," *Journal of the American Dental Association* 69 (1964): 179–80.

52. National Research Council, *Fluoride in Drinking Water,* 236 (n. 6 above).

53. J. Luke, "The Effect of Fluoride on the Physiology of the Pineal Gland," PhD thesis, University of Surrey, Guildford, UK, 1997. Thesis online, with permission of author, at http://fluoridealert.org/luke-1997.pdf.

54. J. Luke, "Fluoride Deposition in the Aged Human Pineal Gland," *Caries Research* 35, no. 2 (2001): 125–28.

55. J. Luke, "The Effect of Fluoride on the Physiology of the Pineal Gland" (n. 53 above).

56. National Research Council, *Fluoride in Drinking Water,* 264 (n. 6 above).

57. E. R. Schlesinger, D. E. Overton, H. C. Chase, and K. T. Cantwell, "Newburgh-Kingston Caries-Fluorine Study XIII. Pediatric Findings after Ten Years," *Journal of the American Dental Association* 52, no. 3 (1956): 296–306.

58. National Research Council, *Fluoride in Drinking Water*, 260 (n. 6 above).

Chapter 17

1. H. C. Hodge, "Safety Factors in Water Fluoridation Based on the Toxicology of Fluorides," *The Proceedings of the Nutrition Society* 22 (1963): 111–17, http://journals .cambridge.org/action/displayFulltext?type=1&fid=784060&jid=PNS&volumeId =22&issueId=01&aid=784052.

2. J. Caffey, "On Fibrous Defects in Cortical Walls: Their Radiological Appearance, Structure, Prevalence, Natural Course, and Diagnostic Significance," in *Advances in Pediatrics*, ed. S. Z. Levin, (New York: Interscience, 1955).

3. E. R. Schlesinger, D. E. Overton, H. C. Chase, and K. T. Cantwell, "Newburgh-Kingston Caries-Fluorine Study XIII. Pediatric Findings after Ten Years," *Journal of the American Dental Association* 52, no. 3 (1956): 296–306.

4. M. T. Alarcón-Herrera, I. R. Martín-Domínguez, R. Trejo-Vázquez, et al., "Well Water Fluoride, Dental Fluorosis, Bone Fractures in the Guadiana Valley of Mexico," *Fluoride* 34, no. 2 (2001): 139–49, http://www.fluoride-journal.com/01-34-2/342-139.pdf.

5. K. E. Heller, S. A. Eklund, and B. A. Burt, "Dental Caries and Dental Fluorosis at Varying Water Fluoride Concentrations," *Journal of Public Health Dentistry* 57, no. 3 (1997): 136–43.

6. E. D. Beltrán-Aguilar, B. F. Gooch, A. Kingman, et al., "Surveillance for Dental Caries, Dental Sealants, Tooth Retention, Edentulism, and Enamel Fluorosis—United States, 1988–1994 and 1999–2002," *Morbidity and Mortality Weekly Report* 54, no. 3 (August 26, 2005): 1–44, http://www.cdc.gov/mmwr/preview/mmwrhtml/ss5403a1.htm.

7. A. Singh, S. S. Jolly, B. C. Bansal, and C. C. Mathur, "Endemic Fluorosis: Epidemiological, Clinical and Biochemical Study of Chronic Fluoride Intoxication in Punjab (India)," *Medicine* 42 (1963): 229–46.

8. J. Franke, F. Rath, H. Runge, et al., "Industrial Fluorosis," *Fluoride* 8, no. 2 (1975): 61–83, http://www.fluoridealert.org/re/franke-1975.pdf.

9. S. P. S. Teotia, M. Teotia, and N. P. S. Teotia, "Symposium on the Non-Skeletal Phase of Chronic Fluorosis: The Joints," *Fluoride* 9, no. 1 (1976): 19–24, http://www.fluoridealert .org/re/teotia-1976.pdf.

10. B. W. Carnow and S. A. Conibear, "Industrial Fluorosis," *Fluoride* 14, no. 4 (1981): 172–81, http://fluoridealert.org/re/carnow.1981.pdf.

11. E. Czerwinski, J. Nowak, D. Dabrowska, et al., "Bone and Joint Pathology in Fluoride-Exposed Workers," *Archives of Environmental Health* 43, no. 5 (1988): 340–43.

12. U.S. Department of Health and Human Services, *Review of Fluoride: Benefits and Risks,* Public Health Service, Washington, DC, February 1991, http://health.gov/environment/ ReviewofFluoride/.

13. B. Hileman, "Fluoridation of Water. Questions about Health Risks and Benefits Remain After More than 40 Years," *Chemical & Engineering News* (August 1, 1988): 26–42.

14. American Medical News, "Arthritis Rates Increase," January 21, 2008, http://www .ama-assn.org/amednews/2008/01/21/hlbf0121.htm.

15. Ibid.

16. National Research Council of the National Academies, *Fluoride in Drinking Water: A Scientific Review of EPA's Standards* (Washington, DC: National Academies Press, 2006),

170–71, http://www.nap.edu/openbook.php?record_id=11571&page=170 and http://www.nap.edu/openbook.php?record_id=11571&page=171.

17. Ibid.,180.

18. P. Connett and M. Connett. Invited presentation to the National Research Council of the National Academies committee reviewing the safety of the U.S. Environmental Protection Agency's maximum contaminant level (MCL) for fluoride in drinking water, 2003. This PowerPoint presentation is at http://www.fluoridealert.org/nrc-final.ppt, and the paper supporting this presentation at http://www.fluoridealert.org/nrc-paper.pdf. See table 2, page 9.

19. H. C. Hodge, "Safety Factors in Water Fluoridation Based on the Toxicology of Fluorides" (n. 1 above).

20. R. Gupta, A. N. Kumar, S. Bandhu, and S. Gupta, "Skeletal Fluorosis Mimicking Seronegative Arthritis," *Scandinavian Journal of Rheumatology* 36, no. 2 (2007): 154–55.

21. J. E. Hallanger Johnson, A. E. Kearns, P. M. Doran, et al., "Fluoride-Related Bone Disease Associated with Habitual Tea Consumption," *Mayo Clinic Proceedings* 82, no. 6 (2007): 719–24. Note: Erratum on dosage error in article text in: *Mayo Clinic Proceedings* 82, no. 8 (2007): 1017, http://www.mayoclinicproceedings.com/content/82/6/719.full.

22. M. P. Whyte, W. G. Totty, V. T. Lim, and G. M. Whitford, "Skeletal Fluorosis from Instant Tea," *Journal of Bone and Mineral Research* 23, no. 5 (2008): 759–69.

23. M. J. Goldacre, S. E. Roberts, and D. Yeates, "Mortality after Admission to Hospital with Fractured Neck of Femur: Database Study," *British Medical Journal* 325, no. 7369 (2002): 868–69.

24. R. A. Marotolli, L. F. Berkman, and L. M. Cooney, "Decline in Physical Function Following Hip Fracture," *Journal of the American Geriatrics Society* 40 (1992): 861–66.

25. R. A. Marotolli, L. F. Berkman, L. Leo-Summers, and L. M. Cooney, "Predictors of Mortality and Institutionalisation after Hip Fracture: The New Haven EPESE Cohort," *American Journal of Public Health* 84 (1994): 1807–12, http://ajph.aphapublications.org/cgi/reprint/84/11/1807.

26. National Research Council, *Fluoride in Drinking Water,* 7, 179–180 (n. 16 above).

27. M. S. McDonagh, P. F. Whiting, P. M. Wilson, et al., "Systematic Review of Water Fluoridation," *British Medical Journal* 321, no. 7265 (2000): 855–59, http://www.bmj.com/cgi/content/full/321/7265/855. Note: The full report that this paper summarizes is commonly known as the York Review and is accessible at http://fluoridealert.org/re/york.review.2000.pdf.

28. National Health and Medical Research Council, *A Systematic Review of the Efficacy and Safety of Fluoridation,* reference no. EH41, Australian Government, December 27, 2007, http://www.nhmrc.gov.au/publications/synopses/eh41syn.htm.

29. Connett and Connett, invited presentation to the National Research Council, table 4, page 17 (n. 18 above).

30. Ibid.

31. Y. Li, C. Liang, C. W. Slemenda, et al., "Effect of Long-Term Exposure to Fluoride in Drinking Water on Risks of Bone Fractures," *Journal of Bone and Mineral Research* 16, no. 5 (2001): 932–39.

32. Ibid.

33. Ibid.

34. World Health Organization, *Fluorides,* Environmental Health Criteria 227, International Programme on Chemical Safety, Geneva, Switzerland, 2002, http://www.inchem.org/documents/ehc/ehc/ehc227.htm.

35. J. Fawell, K. Bailey, J. Chilton, et al., *Fluoride in Drinking-Water*, World Health Organization (London and Seattle: IWA Publishing, 2006).

36. U.S. Department of Health and Human Services, *Review of Fluoride: Benefits and Risks*, table 11, page 17, Public Health Service, Washington, DC, February 1991, http://health.gov/environment/ReviewofFluoride/.

37. Y. Li et al., "Effect of Long-Term Exposure to Fluoride in Drinking Water on Risks of Bone Fractures" (n. 31 above).

38. Ibid.

39. P. Kurttio, N. Gustavsson, T. Vartiainen, and J. Pekkanen, "Exposure to Natural Fluoride in Well Water and Hip Fracture: A Cohort Analysis in Finland," *American Journal of Epidemiology* 150, no. 8 (1999): 817–24.

40. M. T. Alarcón-Herrera et al., "Well Water Fluoride, Dental Fluorosis, Bone Fractures in the Guadiana Valley of Mexico" (n. 4 above).

41. National Research Council, *Fluoride in Drinking Water*, 164 (n. 16 above), http://www.nap.edu/openbook.php?record_id=11571&page=164.

42. National Resource Council, Fluoride in Drinking Water, 10 (n. 16 above), http://www.nap.edu/openbook.php?record_id=11571&page=10.

Chapter 18

1. National Research Council, *Drinking Water and Health*, National Academy of Sciences (Washington DC: National Academy Press, 1977), 388–89.

2. J. Caffey, "On Fibrous Defects in Cortical Walls: Their Radiological Appearance, Structure, Prevalence, Natural Course, and Diagnostic Significance," in: *Advances in Pediatrics*, ed. S. Z. Levin (New York: Interscience, 1955).

3. T. Tsutsui, N. Suzuki, M. Ohmori, and H. Maizumi, "Cytotoxicity, Chromosome Aberrations and Unscheduled DNA Synthesis in Cultured Human Diploid Fibroblasts Induced by Sodium Fluoride," *Mutation Research* 139, no. 4 (1984): 193–98.

4. W. J. Caspary, B. Myhr, L. Bowers, et al., "Mutagenic Activity of Fluorides in Mouse Lymphoma Cells," *Mutation Research* 187, no. 3 (1987): 165–80.

5. K. Kishi and T. Ishida, "Clastogenic Activity of Sodium Fluoride in Great Ape Cells," *Mutation Research* 301, no. 3 (1993): 183–88.

6. M. Mihashi and T. Tsutsui, "Clastogenic Activity of Sodium Fluoride to Rat Vertebral Body-Derived Cells in Culture," *Mutation Research* 368, no. 1 (1996): 7–13.

7. D. Q. Wu and Y. Wu, "Micronucleus and Sister Chromatid Exchange Frequency in Endemic Fluorosis," *Fluoride* 28, no. 3 (1995): 125–27, http://fluoridealert.org/re/wu.1995.pdf.

8. Z. Meng and B. Zhang, "Chromosomal Aberrations and Micronuclei in Lymphocytes of Workers at a Phosphate Fertilizer Factory," *Mutation Research* 393, no. 3 (1997): 283–38.

9. S. Joseph and P. K. Gadhia, "Sister Chromatid Exchange Frequency and Chromosome Aberrations in Residents of Fluoride Endemic Regions of South Gujarat," *Fluoride* 33, no. 4 (2000): 154–58, http://www.fluorideresearch.org/334/files/FJ2000_v33_n4_p154-158.pdf.

10. K. H. Lau, J. R. Farley, T. K. Freeman, and D. J. Baylink, "A Proposed Mechanism of the Mitogenic Action of Fluoride on Bone Cells: Inhibition of the Activity of an Osteoblastic Acid Phosphatase," *Metabolism: Clinical and Experimental* 38, no. 9 (1989): 858–68.

11. J. Caverzasio, G. Palmer, and J. P. Bonjour, "Fluoride: Mode of Action," *Bone* 22, no. 6 (1998): 585–89.

12. National Research Council of the National Academies, *Fluoride in Drinking Water: A Scientific Review of EPA's Standards* (Washington, DC: National Academies Press, 2006), 322, http://www.nap.edu/openbook.php?record_id=11571&page=322.
13. J. Yiamouyiannis and D. Burk, "Cancer from Our Drinking Water?" *Congressional Record*, proceedings and debates of the 94th Congress, First Session 121, no. 186 (December 16, 1975): H12731-34.
14. J. Yiamouyiannis and D. Burk, "Fluoridation and Cancer-Age-Dependence of Cancer Mortality Related to Artificial Fluoridation," *Fluoride* 10, no. 3 (1977): 102–23.
15. R. N. Hoover, F. W. McKay, et al., "Fluoridated Drinking Water and Subsequent Cancer Incidence and Mortality," *Journal of the National Cancer Institute* 57 (1976): 757–68.
16. J. R. Graham, D. Burk, and P. Morin, "A Current Restatement and Continuing Reappraisal Concerning Demographic Variables in American Time-Trend Studies on Water Fluoridation and Human Cancer," *Proceedings of the Pennsylvania Academy of Science* 61 (1987): 138–46.
17. J. R. Graham and P. J. Morin, "Highlights in North American Litigation During the Twentieth Century on Artificial Fluoridation of Public Water Supplies," *Journal of Land Use & Environmental Law* 14, no. 2 (1999): 195–248.
18. P. J. Morin, J. R. Graham, and G. Parent, *La Fluoration: Autopsie d'une Erreur Scientifique* (Québec, Canada: Editions Berger, Eastman, 2005), chapters 6 and 7. Republished in English as *Fluoridation: Autopsy of a Scientific Error,* by the same publisher, in 2010.
19. S. Begley, "Don't Drink the Water?" *Newsweek*, February 5, 1990.
20. National Toxicology Program, "NTP Technical Report on the Toxicology and Carcinogenesis Studies of Sodium Fluoride (CAS no. 7682-49-4) in F344/N Rats and B6C3F1 (Drinking Water Studies)," Technical Report 393, NIH publ. no. 91-2848, National Institutes of Health, Public Health Service, U.S. Department of Health and Human Services, Research Triangle Park, NC, 1990.
21. J. Bucher, "Peer Review of Draft Technical Report of Long-Term Toxicology and Carcinogenesis Studies and Toxicity Study, Sodium Fluoride," pages 30–31, Research Triangle Park, NC, April 26, 1990.
22. J. R. Bucher, M. R. Heitmancik, J. Toft, et al., "Results and Conclusions of the National Toxicology Program's Rodent Carcinogenicity Studies with Sodium Fluoride," *International Journal of Cancer* 48, no. 5 (1991): 733–37.
23. J. K. Maurer, M. C. Cheng, B. G. Boysen, and R. L. Anderson, "Two-Year Carcinogenicity Study of Sodium Fluoride in Rats," *Journal of the National Cancer Institute* 82, no. 13 (1990): 1118–26.
24. Food & Drug Administration, "Dose Determination and Carcinogenicity Studies of Sodium Fluoride in Crl:CD-1 Mice and Crl:CD (Sprague Dawley)BR Rats, June 28, 1990," in: *Review of Fluoride: Benefits and Risks*, pages D1–D7, U.S. Department of Health & Human Services, Public Health Service, Washington, DC, February 1991.
25. Ibid.
26. Ibid.
27. Memorandum from William L. Marcus, PhD, Senior Science Advisor, Criteria & Standards Division, ODW (WH-550D) to Alan B. Hais, Acting Director, Criteria & Standards Division, ODW (WH-550D), U.S. Environmental Protection Agency, May 1, 1990, http://www.fluoridealert.org/health/cancer/ntp/marcus-memo.html.
28. H. Ettel, "Reich Orders EPA to Reinstate Scientist," National Whistleblower Center, February 10, 1994, http://www.fluoridealert.org/health/cancer/ntp/marcus3.html.

29. Memorandum from William L. Marcus, Senior Science Advisor, Criteria & Standards Division, U.S. EPA Office of Drinking Water to Alan B. Hais (n. 27 above).

30. J. W. Hirzy testimony on behalf of the National Treasury Employees Union Chapter 280, before the Subcommittee on Wildlife, Fisheries and Drinking Water, U.S. Senate, Washington DC, June 29, 2000. Video of testimony, "EPA Union Calls for Moratorium on Water Fluoridation," at http://video.google.com/videoplay ?docid=8903910725020792574#, transcript of testimony at http://www.fluoridealert.org/ testimony.htm.

31. Amicus curiae brief of the U.S. Environmental Protection Agency Headquarters Union (Local 2050, National Federation of Federal Employees), in: *Natural Resources Defense Council v. Environmental Protection Agency and Lee M. Thomas, Administrator.* In the Court of Appeals for the District of Columbia Circuit, 1986, http://www.fluoridealert .org/health/epa/nrdc/union-brief1986.pdf; see also http://www.fluoridealert.org/health/ epa/nrdc/index.html. Note: The US EPA's Union for Professionals in Washington, DC, is now called National Treasury Employees Union Chapter 280.

32. G. Lee, "Whistle-Blower Clears the Air," *Washington Post*, March 1, 1994.

33. J. W. Hirzy, "Why EPA's Headquarters Professionals' Union Opposes Fluoridation," National Treasury Employees Union, Chapter 280, May 1, 1999, http://www.fluoride alert.org/hp-epa.htm.

34. National Research Council, *Drinking Water and Health* (n. 1 above).

35. U.S. Department of Health and Human Services, *Review of Fluoride: Benefits and Risks,* Public Health Service, Washington, DC, February 1991, http://health.gov/environment/ ReviewofFluoride/.

36. Ibid., appendix E.

37. Ibid., appendix F.

38. Ibid., appendix E.

39. Ibid., appendix F.

40. Ibid.

41. P. Connett, C. Neurath, and M. Connett, "Revisiting the Fluoride-Osteorsarcoma Connection in the Context of Elise Bassin's Findings: Part I," submission to the National Research Council, National Academies Toxicologic Risk of Fluoride in Drinking Water, March 2, 2005, http://www.fluoridealert.org/health/cancer/fan-nrc.part1.pdf.

42. P. Connett, C. Neurath, and M. Connett, "Revisiting the Fluoride-Osteosarcoma Connection in the Context of Elise Bassin's Findings: Part II." Submission to the National Research Council of the National Academies review panel on the Toxicologic Risk of Fluoride in Drinking Water, March 21, 2005 (revised April 8, 2005), http:// www.fluoridealert.org/health/cancer/fan-nrc.part2.pdf.

43. P. Connett, M. Connett, and C. Neurath, "The Fluoride-Osteosarcoma Connection Revisited," paper presented at the XXVIth conference of the International Society for Fluoride Research, Wiesbaden, Germany, *Fluoride* 38, no. 3 (2005): 227, abstract 10 at http://fluoridealert.org/scher/connett-2005c.pdf.

44. U.S. Department of Health and Human Services, *Review of Fluoride: Benefits and Risks*, abstract, page i (n. 35 above).

45. U.S. Department of Health and Human Services, *Review of Fluoride: Benefits and Risks*, appendix A and A-2 (n. 35 above).

46. S. M. McGuire, E. D. Vanable, M. H. McGuire, J. A. Buckwalter, and C. W. Douglass, "Is There a Link between Fluoridated Water and Osteosarcoma?" *Journal of the American Dental Association* 122, no. 4 (1991): 38–45.

47. Ibid., 39.

48. Ibid., 40.

49. Ibid., 44.

50. Ibid., 45.

51. P. D. Cohn, *An Epidemiologic Report on Drinking Water and Fluoridation,* New Jersey Department of Health, Environmental Health Service, November 8, 1992. Note: The original title of this report was *A Brief Report on the Association of Drinking Water Fluoridation and the Incidence of Osteosarcoma Among Young Males.* The word "osteosarcoma" was deleted from the title soon after the report was released; http://fluoridealert .org/cohn-1992.pdf.

52. Ibid., 11.

53. A. G. Glass and J. F. Fraumeni, "Epidemiology of Bone Cancer in Children," *Journal of the National Cancer Institute* 44, no. 1 (1970): 187–99, as cited by P. D. Cohn (n. 51 above).

54. L. S. Kaminsky, M. C. Mahoney, J. Leach, et al., "Fluoride Benefits and Risks of Exposure," *Critical Reviews in Oral Biology & Medicine* 1, no. 4 (1990): 261–81, as cited by P. D. Cohn (n. 51 above), http://cro.sagepub.com/cgi/reprint/1/4/261.

55. U.S. Department of Health and Human Services, *Review of Fluoride: Benefits and Risks* (n. 35 above), as cited by P. D. Cohn (n. 51 above).

56. S. E. Hrudey, C. L. Soskolne, J. Berkel, and S. Fincham, "Drinking Water Fluoridation and Osteosarcoma," *Canadian Journal of Public Health* 81, no. 6 (1990): 415–16.

57. M. C. Mahoney, P. C. Nasca, W. S. Burnett, and J. M. Meius, "Bone Cancer Incidence Rates in New York State: Time Trends and Fluoridated Drinking Water," *American Journal of Public Health* 81, no. 4 (1991): 475–79, http://ajph.aphapublications.org/cgi/reprint/81/4/475.pdf.

58. S. C. Freni and D. W. Gaylor, "International Trends in the Incidence of Bone Cancer Are Not Related to Drinking Water Fluoridation," *Cancer* 70, no. 3 (1992): 611–18.

59. K. H. Gelberg, E. F. Fitzgerald, S. Hwang, and R. Dubrow, "Fluoride Exposure and Childhood Osteosarcoma: A Case-Control Study," *American Journal of Public Health* 85, no. 12 (1995): 1678–83, http://ajph.aphapublications.org/cgi/reprint/85/12/1678.pdf.

60. M. E. Moss, M. S. Kanarek, H. A. Anderson, et al., "Osteosarcoma, Seasonality, and Environmental Factors in Wisconsin, 1979–1989," *Archives of Environmental Health* 50, no. 3 (1995): 235–41.

61. P. Connett et al., "Revisiting the Fluoride-Osteorsarcoma Connection in the Context of Elise Bassin's Findings: Part I" (n. 41 above).

62. P. Connett et al., "Revisiting the Fluoride-Osteosarcoma Connection in the Context of Elise Bassin's Findings: Part II" (n. 42 above).

63. E. B. Bassin, "Association Between Fluoride in Drinking Water During Growth and Development and the Incidence of Osteosarcoma for Children and Adolescents," DMSc thesis, Harvard School of Dental Medicine, Boston, Massachusetts, 2001.

64. P. D. Cohn, *An Epidemiologic Report on Drinking Water and Fluoridation* (n. 51 above).

65. E. B. Bassin, "Association Between Fluoride in Drinking Water During Growth and Development and the Incidence of Osteosarcoma for Children and Adolescents" (n. 63 above).

66. S. M. McGuire et al., "Is There a Link Between Fluoridated Water and Osteosarcoma?" (n. 46 above).

67. S. Jones and K. Lennon, *One in a Million. The Facts About Fluoridation,* 2nd ed., published by the British Fluoridation Society, UK Public Health Association, British Dental Association, and the Faculty of Public Health, 2004, http://fluoridealert.org/re/uk.bfs.one-in-a-million.2004.pdf.

68. National Research Council, *Fluoride in Drinking Water* (n. 12 above).
69. Report submitted in 2004 by Chester W. Douglass to the National Research Council of the National Academies Committee: Toxicologic Risk of Fluoride in Drinking Water [BEST-K-02-05-A], http://www.fluoridealert.org/harvard/docs/final-report.pdf.
70. S. Begley, "Fluoridation, Cancer: Did Researchers Ask the Right Question?" *Wall Street Journal*, July 22, 2005, page B1.
71. Harvard Medical School Office of Public Affairs, "Statement Concerning the Outcome of the Review into Allegations of Research Misconduct Involving Fluoride Research," News Release, August 15, 2006, http://web.med.harvard.edu/sites/RELEASES/html/8_15Douglass.html.
72. E. B. Bassin, D. Wypij, R. B. Davis, and M. A. Mittleman, "Age-specific Fluoride Exposure in Drinking Water and Osteosarcoma (United States)," *Cancer Causes and Control* 17, no. 4 (May 2006): 421–28.
73. C. W. Douglass and K. Joshipura, "Caution Needed in Fluoride and Osteosarcoma Study" (letter), *Cancer Causes & Control* 17, no. 4 (May 2006): 481–82.
74. Ibid.
75. E. B. Bassin, "Association Between Fluoride in Drinking Water During Growth and Development and the Incidence of Ostosarcoma for Children and Adolescents" (n. 63 above).
76. E. B. Bassin et al., "Age-specific Fluoride Exposure in Drinking Water and Osteosarcoma (United States)" (n. 72 above).
77. C. Neurath and P. Connett, "Current Epidemiological Research on Link between Fluoride and Osteosarcoma," *Fluoride* 41, no. 3 (2008): 241–42 (abstracts from the XXVIIIth Conference of the International Society for Fluoride Research), http://www.fluorideresearch.org/413/files/FJ2008_v41_n3_p233-258.pdf.
78. National Health and Medical Research Council, *A Systematic Review of the Efficacy and Safety of Fluoridation*, reference no. EH41, Australian Government, December 27, 2007, http://www.nhmrc.gov.au/publications/synopses/eh41syn.htm.
79. South Central Strategic Health Authority, "Public Consultation on the Proposal for Water Fluoridation in Southampton and Parts of Southwest Hampshire," September 2008, pages 18–19, http://fluoridealert.org/re/uk.sha.brochure.2008.pdf.
80. Video of the presentation by Dr. Peter Cooney, Chief Dental Officer of Canada, on the case for fluoridation of drinking water in Dryden, Ontario, Canada, April 1, 2008, http://video.google.com/videoplay?docid=4888471756915953833&hl=en.
81. California Office of Environmental Health Hazard Assessment, "Announcement of Chemicals Selected by OEHHA for Consideration for Listing by the Carcinogen Identification Committee and Request for Relevant Information on the Carcinogenic Hazards of These Chemicals," California Environmental Protection Agency, October 15, 2009, http://www.oehha.ca.gov/prop65/CRNR_notices/state_listing/data_callin/sqe101509.html.
82. C. Neurath and P. Connett, "Evidence Supporting Prioritizing Fluoride for Carcinogenicity Hazard Identification," submission to the California Office of Environmental Health Hazard Assessment and Carcinogenicity Identification Committee, Prioritization of Chemicals for Carcinogen Identification Committee Review, California Environmental Protection Agency, May 5, 2009, http://fluoridealert.org/neurath-2009.may5.pdf.
83. Environmental Working Group, "Research on PFOA and Fluoride Carcinogenicity Supports Their High Priority Review for Proposition 65 Listing," submission to the

California Office of Environmental Health Hazard Assessment, Prioritization of Chemicals for Carcinogen Identification Committee Review, California Environmental Protection Agency, May 5, 2009, http://fluoridealert.org/ca/ewg-may2009.pdf.

84. K. M. Thiessen, "Comments on Prioritization of Chemicals for Carcinogen Identification Committee Review. Proposed Chemicals for Committee Consideration and Consultation. March 2009," submission to: Proposition 65 Implementation, Office of Environmental Health Hazard Assessment, California Environmental Protection Agency, from Kathleen M. Thiessen, PhD, SENES Oak Ridge, Inc., Center for Risk Analysis, Oak Ridge, TN, May 5, 2009, http://fluoridealert.org/ca/thiessen-2009.pdf.

85. California Dental Association, "CDA Receives ADA State Public Affairs Program Grants," executive bulletin from the desk of Executive Director Peter DuBois, January 12, 2010.

86. California Office of Environmental Health Hazard Assessment, "Announcement of Chemicals Selected by OEHHA" (n. 81 above).

Chapter 19

1. C. F. Hongslo, J. K. Hongslo, and R. I. Holland, "Fluoride Sensitivity of Cells from Different Organs," *Acta Pharmacologica et Toxicologica* 46, no. 1 (1980): 73–77.

2. J. Ekstrand, "Fluoride Intake," in: *Fluoride in Dentistry,* 2nd ed., ed. O. Fejerskov, J. Ekstrand, and B. Burt (Denmark: Munksgaard, 1996), 40–52.

3. G. M. Whitford, "The Metabolism and Toxicity of Fluoride," in: *Monographs in Oral Science,* vol. 16, 2nd rev. ed. (New York: Karger, 1996).

4. R. I. Mazze, "Methoxyflurane Nephropathy," *Environmental Health Perspectives* 15 (1976): 111–19, http://fluoridealert.org/re/mazze-1976.pdf.

5. J. Marier and D. Rose, *Environmental Fluoride,* Associate Committee on Scientific Criteria for Environmental Quality, NRCC no. 16081, National Research Council of Canada, 1977. A large part of this report can be found at http://www.fluoridealert.org/NRC-Fluoride.htm.

6. M. Nuscheler, P. Conzen, D. Schwender, and K. Peter, "Fluoride-Induced Nephrotoxicity: Fact or Fiction?" (article in German), *Der Anaesthesist* 45, suppl. 1 (1996): S32–40.

7. S. Partanen, "Inhibition of Human Renal Acid Phosphatases by Nephrotoxic Micromolar Concentrations of Fluoride," *Experimental and Toxicologic Pathology* 54, no. 3 (2002): 231–37.

8. R. I. Mazze, "Fluorinated Anesthetic Nephrotoxicity: An Update," *Canadian Anaesthetists' Society Journal* 31 (1984): S16–22.

9. J. A. Varner, K. F. Jensen, W. Horvath, and R. L. Isaacson, "Chronic Administration of Aluminum-Fluoride or Sodium-Fluoride to Rats in Drinking Water: Alterations in Neuronal and Cerebrovascular Integrity," *Brain Research* 784, no. 1–2 (1998): 284–98. Extended excerpts at http://www.fluoride-journal.com/98-31-2/31291-95.htm.

10. C. M. McCay, W. F. Ramseyer, and C. A. Smith, "Effect of Sodium Fluoride Administration on Body Changes in Old Rats," *Journal of Gerontology* 12, no. 1 (1957): 14–19.

11. S. L. Manocha, H. Warner, and Z. L. Olkowski, "Cytochemical Response of Kidney, Liver and Nervous System to Fluoride Ions in Drinking Water," *Histochemical Journal* 7, no. 4 (1975): 343–55.

12. J. L. Borke and G. M. Whitford, "Chronic Fluoride Ingestion Decreases 45Ca Uptake by Rat Kidney Membranes," *Journal of Nutrition* 129 (1999): 1209–13, http://jn.nutrition.org/cgi/content/full/129/6/1209.

13. M. Ando, M. Tadano, S. Yamamoto, et al., "Health Effects of Fluoride Pollution Caused by Coal Burning," *Science of the Total Environment* 271, no. 1–3 (2001): 107–16.

14. O. M. Derryberry, M. D. Bartholomew, and R. B. Fleming, "Fluoride Exposure and Worker Health. The Health Status of Workers in a Fertilizer Manufacturing Plant in Relation to Fluoride Exposure," *Archives of Environmental Health* 6 (1963): 503–14.

15. S. P. Kumar and R. A. Harper, "Fluorosis in Aden," *British Journal of Radiology* 36 (1963): 497–502.

16. O. Lantz, M. H. Jouvin, M. C. De Vernejoul, and P. Druet, "Fluoride-Induced Chronic Renal Failure," *American Journal of Kidney Diseases* 10, no. 2 (1987): 136–39.

17. M. Reggabi, K. Khelfat, M. T. Aoul, et al., "Renal Function in Residents of an Endemic Fluorosis Area in Southern Algeria," *Fluoride* 17, no. 1 (1984): 35–41, http://www.fluoridealert.org/re/reggabi-1984.pdf.

18. H. E. Shortt, G. R. McRobert, T. W. Barnard, and A. S. M. Nayar, "Endemic Fluorosis in the Madras Presidency," *Indian Journal of Medical Research* 25, no. 2 (1937): 553–68.

19. A. H. Siddiqui, "Fluorosis in Nalgonda District, Hyderabad-Deccan," *British Medical Journal* 2, no. 4953 (1955): 1408–13.

20. A. Singh, S. S. Jolly, B. C. Bansal, and C. C. Mathur, "Endemic Fluorosis: Epidemiological, Clinical and Biochemical Study of Chronic Fluoride Intoxication in Punjab (India)," *Medicine* 42 (1963): 229–46.

21. V. P. Singla, G. L. Garg, and S. S. Jolly, "The Kidneys," *Fluoride* 9, no. 1 (1976): 33–35.

22. S. S. Jolly, O. P. Sharma, G. Garg, and R. Sharma, "Kidney Changes and Kidney Stones in Endemic Fluorosis," *Fluoride* 13, no. 1 (1980): 10–16, http://www.fluoridealert.org/re/jolly-1980.pdf.

23. J. L. Liu, T. Xia, Y. Y. Yu, et al., "The Dose-Effect Relationship of Water Fluoride Levels and Renal Damage in Children" (article in Chinese), *Wei Sheng Yan Jiu* 34, no. 3 (2005): 287–88.

24. W. Johnson et al., "Fluoridation and Bone Disease in Renal Patients," pages 275–93, in: *Continuing Evaluation of the Use of Fluorides,* ed. E. Johansen, D. R. Taves, and T. O. Olsen, AAAS Selected Symposium (Boulder, Colorado: Westview Press, 1979).

25. L. I. Juncos and J. V. Donadio, "Renal Failure and Fluorosis," *Journal of the American Medical Association* 222, no. 7 (1972): 783–85.

26. National Research Council of the National Academies, *Fluoride in Drinking Water: A Scientific Review of EPA's Standards* (Washington, DC: National Academies Press, 2006), 280, http://www.nap.edu/openbook.php?record_id=11571&page=280.

27. Ibid., 281, http://www.nap.edu/openbook.php?record_id=11571&page=281.

28. Ibid.

29. Ibid., 303, http://www.nap.edu/openbook.php?record_id=11571&page=303.

30. Ibid, chapters 6 and 9.

31. S. C. Freni, "Exposure to High Fluoride Concentrations in Drinking Water Is Associated with Decreased Birth Rates," *Journal of Toxicology and Environmental Health* 42, no. 1 (1994): 109–21.

32. H. Long, Y. Jin, M. Lin, et al., "Fluoride Toxicity in the Male Reproductive System," *Fluoride* 42, no. 4 (2009): 260–76, http://www.fluorideresearch.org/424/files/FJ2009_v42_n4_p260-276.pdf.

33. E. Varol, S. Akcay, I. H. Ersoy, et al., "Impact of Chronic Fluorosis on Left Ventricular Diastolic and Global Functions," *The Science of the Total Environment* 408, no. 11 (2010): 2295–98.

34. E. Varol, S. Akcay, I. H. Ersoy, et al., "Aortic Elasticity Is Impaired in Patients with Endemic Fluorosis," *Biological Trace Element Research* 133, no. 2 (2010): 121–27.

Chapter 20

1. National Health and Medical Research Council, *A Systematic Review of the Efficacy and Safety of Fluoridation*, reference no. EH41, Australian Government, December 27, 2007, http://www.nhmrc.gov.au/publications/synopses/eh41syn.htm.

2. Video of the presentation by Dr. Peter Cooney, Chief Dental Officer of Canada, on the case for fluoridation of drinking water in Dryden, Ontario, Canada, April 1, 2008, http://video.google.com/videoplay?docid=4888471756915953833&hl=en.

3. Presentations by Barry Cockcroft, Chief Dental Officer for England, at "Question Time on Fluoridation" held on October 20, November 18, and December 3, 2008. Organized by the South Central Strategic Health Authority Southampton, UK.

4. Bazian Ltd., "Critical Appraisal of 'Fluoride in Drinking Water: A Scientific Review of EPA's standards.'" A report for South Central Strategic Health Authority, UK, delivery date: February 11, 2009, http://fluoridealert.org/sha.basian.nrc.feb09.pdf.

5. American Dental Association, "Statement on Fluoride in Drinking Water: A Scientific Review of EPA's Standards [the NRC 2006 report]," news release, March 22, 2006.

6. Centers for Disease Control and Prevention, "Statement on the 2006 National Research Council Report, Fluoride in Drinking Water: A Scientific Review of EPA's Standards," Division of Oral Health. Posted originally on March 28, 2006. Date last updated: August 24, 2009, http://www.cdc.gov/FLUORIDATION/safety/nrc_report.htm.

7. National Research Council of the National Academies, *Fluoride in Drinking Water: A Scientific Review of EPA's Standards* (Washington, DC: National Academies Press, 2006), http://books.nap.edu/openbook.php?record_id=11571.

8. Ibid.

9. R. J. Carton, "Review of the 2006 National Research Council Report: Fluoride in Drinking Water," *Fluoride* 39, no. 3 (2006): 163–72, http://www.fluorideresearch.org/393/files/FJ2006_v39_n3_p163-172.pdf.

10. National Research Council, *Fluoride in Drinking Water* (n. 7 above).

11. P. P. Bachinskii, O. A. Gutsalenko, N. D. Naryzhniuk, et al., "Action of Fluoride on the Function of the Pituitary-thyroid System of Healthy Persons and Patients with Thyroid Disorders" (article in Russian), *Problemy Endokrinologii (Mosk)* 31, no. 6 (1985): 25–29, English translation at http://www.fluoridealert.org/bachinskii.1985.pdf.

12. Q. Xiang, Y. Liang, L. Chen, et al., "Effect of Fluoride in Drinking Water on Children's Intelligence," *Fluoride* 36, no. 2 (2003): 84–94, http://www.fluorideresearch.org/362/files/FJ2003_v36_n2_p84-94.pdf.

13. Q. Xiang, Y. Liang, M. Zhou, and H. Zang, "Blood Lead of Children in Wamiao-Xinhuai Intelligence Study" (letter), *Fluoride* 36, no. 3 (2003): 198–99, http://www.fluorideresearch.org/363/files/FJ2003_v36_n3_p198-199.pdf.

14. F. F. Lin, Aihaiti, H. X. Zhao, et al., "The Relationship of a Low-Iodine and High-Fluoride Environment to Subclinical Cretinism in Xinjiang," Xinjiang Institute for Endemic Disease Control and Research; Office of Leading Group for Endemic Disease Control of Hetian Prefectural Committee of the Communist Party of China; and County Health and Epidemic Prevention Station, Yutian, Xinjiang, *Iodine Deficiency Disorder Newsletter* 7 (1991): 3, http://fluoridealert.org/scher/lin-1991.pdf; also see http://www.fluoridealert.org/IDD.htm.

15. P. Kurttio, N. Gustavsson, T. Vartiainen, and J. Pekkanen, "Exposure to Natural Fluoride in Well Water and Hip Fracture: A Cohort Analysis in Finland," *American Journal of Epidemiology* 150, no. 8 (1999): 817–24.

16. Y. Li, C. Liang, C. W. Slemenda, et al., "Effect of Long-term Exposure to Fluoride in Drinking Water on Risks of Bone Fractures," *Journal of Bone and Mineral Research* 16, no. 5 (2001): 932–39.

17. B. C. Nesin, "A Water Supply Perspective of the Fluoridation Discussion," *Journal of the Maine Water Utilities Association* 32 (1956): 33–47.

18. U.S. Environmental Protection Agency, "National Primary Drinking Water Regulations; Fluoride. Final Rule," *Federal Register*, 40 CM Part 104 [WH-FRL-2913-8(b)], November 14, 1985. Note: The MCL established on April 2, 1986 [51 FR 11396], finalizes regulations proposed in the Federal Register of May 14, 1985 (50 FR 20164)]; http://fluoridealert.org/scher/epa-1985.pdf.

19. U.S. Environmental Protection Agency. 2004: First Human Health Risk Assessment for Sulfuryl Fluoride and Fluoride Anion: "Human Health Risk Assessment for Sulfuryl Fluoride and Fluoride Anion Addressing the Section 3 Registration of Sulfuryl Fluoride Post-Harvest Fumigation of Stored Cereal Grains, Dried Fruits and Tree Nuts and Pest Control in Grain Processing Facilities. PP# 1F6312." This assessment is preceded by a memorandum from Michael Doherty, chemist, and Edwin Budd, toxicologist, Registration Action Branch 2, Health Effects Division (7509C), and Becky Daiss, environmental health scientist, Reregistration Branch 4, Health Effects Division (7509C), Office of Prevention, Pesticides and Toxic Substances, Washington, DC, January 20, 2004, http://www.fluoridealert.org/pesticides/sf.jan.20.2004.epa.docket.pdf.

20. Comments on reevaluating the fluoride in drinking water standard by Robert J. Carton, PhD, vice president, Local 2050 of the National Federation of Federal Employees, before the Drinking Water Committee of the Science Advisory Board of the U.S. Environmental Protection Agency, Arlington, VA, November 1, 1991.

21. P. Galletti and G. Joyet, "Effect of Fluorine on Thyroidal Iodine Metabolism in Hyperthyroidism," *Journal of Clinical Endocrinology* 18, no. 10 (1958): 1102–10. Full study at http://www.slweb.org/galletti.html

22. P. P. Bachinskii, O. A. Gutsalenko, N. D. Naryzhniuk, et al., "Action of Fluoride on the Function of the Pituitary-thyroid System of Healthy Persons and Patients with Thyroid Disorders" (n. 11 above).

23. S. Bang, G. Boivin, J. C. Gerster, and C. A. Baud, "Distribution of Fluoride in Calcified Cartilage of a Fluoride-treated Osteoporotic Patient," *Bone* 6, no. 4 (1985): 207–10.

24. B. S. Bhavsar, V. K. Desai, N. R. Mehta, R. T. Vashi, K. A. V. R. Krishnamachari, "Neighborhood Fluorosis in Western India Part II: Population Study," *Fluoride* 18, no 2 (1985): 86–92.

25. B. W. Carnow and S. A. Conibear, "Industrial Fluorosis," *Fluoride* 14, no. 4 (1981): 172–81, http://fluoridealert.org/re/carnow.1981.pdf.

26. M. A. Boillat, J. Garcia and L. Velebit, "Radiological Criteria of Industrial Fluorosis," *Skeletal Radiology* 5, no. 3 (1980): 161–65.

27. H. C. Hodge and F. A. Smith, "Occupational Fluoride Exposure," Journal of Occupational Medicine 19, no. 1 (1977): 12–39.

28. E. Czerwinski and W. Lankosz, "Fluoride-induced Changes in 60 Retired Aluminum Workers," *Fluoride* 10, no. 3 (1977): 125–36.

29. National Research Council, Fluoride in Drinking Water, 179 (n. 7 above).

30. E. R. Schlesinger, D. E. Overton, H. C. Chase, and K. T. Cantwell, "Newburgh-Kingston Caries-Fluorine Study XIII. Pediatric Findings after Ten Years," *Journal of the American Dental Association* 52, no. 3 (1956): 296–306.

31. Ibid.

32. P. P. Bachinskii, O. A. Gutsalenko, N. D. Naryzhniuk, et al., "Action of Fluoride on the Function of the Pituitary-thyroid System of Healthy Persons and Patients with Thyroid Disorders" (n. 11 above).

33. Ibid.

34. K. Baetcke, J. Blondell, W. Burnam, et al., "A Preliminary Evaluation of Articles Related to Fluoride Cited by the Fluoride Action Network (FAN) as Objections to the Sulfuryl Fluoride Pesticide Tolerance Rule," U.S. Environmental Protection Agency, Office of Prevention, Pesticides and Toxic Substances, Health Effects Division, November 18, 2003, http://www.fluoridealert.org/pesticides/sf.nov.18.2003.epa.docket.pdf.

35. E. R. Schlesinger, D. E. Overton, H. C. Chase, and K. T. Cantwell, "Newburgh-Kingston Caries-Fluorine Study XIII. Pediatric Findings after Ten Years," *Journal of the American Dental Association* 52, no. 3 (1956): 296–306.

36. U.S. Department of Health and Human Services, *Review of Fluoride: Benefits and Risks*, Public Health Service, Washington, DC, February 1991, http://health.gov/environment/ReviewofFluoride/.

37. Ibid.

38. J. Franke, F. Rath, H. Runge, et al., "Industrial Fluorosis," *Fluoride* 8, no. 2 (1975): 61–83, http://www.fluoridealert.org/re/franke-1975.pdf.

39. National Research Council, *Fluoride in Drinking Water*, 179 (n. 7 above).

40. C. G. Pandit, T. N. S. Raghavachari, D. S. Rao, and V. Krishnamurti, "Endemic Fluorosis in South India," *Indian Journal of Medical Research* 28, no. 2 (1940): 533–58.

41. K. Roholm, *Fluorine Intoxication: A Clinical-Hygienic Study, with a Review of the Literature and Some Experimental Investigations* (Copenhagen: Nyt Nordisk Forlag; London: H. K. Lewis and Co. Ltd., 1937), http://www.scribd.com/doc/11757791/Fluorine-Intoxication-Kaj-Roholm-1937-Copenhagen.

42. U.S. Environmental Protection Agency, 2004: First Human Health Risk Assessment for Sulfuryl Fluoride and Fluoride Anion (n. 19 above).

43. Presentation by Joyce Donahue, PhD, toxicologist, Office of Science and Technology, U.S. EPA Office of Drinking Water, to the National Research Council Committee: Toxicologic Risk of Fluoride in Drinking Water [BEST-K-02-05-A], August 12, 2003, http://www.fluoridealert.org/pesticides/nrc.aug.2003.epa..html.

44. National Research Council, *Fluoride in Drinking Water* (n. 7 above).

45. Institute of Medicine of the National Academies, *Dietary Reference Intakes: Water, Potassium, Sodium, Chloride, and Sulfate*, Food and Nutrition Board (Washington, DC: The National Academies Press, February 2004), http://books.nap.edu/openbook.php?record_id=10925.

46. Ibid., appendix E.

47. M. C. Kiritsy, S. M. Levy, J. J. Warren, et al., "Assessing Fluoride Concentrations of Juices and Juice-Flavored Drinks," *Journal of the American Dental Association* 127, no. 7 (1996): 895–902.

48. J. R. Heilman, M. C. Kiritsy, S. M. Levy, and J. S. Wefel, "Assessing Fluoride Levels of Carbonated Soft Drinks," *Journal of the American Dental Association* 130, no. 11 (1999): 1593–99.

49. J. G. Stannard, Y. S. Shim, M. Kritsineli, et al., "Fluoride Levels and Fluoride Contamination of Fruit Juices," *Journal of Clinical Pediatric Dentistry* 16, no. 1 (1991): 38–40.

50. U.S. Department of Agriculture, "USDA National Fluoride Database of Selected Beverages and Foods," prepared by Nutrient Data Laboratory, Beltsville Human Nutrition

Research Center, Agricultural Research Service, USDA; in collaboration with University of Minnesota, Nutrition Coordinating Center; University of Iowa, College of Dentistry; Virginia Polytechnic Institute and State University, Food Analysis Laboratory Control Center; National Agricultural Statistics Service, CSREES, USDA; and Food Composition Laboratory, Beltsville Human Nutrition Research Center, Agricultural Research Service, 2004, http://www.fluoridealert.org/pesticides/fluoride.food.levels.2004.pdf.

51. E. M. Bentley, R. P. Ellwood, and R. M. Davies, "Fluoride Ingestion from Toothpaste by Young Children," *British Dental Journal* 186, no. 9 (1999): 460–62.

52. S. M. Levy and N. Guha-Chowdhury, "Total Fluoride Intake and Implications for Dietary Fluoride Supplementation," *Journal of Public Health Dentistry* 59, no. 4 (1999): 211–23.

53. N. J. Fein and F. L. Cerklewski, "Fluoride Content of Foods Made with Mechanically Separated Chicken," *Journal of Agricultural and Food Chemistry* 49, no. 9 (2001): 4284–86.

54. P. Pehrsson, R. Cutrufelli, K. Patterson, et al., "The Fluoride Content of Brewed and Microwave Brewed Black Teas," U.S. Department of Agriculture, Agricultural Research Service, 2005, http://fluoridealert.org/re/pehrsson-2005.usda.pdf.

55. M. P. Whyte, "Fluoride Levels in Bottled Teas," *The American Journal of Medicine* 119, no. 2 (2006): 189–90.

56. M. P. Whyte, W. G. Totty, V. T. Lim, and G. M. Whitford, "Skeletal Fluorosis from Instant Tea," *Journal of Bone and Mineral Research* 23, no. 5 (2008): 759–69.

57. J. E. Hallanger Johnson, A. E. Kearns, P. M. Doran, et al., "Fluoride-Related Bone Disease Associated with Habitual Tea Consumption," *Mayo Clinic Proceedings* 82, no. 6 (2007): 719–24. Note: Erratum on dosage error in article text in: *Mayo Clinic Proceedings* 82, no. 8 (2007): 1017, http://www.mayoclinicproceedings.com/content/82/6/719.full.

58. U.S. Department of Agriculture, "USDA National Fluoride Database of Selected Beverages and Foods" (n. 39 above).

59. A. W. Burgstahler and M. A. Robinson, "Fluoride in California Wines and Raisins," *Fluoride* 30, no. 3 (1997): 142–46, http://fluoridealert.org/re/burgstahler-1997.pdf.

60. G. S. Ostrom, "Cryolite on Grapes/Fluoride in Wines—A Guide for Growers and Vintners to Determine Optimum Cryolite Applications on Grapevines," CATI Viticulture and Enology Research Center, California State University, Fresno, published by the California Agricultural Technology Institute, CATI Publication #960601, June, 1996.

61. Amicus curiae brief of the U.S. Environmental Protection Agency Headquarters Union (Local 2050, National Federation of Federal Employees), in: *Natural Resources Defense Council v. Environmental Protection Agency and Lee M. Thomas, Administrator*. In the Court of Appeals for the District of Columbia Circuit, 1986, http://www.fluoridealert .org/health/epa/nrdc/union-brief1986.pdf; see also http://www.fluoridealert.org/health/ epa/nrdc/index.html.

62. National Research Council, *Fluoride in Drinking Water* (n. 7 above).

63. Institute of Medicine, *Dietary Reference Intakes for Calcium, Phosphorus, Magnesium, Vitamin D, and Fluoride* (Washington, DC: Standing Committee on the Scientific Evaluation of Dietary Reference Intakes, Food and Nutrition Board, 1997), http://www .nap.edu/openbook.php?record_id=5776.

64. Centers for Disease Control and Prevention, "Achievements in Public Health, 1900–1999: Fluoridation of Drinking Water to Prevent Dental Caries," *Mortality and Morbidity Weekly Review* 48, no. 41 (October 22, 1999): 933–40, http://www.cdc.gov/ mmwr/preview/mmwrhtml/mm4841a1.htm. Note: The authors of this report were Scott

Tomar and Susan Griffin, as cited in Tomar's curriculum vitae, paper number 27 on page 27, http://fluoridealert.org/re/tomar.scott.cv.ref.27.pdf.

65. Centers for Disease Control and Prevention, "Recommendations for Using Fluoride to Prevent and Control Dental Caries in the United States," *Morbidity and Mortality Weekly Report* 50, no. RR14 (August 17, 2001): 1–42, http://www.cdc.gov/mmwr/preview/mmwrhtml/rr5014a1.htm.

66. Letter coauthored by Bruce Alberts, president of the National Academy of Sciences, and Kenneth Shine, president of the Institute of Medicine, to Albert W. Burgstahler and others, November 20, 1998, http://www.fluoridation.com/fraud.htm.

67. Institute of Medicine, *Dietary Reference Intakes for Calcium, Phosphorus, Magnesium, Vitamin D, and Fluoride*, 309 (n. 52 above).

68. *Forum on Fluoridation* (Dublin, Ireland: Stationery Office, 2002), page 110, http://fluoridealert.org/re/fluoridation.forum.2002.pdf.

69. U.S. Environmental Protection Agency, 2004: First Human Health Risk Assessment for Sulfuryl Fluoride and Fluoride Anion (n. 19 above).

70. U.S. Environmental Protection Agency, 2005: Second Human Health Risk Assessment for Sulfuryl Fluoride and Fluoride Anion: "Draft. Human Health Risk Assessment for Sulfuryl Fluoride and Fluoride Anion Addressing the Section 3 Registration of Sulfuryl Fluoride Fumigation of Food Processing Facilities. PP# 3F6573," Office of Prevention, Pesticides and Toxic Substances, June 2, 2005, http://www.fluoridealert.org/pesticides/sf.hra-june2.2005.pdf.

71. U.S. Environmental Protection Agency, 2006: Third Human Health Risk Assessment for Sulfuryl Fluoride and Fluoride Anion: "Final. Human Health Risk Assessment for Sulfuryl Fluoride and Fluoride Anion Addressing the Section 3 Registration of Sulfuryl Fluoride Fumigation of Food Processing Facilities. PP# 3F6573," Office of Prevention, Pesticides and Toxic Substances, January 18, 2006, http://www.fluoridealert.org/pesticides/sf.hra-jan18.2006.pdf.

72. Ibid.

73. Fluoride Action Network Pesticide Project, "Fluoride Residue Tolerances Approved for Food by US EPA as of July 15, 2005," http://www.fluoridealert.org/pesticides/fluoride.tols.july.2005.html.

Chapter 21

1. J. Tickner and M. Coffin, "What Does the Precautionary Principle Mean for Evidence-Based Dentistry?" *Journal of Evidence Based Dental Practice* 6, no. 1 (2006): 6–15.

2. C. Raffensperger and J. Tickner, *Protecting Public Health and the Environment: Implementing the Precautionary Principle* (Washington, DC: Island Press, 1999).

3. R. Bailey, "Precautionary Tale: The Latest Environmentalist Concept—The Precautionary Principle—Seeks to Stop Innovation Before It Happens. Very Bad Idea," *Reason Magazine*, April 1999, http://reason.com/archives/1999/04/01/precautionary-tale.

4. R. Bailey, "Are Chemicals Killing Us? Hit & Run," *Reason Magazine*, May 21, 2009, http://reason.com/blog/2009/05/21/are-chemicals-killing-us.

5. J. D. Graham, "The Perils of the Precautionary Principle: Lessons from the American and European Experience," The Heritage Foundation, Policy and Research Analysis, January 15, 2004, http://www.heritage.org/Research/Regulation/hl818.cfm.

6. National Research Council of the National Academies, *Fluoride in Drinking Water: A Scientific Review of EPA's Standards* (Washington, DC: National Academies Press, 2006), http://books.nap.edu/openbook.php?record_id=11571.

7. J. Tickner and M. Coffin, "What Does the Precautionary Principle Mean for Evidence-Based Dentistry?" (n. 1 above).
8. Ibid.

Chapter 22

1. National Health and Medical Research Council, *The Effectiveness of Water Fluoridation* (Canberra: Australian Government Publishing Service, 1991), 142.
2. P. Mansfield, "The Distribution of Urinary Fluoride Concentration in the UK," *Fluoride* 32, no. 1 (1999): 27–32.
3. Open Letter by Professor Trevor Sheldon, DSc, FMedSci, of the University of York, Department of Health Sciences, Heslington, York, UK, January 3, 2001, http://www.appgaf.org.uk/archive/archive_letter_shel/.
4. D. Fagin, "Second Thoughts on Fluoride," *Scientific American* 298, no. 1 (January 2008): 74–81. Excerpts at http://www.fluoridealert.org/sc.am.jan.2008.html.
5. J. A. Varner, K. F. Jensen, W. Horvath, and R. L. Isaacson, "Chronic Administration of Aluminum-Fluoride and Sodium-Fluoride to Rats in Drinking Water: Alterations in Neuronal and Cerebrovascular Integrity," *Brain Research* 784, no. 1–2 (1998): 284–98. Extended excerpts at http://www.fluoride-journal.com/98-31-2/31291-95.htm.
6. E. R. Schlesinger, D. E. Overton, H. C. Chase, and K. T. Cantwell, "Newburgh-Kingston Caries-Fluorine Study XIII. Pediatric Findings After Ten Years," *Journal of the American Dental Association* 52, no. 3 (1956): 296–306.
7. M. T. Alarcón-Herrera, I. R. Martín-Domínguez, R. Trejo-Vázquez, et al., "Well Water Fluoride, Dental Fluorosis, Bone Fractures in the Guadiana Valley of Mexico," *Fluoride* 34, no. 2 (2001): 139–49, http://www.fluoride-journal.com/01-34-2/342-139.pdf.
8. J. Luke, "Fluoride Deposition in the Aged Human Pineal Gland," *Caries Research* 35, no. 2 (2001): 125–28.
9. J. Luke, "The Effect of Fluoride on the Physiology of the Pineal Gland," PhD thesis, University of Surrey, Guildford, UK, 1997. Thesis online, with permission of author, at http://fluoridealert.org/luke-1997.pdf.
10. M. T. Alarcón-Herrera et al., "Well Water Fluoride, Dental Fluorosis, Bone Fractures in the Guadiana Valley of Mexico" (n. 7 above).
11. L. Morgan, E. Allred, M. Tavares, D. Bellinger, and H. Needleman, "Investigation of the Possible Associations between Fluorosis, Fluoride Exposure, and Childhood Behavior Problems," *Pediatric Dentistry* 20, no. 4 (1998): 244–52.
12. National Research Council of the National Academies, *Fluoride in Drinking Water: A Scientific Review of EPA's Standards* (Washington, DC: National Academies Press, 2006), http://books.nap.edu/openbook.php?record_id=11571.
13. M. S. McDonagh, P. F. Whiting, P. M. Wilson, et al., "Systematic Review of Water Fluoridation," *British Medical Journal* 321, no. 7265 (2000): 855–59, http://www.bmj.com/cgi/content/full/321/7265/855. Note: The full report that this paper summarizes is commonly known as the York Review and is accessible at http://fluoridealert.org/re/york.review.2000.pdf.
14. Medical Research Council, *Water Fluoridation and Health*, Working Group Report, UK, September 2002, http://fluoridealert.org/re/mrc-2002.pdf.
15. F. F. Lin, Aihaiti, H. X. Zhao, et al., "The Relationship of a Low-Iodine and High-Fluoride Environment to Subclinical Cretinism in Xinjiang," Xinjiang Institute for Endemic Disease Control and Research; Office of Leading Group for Endemic Disease

Control of Hetian Prefectural Committee of the Communist Party of China; and County Health and Epidemic Prevention Station, Yutian, Xinjiang, *Iodine Deficiency Disorder Newsletter* 7 (1991): 3, http://fluoridealert.org/scher/lin-1991.pdf; also see http://www.fluoridealert.org/IDD.htm.

16. X. S. Li , J. L. Zhi, and R. O. Gao, "Effect of Fluoride Exposure on Intelligence in Children," *Fluoride* 28, no. 4 (1995): 189–92, http://fluoridealert.org/scher/li-1995.pdf.

17. L. B. Zhao, G. H. Liang, D. N. Zhang, and X. R. Wu, "Effect of High-Fluoride Water Supply on Children's Intelligence," *Fluoride* 29, no. 4 (1996): 190–92, http://fluoridealert .org/scher/zhao-1996.pdf.

18. Y. Lu, Z. R. Sun, L. N. Wu, et al., "Effect of High-Fluoride Water on Intelligence in Children," *Fluoride* 33, no. 2 (2000): 74–78, http://fluoridealert.org/re/lu-2000.pdf.

19. J. Luke, "Fluoride Deposition in the Aged Human Pineal Gland" (n. 8 above).

20. J. Luke, "The Effect of Fluoride on the Physiology of the Pineal Gland" (n. 9 above).

21. National Research Council, *Fluoride in Drinking Water* (n. 12 above).

22. Bazian Ltd., "Critical Appraisal of 'Fluoride in Drinking Water: A Scientific Review of EPA's standards.'" A report for South Central Strategic Health Authority, UK, delivery date: February 11, 2009, http://fluoridealert.org/sha.basian.nrc.feb09.pdf.

23. Bazian Ltd., "Independent Critical Appraisal of Selected Studies Reporting an Association between Fluoride in Drinking Water and IQ." A report for South Central Strategic Health Authority, UK, delivery date: February 11, 2009, http://fluoridealert .org/iq.bazian.feb09.pdf.

24. National Health and Medical Research Council, *The Effectiveness of Water Fluoridation* (n. 1 above).

25. J. Luke, "Fluoride Deposition in the Aged Human Pineal Gland" (n. 8 above).

26. J. Luke, "The Effect of Fluoride on the Physiology of the Pineal Gland" (n. 9 above).

27. Y. Li, C. Liang, C. W. Slemenda, et al., "Effect of Long-term Exposure to Fluoride in Drinking Water on Risks of Bone Fractures," *Journal of Bone and Mineral Research* 16, no. 5 (2001): 932–39.

28. E. B. Bassin, D. Wypij, R. B. Davis, and M. A. Mittleman, "Age-specific Fluoride Exposure in Drinking Water and Osteosarcoma (United States)," *Cancer Causes and Control* 17, no. 4 (May 2006): 421–28.

29. G. L. Waldbott, A. W. Burgstahler, and H. L. McKinney, *Fluoridation: The Great Dilemma* (Lawrence, Kansas: Coronado Press, 1978).

30. W. Wagner and R. Steinzer (eds.), *Rescuing Science from Politics: Regulation and the Distortion of Scientific Research* (UK: Cambridge University Press, 2006).

31. American Dental Association, "Fluoridation Facts," an update commemorating the sixtieth anniversary of community water fluoridation, 2005, https://www.ada.org/ sections/professionalResources/pdfs/fluoridation_facts.pdf.

32. U.S. Department of Health and Human Services, *Review of Fluoride: Benefits and Risks,* Public Health Service, Washington, DC, February 1991, http://health.gov/environment/ ReviewofFluoride/.

33. S. C. Freni, "Exposure to High Fluoride Concentrations in Drinking Water Is Associated with Decreased Birth Rates," *Journal of Toxicology and Environmental Health* 42, no. 1 (1994): 109–21.

34. American Dental Association, *Fluoridation Facts* (n. 31 above). Reference 271 refers to Freni's paper (n. 33 above).

35. P. Connett, personal communication with Stan Freni, 2004.

36. National Research Council, *Fluoride in Drinking Water* (n. 12 above).

37. American Dental Association, "Statement on Fluoride in Drinking Water: A Scientific Review of EPA's Standards [the NRC 2006 report]," news release, March 22, 2006.

38. Centers for Disease Control and Prevention, "Statement on the 2006 National Research Council Report, Fluoride in Drinking Water: A Scientific Review of EPA's Standards," Division of Oral Health. Posted originally on March 28, 2006. Date last updated: August 24, 2009, http://www.cdc.gov/FLUORIDATION/safety/nrc_report.htm.

39. J. W. Knutson, "The Case for Water Fluoridation," *New England Journal of Medicine* 246, no. 19 (1952): 737–43.

40. H. C. Hodge, "Safety Factors in Water Fluoridation Based on the Toxicology of Fluorides," *The Proceedings of the Nutrition Society* 22 (1963): 111–17, http://journals .cambridge.org/action/displayFulltext?type=1&fid=784060&jid=PNS&volumeId =22&issueId=01&aid=784052.

41. Video of the presentation by Dr. Peter Cooney, Chief Dental Officer of Canada, on the case for fluoridation of drinking water in Dryden, Ontario, Canada, April 1, 2008, http://video.google.com/videoplay?docid=4888471756915953833&hl=en.

Chapter 23

1. P. Connett, "50 Reasons to Oppose Fluoridation" (updated April 12, 2004). Reprinted in *Medical Veritas* 1:70–80, http://www.fluoridealert.org/50reasons.htm.

2. American Dental Association, "Fluoridation Facts," an update commemorating the sixtieth anniversary of community water fluoridation, 2005, https://www.ada.org/ sections/professionalResources/pdfs/fluoridation_facts.pdf.

3. Centers for Disease Control and Prevention, "Ten Great Public Health Achievements: United States, 1900–1999," *Morbidity and Mortality Weekly Report* 48, no. 12 (April 2, 1999): 241–43, http://www.cdc.gov/mmwr/preview/mmwrhtml/00056796.htm.

4. Centers for Disease Control and Prevention, "Achievements in Public Health, 1900–1999: Fluoridation of Drinking Water to Prevent Dental Caries," *Mortality and Morbidity Weekly Review* 48, no. 41 (October 22, 1999): 933–40, http://www.cdc.gov/ mmwr/preview/mmwrhtml/mm4841a1.htm. Note: The authors of this report were Scott Tomar and Susan Griffin, as cited in Tomar's curriculum vitae, paper number 27 on page 27, http://fluoridealert.org/re/tomar.scott.cv.ref.27.pdf.

5. P. Connett and M. Connett, "The Emperor Has No Clothes: A Critique of the CDC's Promotion of Fluoridation," *Waste Not,* no. 468, September 2000 (revised October 3). Published by Work on Waste, USA, 82 Judson Street, Canton, NY 13617, http://www .fluoridealert.org/cdc.htm.

6. National Research Council, *Health Effects of Ingested Fluoride* (Washington, DC: National Academy Press, 1993), http://www.nap.edu/openbook.php?isbn=030904975X.

7. American Dental Association, "White Paper on Fluoridation," Council on Dental Health and Health Planning, 1979, http://fluoridealert.org/ada.white.paper.1979.html.

8. Ibid., 13–14.

9. S. Barrett, "Fluoridation: Poison-mongers Delaying Health for Millions?" *Journal of the American Dental Association* 93, no. 5 (1976): 880, as cited in *Scientific Knowledge in Controversy: The Social Dynamics of the Fluoridation Debate*, by Brian Martin (State University of New York, 1991).

10. M. W. Easley, "Community Fluoridation in America: The Unprincipled Opposition," 1999, posted on Dental Watch as of March 21, 2010, http://www.dentalwatch.org/fl/ opposition.pdf.

11. Ibid.

12. P. Connett and E. Connett, "The Fluoridation of Drinking Water: A House of Cards Waiting to Fall. Part 1: The Science," *Waste Not*, no. 373, November 1996. Published by Work on Waste USA, 82 Judson Street, Canton, NY 13617.

13. E-mail from Colleen Wulf of the Ohio Department of Health, Bureau of Oral Health Services, to Councilor Elahu Goselin, Athens, Ohio, October 9, 2009.

14. Department of Human Services, "Water Fluoridation: Questions and Answers," pamphlet distributed by the Department of Human Services, Melbourne, Australia, February, 2009, http://fluoridealert.org/re/australia.2009.victoria.pamphlet.pdf.

15. A. W. Burgstahler et al., "Citizens Are Being Misled. Opinion," *Sunraysia Daily* (Australia), September 18, 2009.

16. American Dental Association, "White Paper on Fluoridation," pages 10–11, Council on Dental Health and Health Planning, 1979, http://fluoridealert.org/ada.white.paper.1979 .html.

17. Video statement of Dr. Poul Erik Petersen, Chief, Oral Health Director for the World Health Organization's Department of Chronic Diseases and Health Promotion, to the attendees of a meeting celebrating the sixtieth anniversary of fluoridation, hosted by the American Dental Association and the U.S. Centers for Disease Control in Chicago, Illinois, July 2005, http://terrance.who.int/mediacentre/videos/ Dr_Petersen.mpg.

18. M. Diesendorf, "The Mystery of Declining Tooth Decay," *Nature* 322, no. 6075 (1986): 125–29.

19. B. Hileman, "Fluoridation of Water. Questions About Health Risks and Benefits Remain after More Than 40 years," *Chemical & Engineering News*, August 1, 1988.

20. D. Fagin, "Second Thoughts on Fluoride," *Scientific American* 298, no. 1 (January 2008): 74–81; excerpts at http://www.fluoridealert.org/sc.am.jan.2008.html.

21. The journal *Fluoride* is published by the International Society for Fluoride Research. Back issues available at http://www.fluorideresearch.org/backissues.pdf.

22. Agency for Toxic Substances and Disease Registry, *Toxicological Profile for Fluorides, Hydrogen Fluoride and Fluorine* (Atlanta, GA: U.S. Department of Health and Human Services, Public Health Service, September 2003), http://www.atsdr.cdc.gov/toxprofiles/ tp11.pdf.

23. National Research Council of the National Academies, *Fluoride in Drinking Water: A Scientific Review of EPA's Standards* (Washington, DC: National Academies Press, 2006), http://books.nap.edu/openbook.php?record_id=11571.

24. TOXNET is an online search site hosted by the U.S. Library of Medicine and the National Institutes of Health, http://toxnet.nlm.nih.gov/.

25. National Research Council, *Fluoride in Drinking Water* (n. 23 above).

26. Back copies of *Dentistry Today* can be viewed at http://www.dentistrytoday.com/ME2/ Default.asp.

27. J. Monahan, "Dental Health Remains Prime Goal," *The Telegram & Gazette* (Worcester, Massachusetts), November 7, 2001.

28. M. Roosevelt, "Not in My Water Supply," *Time Magazine*, October 17, 2005, http:// www.time.com/time/magazine/article/0,9171,1118379-3,00.html.

29. P. Forgey, "Pro-Fluoride Campaign Nets $151,623," *Juneau Empire* (Alaska), September 30, 2007, http://juneauempire.com/stories/093007/loc_20070930051.shtml.

30. W. Blackwell, "LDA Urges Louisiana to 'Tap into a Healthier Smile!'" Louisiana Dental Association (LDA), undated (2007–2008). Note: Ward Blackwell is executive director of the LDA, http://www.ladental.org/cms/content/view/113/35/.

31. See news items on fluoridation from Australia at Fluoride Action Network, http://www2.fluoridealert.org/Alert/Australia.

32. W. Varney, *Fluoride in Australia: A Case to Answer* (Sydney: Hale and Iremonger, 1986).

33. W. Varney, "Troubled Waters, Little Transparency: Fluoridation in Australia," April 2010, http://fluoridealert.org/varney.html.

34. J. Meikle, "Fluoridation Scheme Could Go England-Wide," *The Guardian* (London), February 27, 2009, http://www.guardian.co.uk/society/2009/feb/27/fluoridation-southampton-health.

35. J. Reeve, "Daily Echo Backs Calls for a Referendum on Fluoride Issue," *Daily Echo* (UK), June 27, 2009, http://www.dailyecho.co.uk/news/4462636.Daily_Echo_backs_calls_for_a_referendum_on_fluoride_issue/.

36. Bazian Ltd., "Critical Appraisal of 'Fluoride in Drinking Water: A Scientific Review of EPA's Standards.'" A report for South Central Strategic Health Authority, UK, delivery date: February 11, 2009, http://fluoridealert.org/sha.basian.nrc.feb09.pdf.

37. Bazian Ltd., "Independent Critical Appraisal of Selected Studies Reporting an Association between Fluoride in Drinking Water and IQ." A report for South Central Strategic Health Authority, UK, delivery date: February 11, 2009, http://fluoridealert.org/iq.bazian.feb09.pdf.

38. J. Reeve, "Southampton Civic Bosses Call for Fluoride Referendum," *Daily Echo* (UK), March 17, 2010, http://www.dailyecho.co.uk/news/5067065.Call_for_fluoride_referendum/.

39. See news items on the fluoridation issue from England at Fluoride Action Network, http://www2.fluoridealert.org/Alert/United-Kingdom/England.

40. R. Nadler-Olenick, "One for the Hall of Shame; Del Rio, Texas. Pt 1. Fluoride Follies," 2006, http://blog.fluoridefreeaustin.com/2009/03/22/del-rio-texas-pt-i---one-for-the-hall-of-shame.aspx.

Chapter 24

1. R. A. Freeze and J. A. Lehr, *The Fluoride Wars: How a Modest Public Health Measure Became America's Longest-Running Political Melodrama* (Hoboken, NJ: John Wiley, 2009).

2. U.S. Department of Health and Human Services, *Review of Fluoride: Benefits and Risks*, Public Health Service, Washington, DC, February 1991, http://health.gov/environment/ReviewofFluoride/.

3. *Forum on Fluoridation* (Dublin, Ireland: Stationery Office, 2002), http://fluoridealert.org/re/fluoridation.forum.2002.pdf.

4. National Health and Medical Research Council, *A Systematic Review of the Efficacy and Safety of Fluoridation*, reference no. EH41, Australian Government, December 27, 2007, http://www.nhmrc.gov.au/publications/synopses/eh41syn.htm.

5. Health Canada, "Findings and Recommendations of the Fluoride Expert Panel (January 2007)," April 2008, http://fluoridealert.org/re/canada.fluoride.expert.panel.2007.pdf.

6. Health Canada, *Fluoride in Drinking Water*. Document for public comment. Guidelines for Canadian Drinking Water Quality: Guideline Technical Document. Prepared by the Federal-Provincial-Territorial Committee on Drinking Water, September 2009, http://fluoridealert.org/canada.2009.report.pdf.

7. *Forum on Fluoridation* (n. 3 above).

8. P. Connett, "50 Reasons to Oppose Fluoridation" (updated April 12, 2004). Reprinted in *Medical Veritas* 1:70–80, http://www.fluoridealert.org/50reasons.htm.

9. Y. Li, C. Liang, C. W. Slemenda, et al., "Effect of Long-Term Exposure to Fluoride in

Drinking Water on Risks of Bone Fractures," *Journal of Bone and Mineral Research* 16, no. 5 (2001): 932–39.

10. A. Burgstahler, R. J. Carton, P. Connett, et al., "A Scientific Critique of the Fluoridation Forum Report, Ireland," 2002, http://www.fluoridealert.org/irish.forum-critique.htm.

11. Anonymous, "A critical appraisal of, and commentary on,'50 Reasons to Oppose Fluoridation,'" posted May 5, 2005, on Ireland's Department of Health Web site, http://www.dohc.ie/other_health_issues/dental_research/critical_fifty.pdf?direct=1.

12. Letter from Paul Connett to John Moloney, TD, chairman, Oireachtas Joint Committee on Health & Children, Dublin, Ireland, in response to the critique of his "50 Reasons to Oppose Fluoridation" posted on Ireland's Department of Health's Web site, January 20, 2006, http://www.fluoridealert.org/50reasons.ireland.pdf.

13. National Health and Medical Research Council, *A Systematic Review of the Efficacy and Safety of Fluoridation* (n. 4 above).

14. M. McDonagh, P. Whiting, M. Bradley, et al., "A Systematic Review of Water Fluoridation," NHS Centre for Reviews and Dissemination, The University of York, Report 18 (this report is commonly known as the York Review), http://fluoridealert.org/re/york.review.2000.pdf.

15. Open letter by Professor Trevor Sheldon, DSc, FMedSci, of the University of York, Department of Health Sciences, Heslington, York, UK, January 3, 2001, http://www.appgaf.org.uk/archive/archive_letter_shel/.

16. National Research Council of the National Academies, *Fluoride in Drinking Water: A Scientific Review of EPA's Standards* (Washington, DC: National Academies Press, 2006), http://books.nap.edu/openbook.php?record_id=11571.

17. National Health and Medical Research Council, *A Systematic Review of the Efficacy and Safety of Fluoridation,* 15 (n. 4 above).

18. National Research Council, *Fluoride in Drinking Water* (n. 16 above).

19. C. W. Douglass and K. Joshipura, "Caution Needed in Fluoride and Osteosarcoma Study" (letter), *Cancer Causes & Control* 17, no. 4 (May 2006): 481–82.

20. B. Bassin, D. Wypij, R. B. Davis, and M. A. Mittleman, "Age-Specific Fluoride Exposure in Drinking Water and Osteosarcoma (United States)," *Cancer Causes and Control* 17, no. 4 (May 2006): 421–28.

21. Letter from Anna Bligh, MP, Premier of Queensland (Australia), to constituent J Lewis, May 15, 2009, http://fluoridealert.org/au.bligh.may15.2009.letter.html.

22. Health Canada, "Findings and Recommendations of the Fluoride Expert Panel (January 2007)" (n. 5 above).

23. Health Canada, *Fluoride in Drinking Water* (n. 6 above).

24. M. Levy and F. Corbeil, *Water Fluoridation: An Analysis of the Health Benefits and Risks,* Scientific Advisory, Développement des Individues et des Communautés, Institut National de Santé Publique, Québec, Canada, June 2007, http://fluoridealert.org/re/levy-2007.canada.pdf.

25. National Research Council, *Fluoride in Drinking Water* (n. 16 above).

26. Health Canada, "Findings and Recommendations of the Fluoride Expert Panel (January 2007)" (n. 5 above).

27. C. W. Douglass and K. Joshipura, "Caution Needed in Fluoride and Osteosarcoma Study" (n. 19 above).

28. Health Canada, *Fluoride in Drinking Water* (n. 6 above).

29. World Health Organization, *Fluorides,* Environmental Health Criteria 227, International Programme on Chemical Safety, Geneva, Switzerland, 2002, http://www.inchem.org/documents/ehc/ehc/ehc227.htm.

30. Agency for Toxic Substances and Disease Registry, *Toxicological Profile for Fluorides, Hydrogen Fluoride and Fluorine* (Atlanta, GA: U.S. Department of Health and Human Services, Public Health Service, September 2003), http://www.atsdr.cdc.gov/toxprofiles/tp11.pdf.
31. National Research Council, *Fluoride in Drinking Water* (n. 16 above).
32. "Dental Experts Defend Fluoride in Water; Activists Claim Link to Brain Damage," *Canadian Press*, August 8, 2008.
33. "Experts Disagree on Fluoride in Drinking Water," *CTV-News* (Canadian Television), August 7, 2008, http://www2.fluoridealert.org/Alert/Canada/Ontario/Experts-disagree-on-fluoride-in-drinking-water.

Chapter 25

1. National Research Council of the National Academies, *Fluoride in Drinking Water: A Scientific Review of EPA's Standards* (Washington, DC: National Academies Press, 2006), 33, 36, 40, http://books.nap.edu/openbook.php?record_id=11571.
2. G. M. Whitford, "Fluoride in Dental Products: Safety Considerations," *Journal of Dental Research* 66, no. 5 (1987): 1056–60.
3. Q. Xiang, Y. Liang, L. Chen, et al., "Effect of Fluoride in Drinking Water on Children's Intelligence," *Fluoride* 36, no. 2 (2003): 84–94, http://www.fluorideresearch.org/362/files/FJ2003_v36_n2_p84-94.pdf.
4. Y. Li, C. Liang, C. W. Slemenda, et al., "Effect of Long-Term Exposure to Fluoride in Drinking Water on Risks of Bone Fractures," *Journal of Bone and Mineral Research* 16, no. 5 (2001): 932–39.
5. Centers for Disease Control and Prevention, "Ten Great Public Health Achievements: United States, 1900–1999," *Morbidity and Mortality Weekly Report* 48, no. 12 (April 2, 1999): 241–43, http://www.cdc.gov/mmwr/preview/mmwrhtml/00056796.htm.
6. Centers for Disease Control and Prevention, "Achievements in Public Health, 1900–1999: Fluoridation of Drinking Water to Prevent Dental Caries," *Mortality and Morbidity Weekly Review* 48, no. 41 (October 22, 1999): 933–40, http://www.cdc.gov/mmwr/preview/mmwrhtml/mm4841a1.htm. Note: The authors of this report were Scott Tomar and Susan Griffin, as cited in Tomar's curriculum vitae, paper number 27 on page 27, http://fluoridealert.org/re/tomar.scott.cv.ref.27.pdf.
7. S. O. Griffin, K. Jones, and S. L. Tomar, "An Economic Evaluation of Community Water Fluoridation," *Journal of Public Health Dentistry* 61, no. 2 (2001): 78–86.
8. M. S. McDonagh, P. F. Whiting, P. M. Wilson, et al., "Systematic Review of Water Fluoridation," *British Medical Journal* 321, no. 7265 (2000): 855–59, http://www.bmj.com/cgi/content/full/321/7265/855. Note: The full report that this paper summarizes is commonly known as the York Review and is accessible at http://fluoridealert.org/re/york.review.2000.pdf.
9. Fluoride Action Network, "Professionals' Statement Calling for an End to Fluoridation," http://fluoridealert.org/professionals.statement.html.
10. P. P. Bachinskii, O. A. Gutsalenko, N. D. Naryzhniuk et al., "Action of Fluoride on the Function of the Pituitary-thyroid System of Healthy Persons and Patients with Thyroid Disorders" (article in Russian), *Problemy Endokrinologii (Mosk)* 31, no. 6 (1985): 25–29. English translation at http://www.fluoridealert.org/bachinskii.1985.pdf.
11. F. F. Lin, Aihaiti, H. X. Zhao, et al., "The Relationship of a Low-Iodine and High-Fluoride Environment to Subclinical Cretinism in Xinjiang," Xinjiang Institute for Endemic Disease Control and Research; Office of Leading Group for Endemic Disease

Control of Hetian Prefectural Committee of the Communist Party of China; and County Health and Epidemic Prevention Station, Yutian, Xinjiang, *Iodine Deficiency Disorder Newsletter* 7 (1991): 3, http://fluoridealert.org/scher/lin-1991.pdf; also see http://www.fluoridealert.org/IDD.htm.

12. Y. Li et al., "Effect of Long-Term Exposure to Fluoride in Drinking Water on Risks of Bone Fractures" (n. 4 above).

13. E. B. Bassin, D. Wypij, R. B. Davis, and M. A. Mittleman, "Age-specific Fluoride Exposure in Drinking Water and Osteosarcoma (United States)," *Cancer Causes and Control* 17, no. 4 (May 2006): 421–28.

14. C. W. Douglass and K. Joshipura, "Caution Needed in Fluoride and Osteosarcoma Study" (letter), *Cancer Causes & Control* 17, no. 4 (May 2006): 481–82.

15. F. T. Shannon, D. M. Fergusson, and L. J. Horwood, "Exposure to Fluoridated Water Supplies and Child Behaviour," *New Zealand Medical Journal* 99, no. 803 (1986): 416–18.

16. K. E. Heller, S. A. Eklund, and B. A. Burt, "Dental Caries and Dental Fluorosis at Varying Water Fluoride Concentrations," *Journal of Public Health Dentistry* 57, no. 3 (1997): 136–43.

17. E. Dincer, "Why Do I Have White Spots on My Front Teeth," *New York State Dental Journal* 74, no. 1 (2008): 58–60, http://www.nysdental.org/img/current-pdf/JrnlJan2008 .pdf.

18. Centers for Disease Control and Prevention, "Fluoridation Census 1992," page iv, U.S. Department of Health & Human Services, Public Health Service, National Center for Prevention Services, Division of Oral Health, Atlanta, Georgia, 1993, http://fluoride alert.org/cdc.f.census.1992.html.

19. E. D. Beltrán-Aguilar, B. F. Gooch, A. Kingman, et al., "Surveillance for Dental Caries, Dental Sealants, Tooth Retention, Edentulism, and Enamel Fluorosis—United States, 1988–1994 and 1999–2002," *Morbidity and Mortality Weekly Report* 54, no. 3 (August 26, 2005): 1–44, http://www.cdc.gov/mmwr/preview/mmwrhtml/ss5403a1.htm.

20. K. E. Heller et al., "Dental Caries and Dental Fluorosis at Varying Water Fluoride Concentrations" (n. 16 above).

21. National Research Council, *Fluoride in Drinking Water*, 177 (n. 1 above).

22. S. Barrett, "Fluoridation: Poison-mongers Delaying Health for Millions?" *Journal of the American Dental Association* 93, no. 55 (1976): 880, as cited by Brian Martin in *Scientific Knowledge in Controversy: The Social Dynamics of the Fluoridation Debate* (State University of New York Press, 1991).

23. B. Sprague, M. Bernhardt, and S. Barrett, "Fluoridation: Don't Let the Poisonmongers Scare You" (undated), online at QuackWatch, http://www.quackwatch.com/03Health Promotion/fluoride.html.

24. M. Crichton, "'Aliens Cause Global Warming'. From a lecture delivered by the late Michael Crichton at the California Institute of Technology on Jan. 17, 2003," *Wall Street Journal*, November 7, 2008, http://online.wsj.com/article/SB122603134258207975.html.

Chapter 26

1. B. Martin, *Scientific Knowledge in Controversy: The Social Dynamics of the Fluoridation Debate* (State University of New York Press, 1991).

2. E. Groth, "The Fluoridation Controversy; Which Side is Science On?" A commentary in *Scientific Knowledge in Controversy: The Social Dynamics of the Fluoridation Debate* by Brian Martin (State University of New York Press, 1991), 169–92.

3. Ibid., 174–75.

4. B. Osmunson, personal communication with Paul Connett, 2008.

5. J. Colquhoun, "Education and Fluoridation in New Zealand: An Historical Study," PhD diss., University of Auckland, New Zealand, 1987.

6. J. Colquhoun, "Why I Changed My Mind about Fluoridation," *Perspectives in Biology and Medicine* 41 (1997): 29–44. Reprinted in *Fluoride* 31, no. 2 (1998): 103–18, http:// www.fluoride-journal.com/98-31-2/312103.htm.

7. T. S. Kuhn, *The Structure of Scientific Revolutions* (The University of Chicago Press, 1962).

8. B. C. Nesin, "A Water Supply Perspective of the Fluoridation Discussion," *Journal of the Maine Water Utilities Association* 32 (1956): 33–47.

9. Centers for Disease Control and Prevention, "Achievements in Public Health, 1900–1999: Fluoridation of Drinking Water to Prevent Dental Caries," *Mortality and Morbidity Weekly Review* 48, no. 41 (October 22, 1999): 933–40, http://www.cdc.gov/ mmwr/preview/mmwrhtml/mm4841a1.htm.

10. Centers for Disease Control and Prevention, "Ten Great Public Health Achievements: United States, 1900–1999," *Morbidity and Mortality Weekly Report* 48, no. 12 (April 2, 1999): 241–43, http://www.cdc.gov/mmwr/preview/mmwrhtml/00056796.htm.

11. "Rethinking Fluoridation: EPA Headquarters Union Calls for Moratorium," a video interview with Bill Hirzy, Ph.D., a risk assessment scientist for the U. S. Environmental Protection Agency. Produced by Michael Connett for Grass Roots & Global Video, a project of the American Environmental Health Studies Project in association with Fluoride Action Network, May 2001.

12. C. Bryson, *The Fluoride Deception* (New York: Seven Stories Press, 2004).

13. M. Connett and P. Connett, "The Fluoride Deception: An Interview with Christopher Bryson" (video, 28:30 min.), 2004, http://video.google.com/ videoplay?docid=-3949434744498031545&hl=en#.

14. SourceWatch, "American Council on Science and Health," The Center for Media and Democracy, http://www.sourcewatch.org/index.php?title=American_Council_on _Science_and_Health.

15. Ibid.

16. B. Moyers, "PR Strategies. Trade Secrets: A Moyers Report," PBS-TV (Public Broadcasting Service), produced by Public Affairs Television, Inc., 2001, http://www .pbs.org/tradesecrets/evidence/secrecy_pop03.html, and http://www.pbs.org/tradesecrets/ transcript.html.

17. "ACSH Considers Legal Action Against Attempts to Reclassify Fluoride," *Food Chemical News*, April 30, 1990.

18. F. B. Exner and G. L. Waldbott, *The American Fluoridation Experiment* (New York: Devin-Adair, 1957).

19. G. Caldwell and P. E. Zanfagna, *Fluoridation and Truth Decay* (Massachusetts: Top-Ecol Press, 1974).

20. W. Varney, *Fluoride in Australia: A Case to Answer* (Sydney: Hale and Iremonger, 1986).

21. F. B. Exner and G. L. Waldbott, *The American Fluoridation Experiment*, 8 (n. 18 above).

22. W. Varney, *Fluoride in Australia*, 69 (n. 20 above).

23. T. Cambanis, "Dr. Frederick J. Stare, 91, Pioneer in Nutrition Studies," *Boston Globe* (Massachusetts), April 6, 2002, page B7.

24. G. Caldwell and P. E. Zanfagna, *Fluoridation and Truth Decay*, 11 (n. 19 above).

25. W. Varney, *Fluoride in Australia*, 70 (n. 20 above).

26. Ibid.

27. G. Caldwell and P. E. Zanfagna, *Fluoridation and Truth Decay,* 10 (n. 19 above).

28. Ibid., 244.

29. D. S. Bernstein, D. M. Hegsted, C. D. Guri, and F. J. Stare, "Prevalence of Osteoporosis in High- and Low-fluoride Areas in North Dakota," *Journal of the American Medical Association* 198, no. 5 (1966): 85–90.

30. H. E. Meema, "Fluorides and Osteoporosis" (letter), *The Lancet,* February 25, 1967.

31. E. Hedderberg, "Fluoride Is Called Helpful to the Elderly," *St. Petersburg Times* (Florida), September 9, 1969.

32. "ACSH Considers Legal Action Against Attempts to Reclassify Fluoride" (n. 17 above).

33. Ibid.

34. C. Bryson, *The Fluoride Deception* (n. 12 above).

35. Ibid., 209.

36. J. Barzun, *Science: The Glorious Entertainment* (New York, Evanston, and London: Harper & Row, 1964), 71–72.

Review and Conclusion

1. J. A. Brunelle and J. P. Carlos, "Recent Trends in Dental Caries in U.S. Children and the Effect of Water Fluoridation," *Journal of Dental Research* 69 (1990): 723–27.

2. D. Fagin, "Second Thoughts on Fluoride," *Scientific American* 298, no. 1 (January 2008): 74–81. Excerpts at http://www.fluoridealert.org/sc.am.jan.2008.html.

3. "The Professionals' Statement Calling for an End to Water Fluoridation," Fluoride Action Network, http://fluoridealert.org/prof-statement.pdf.

4. M. Tavares and V. Chomitz, "A Healthy Weight Intervention for Children in a Dental Setting," *Journal of the American Dental Association* 140, no. 3 (2009): 313–16.

About the Authors

Paul Connett obtained his bachelor's degree from Cambridge, England, and his PhD in chemistry from Dartmouth College in the United States. He retired from a full professorship at St. Lawrence University in Canton, New York, in May 2006. He is currently the director of the Fluoride Action Network. His specialty at St. Lawrence was environmental chemistry and toxicology. For twenty-five years, he has been involved in waste management, an issue that has led him to give over two thousand pro bono presentations in forty-nine U.S. states and fifty-two other countries. In 2010, he gave two presentations on *Zero Waste and Sustainability* to the United Nations Commission for Sustainable Development in New York City. At the urging of his wife, Ellen, he 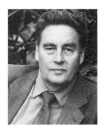 began researching the issues of fluoride's toxicity and the water fluoridation debate in July 1996. Before Professor Connett began reading the literature on fluoride, he had accepted the prevailing American perception that people opposed to fluoridation were scientifically ill informed. After fourteen years of reviewing the primary literature his perception has dramatically changed. Paul and Ellen Connett were included in *American Environmental Leaders from Colonial Times to the Present* by Anne Becher and Joseph Richey (Grey House Publishing, 2008)

James S. Beck, who holds doctorates in medicine (Washington University School of Medicine, St. Louis, Missouri) and biophysics (University of 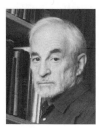 California, Berkeley), was urged nine years ago to look at the issue of fluoridation in the city of Calgary, Canada, by a family physician who opposed it. He was appalled at the ethics of the practice, joined a small committee of one physician and five dentists trying to stop fluoridation in the city, and began a study of the scientific literature on fluoride's purported efficacy as preventive of caries and on its myriad toxicities. He has lobbied city councils and engaged in public debate since. He is currently professor emeritus of medical biophysics at the University of Calgary, Canada.

H. Spedding Micklem is an emeritus professor in the School of Biological Sciences, University of Edinburgh, UK. He graduated DPhil from the University of Oxford and worked on the scientific staff of the Medical Research Council at Harwell for eight years before moving to the Department of Zoology at Edinburgh, where he engaged in teaching and research for twenty-five years, publishing mainly in the fields of stem cell biology and immunology. He held visiting research fellowships for several periods at l'Institut Pasteur in Paris, Stanford University, and New York University School of Medicine. 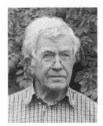 He became interested in fluoride about seven years ago and soon realized that fluoridation of the public water supply was not the sensible public health measure that he had always supposed.

Peter Meiers, author of *Zur Toxizität von Fluorverbindungen* (Heidelberg: Verlag für Medizin, 1984) and owner of the Web site www.fluoride-history .de, became aware of the fluoride debate late in 1981, when the possible carcinogenic effects of fluoride were mentioned by Hans Alfred Nieper, MD, in a letter to the editor of a weekly medical magazine. Though he has no academic degrees, Meiers began a critical study of the available medical literature and approached health officers, as well as community-administered local kindergarten leaders, who then used to distribute fluoride tablets to children, to draw their attention to the issue. The distribution of fluoride tablets by local kindergartens was stopped in 1984, yet a new challenge arose with plans to fluoridate the drinking water of the city of Berlin (later defeated by public vote). Another key event leading to Meiers's special interest in the history of fluoridation was his participation in a TV discussion during which the representative of a dental organization argued in favor of fluoride. As soon as the cameras went off, this dentist said, "In a few years we dentists will ask, 'How could we have ever gotten involved in this fluoride matter?'"

Index

the politics and practice of sustainable living

CHELSEA GREEN PUBLISHING

Chelsea Green Publishing sees books as tools for effecting cultural change and seeks to empower citizens to participate in reclaiming our global commons and become its impassioned stewards. If you enjoyed *The Case Against Fluoride*, please consider these other great books related to health and safety.

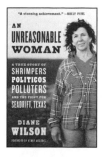

AN UNREASONABLE WOMAN
A True Story of Shrimpers, Politicos, Polluters, and the Fight for Seadrift, Texas
DIANE WILSON
ISBN 9781933392271
Paperback • $18.00

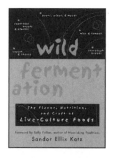

WILD FERMENTATION
The Flavor, Nutrition, and Craft of Live-Culture Foods
SANDOR ELLIX KATZ
ISBN 9781931498234
Paperback • $25.00

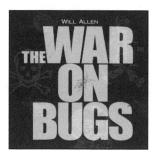

THE WAR ON BUGS
Will Allen
ISBN 9781933392462
Paperback • $35.00

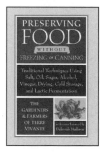

PRESERVING FOOD WITHOUT FREEZING OR CANNING
THE GARDENERS & FARMERS OF TERRE VIVANTE
ISBN 9781933392592
Paperback • $25.00

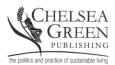

CHELSEA GREEN PUBLISHING
the politics and practice of sustainable living

For more information or to request a catalog, visit **www.chelseagreen.com** or call toll-free **(800) 639-4099**.

the politics and practice of sustainable living

CHELSEA GREEN PUBLISHING

Chelsea Green Publishing sees books as tools for effecting cultural change and seeks to empower citizens to participate in reclaiming our global commons and become its impassioned stewards. If you enjoyed *The Case Against Fluoride*, please consider these other great books related to health and safety.

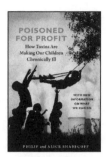

POISONED FOR PROFIT
How Toxins Are Making Our
Children Chronically Ill
PHILIP SHABECOFF, ALICE SHABECOFF
ISBN 9781603582568
Paperback • $17.95

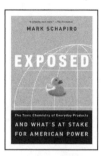

EXPOSED
The Toxic Chemistry of Everyday Products
and What's at Stake for American Power
MARK SHAPIRO
ISBN 9781603580588
Paperback • $16.95

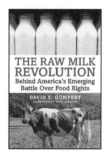

RAW MILK REVOLUTION
Behind America's Emerging
Battle Over Food Rights
DAVID E. GUMPERT
ISBN 9781603582193
Paperback • $19.95

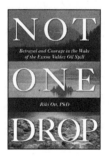

NOT ONE DROP
Betrayal and Courage in the
Wake of the Exxon Valdez Oil Spill
RIKI OTT
ISBN 9781933392585
Paperback • $21.95

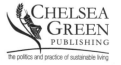

CHELSEA GREEN PUBLISHING
the politics and practice of sustainable living

For more information or to request a catalog,
visit **www.chelseagreen.com** or
call toll-free **(800) 639-4099**.